CLINICAL CHALLENGES AND
Complications
OF **IBD**

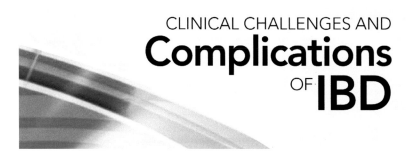

CLINICAL CHALLENGES AND
Complications
OF **IBD**

Edited by

Miguel D. Regueiro, MD

Professor of Medicine
University of Pittsburgh School of Medicine
Associate Chief, Education
Clinical Head and Co-Director, Inflammatory Bowel Disease Center
Director, Gastroenterology, Hepatology, and Nutrition Fellowship
Pittsburgh, Pennsylvania

Jason M. Swoger, MD, MPH

Assistant Professor of Medicine
University of Pittsburgh Medical Center
Associate Program Director, Gastroenterology
Fellowship Program
Pittsburgh, Pennsylvania

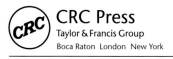

CRC Press
Taylor & Francis Group
Boca Raton London New York

CRC Press is an imprint of the
Taylor & Francis Group, an **informa** business

First published 2013 by SLACK Incorporated

Published 2024 by CRC Press
2385 NW Executive Center Drive, Suite 320, Boca Raton FL 33431

and by CRC Press
4 Park Square, Milton Park, Abingdon, Oxon, OX14 4RN

CRC Press is an imprint of Taylor & Francis Group, LLC

Library of Congress Cataloging-in-Publication Data

Clinical challenges and complications of IBD / [edited by] Miguel Regueiro,
Jason Swoger.
       p. ; cm.
  Includes bibliographical references.
  ISBN 978-1-55642-980-4 (hardcover : alk. paper)
  I. Regueiro, Miguel. II. Swoger, Jason.
  [DNLM: 1. Inflammatory Bowel Diseases—complications. 2. Inflammatory
Bowel Diseases—therapy. WI 420]
  616.3'44—dc23
                        2012006221

ISBN: 9781556429804 (hbk)
ISBN: 9781003523017 (ebk)

DOI: 10.1201/9781003523017

DEDICATION

I would like to dedicate the book to my patients who have taught me the most about inflammatory bowel disease and to my family, Carol, Matt, and Jack.

—Miguel D. Regueiro, MD

I would like to dedicate the book to Lisa, Mütter, and the Silver Fox.

—Jason M. Swoger, MD, MPH

CONTENTS

ACKNOWLEDGMENTS

We would like to acknowledge all the authors who generously gave their time and expertise in contributing to the book.

I (Miguel) would like to acknowledge Carrie Kotlar from SLACK Incorporated for her guidance, patience, and professionalism. I would also like to recognize Jason Swoger, MD, for his dedication, tireless work ethic, and attention to detail in creating such a comprehensive clinical IBD book.

I (Jason) would like to especially acknowledge Ed Loftus and Susie Kane, not only for their valuable contributions to the book, but for their ongoing mentoring and friendship. I would also like to acknowledge Miguel Regueiro, MD, for inspiring the book and continually supporting and guiding my career.

ABOUT THE EDITORS

Miguel D. Regueiro, MD, is Professor of Medicine at the University of Pittsburgh School of Medicine, Head of the Clinical Inflammatory Bowel Disease Program, and Co-Director of the Inflammatory Bowel Disease Center at the University of Pittsburgh Medical Center. He is also the Associate Chief for Education and Director of the Gastroenterology, Hepatology, and Nutrition Fellowship Training Program at the University of Pittsburgh. Dr. Regueiro's primary clinical and research interest is inflammatory bowel disease (IBD), with a focus on Crohn's disease and ulcerative colitis. Dr. Regueiro has published extensively on the prevention and management of postoperative Crohn's disease and genotype–phenotype correlations in IBD. He is the principal investigator on several multicenter, international research trials and conducts clinical research that defines the natural course and phenotypes of IBD. Dr. Regueiro has developed a multidisciplinary IBD Center that operates as a state-of-the-art clinic for patients with Crohn's disease and ulcerative colitis. Dr. Regueiro received his BA at the University of Pennsylvania and earned his medical degree at Hahnemann University. He completed his internal medicine internship and residency and clinical and research fellowship training in gastroenterology at Harvard Medical School's Beth Israel Hospital. Dr. Regueiro has received several honors, including membership in several professional and scientific societies, including the Alpha Omega Alpha Honor Society, the Joan Komblum Memorial Prize for Excellence in Internal Medicine, the Clinical Investigator Training Award from Harvard/MIT Health Sciences, the Crohn's Colitis Foundation of America Physician of the Year, the National Research Excellence in Gastroenterology Disease Award, and American Gastroenterology Association and American College of Gastroenterology Fellowships.

Jason M. Swoger, MD, MPH, is Assistant Professor of Medicine in the Division of Gastroenterology, Hepatology, and Nutrition at the University of Pittsburgh Medical Center. He is Associate Program Director of the Gastroenterology Fellowship Program. Prior to attending medical school, he completed a Master's of Public Health, with a focus on epidemiology, at the University of Illinois at Chicago. Dr. Swoger received his medical degree from Eastern Virginia Medical School, in Norfolk, VA, where he was a member of the Alpha Omega Alpha Honor Society. He then went on to complete his internal medicine residency training at the Cleveland Clinic Foundation. His fellowship training in gastroenterology was pursued at the Mayo Clinic, in Rochester, MN, where he developed an interest in inflammatory bowel disease, as well as in clinical research. His current research interests include the epidemiology and therapeutics of inflammatory bowel disease, as well as clinical trials. Dr. Swoger is a member of several professional and scientific societies, including the American Gastroenterological Association, the American College of Gastroenterology, and the Crohn's & Colitis Foundation of America (CCFA), and he is a member of the CCFA Research Alliance. He lives in Pittsburgh with his wife, Lisa.

Contributing Authors

Ashwin N. Ananthakrishnan, MD, MPH
(Chapter 6)
Assistant in Medicine
Crohn's and Colitis Center
Massachusetts General Hospital
Boston, Massachusetts

Jemilat O. Badamas, MD (Chapter 1)
Internal Medicine
Johns Hopkins
Bayview Medical Center
Baltimore, Maryland

Aaron S. Bancil, BSc (Hons) (Chapter 9)
Department of Gastroenterology
    and Hepatology
Imperial College
London, United Kingdom

David Benhayon, MD, PhD
(Chapter 14)
Research Fellow in Gastroenterology
Departments of Gastroenterology
    and Behavioral Health
Children's Hospital of Pittsburgh
Pittsburgh, Pennsylvania

Adam S. Cheifetz, MD (Chapter 4)
Clinical Director
Center for Inflammatory Bowel
    Disease
Beth Israel Deaconess Medical Center
Assistant Professor of Medicine
Harvard Medical School
Boston, Massachusetts

Garret Cullen, MD (Chapter 4)
Inflammatory Bowel Disease Fellow
Division of Gastroenterology
Beth Israel Deaconess Medical Center
Boston, Massachusetts

Omer J. Deen, MD (Chapter 12)
Clinical Associate
Center for Human Nutrition
Digestive Disease Institute
Cleveland, Ohio

Monika Fischer, MD, MSCR
(Chapter 11)
Assistant Professor of Clinical
    Medicine
Division of Gastroenterology
    and Hepatology
Indiana University
Indianapolis, Indiana

Mark E. Gerich, MD (Chapter 10)
Assistant Professor of Medicine
Division of Gastroenterology and
Hepatology
University of Colorado—Denver
Aurora, Colorado

Leyla J. Ghazi, MD (Chapter 3)
Assistant Professor of Medicine
Department of Medicine
Division of Gastroenterology
    and Hepatology
University of Maryland School of
    Medicine
Baltimore, Maryland

Lisa M. Grandinetti, MD, FAAD, MMS
(Chapter 8)
Assistant Professor of Dermatology
Associate Dermatology Residency
Program Director
University of Pittsburgh
Department of Dermatology
Pittsburgh, Pennsylvania

Peter D.R. Higgins, MD, PhD, MSc
(Chapter 2)
Assistant Professor in
    Gastroenterology
Division of Gastroenterology and
    Hepatology
Department of Internal Medicine
University of Michigan
Ann Arbor, Michigan

Kim L. Isaacs, MD, PhD (Chapter 7)
Professor of Medicine
Division of Gastroenterology
   and Hepatology
University of North Carolina
Chapel Hill, North Carolina

*Sunanda Kane, MD, MSPH
(Chapter 11)*
Professor of Medicine
Division of Gastroenterology and
   Hepatology
Mayo Clinic College of Medicine
Rochester, Minnesota

*Donald F. Kirby, MD, FACP, FACN,
FACG, AGAF, CNSC, CPNS
 (Chapter 12)*
Professor of Medicine
Director, Center for Human Nutrition
Medical Director
Intestinal Transplant Program
Cleveland, Ohio

Mark Lazarev, MD (Chapter 1)
Assistant Professor of Medicine
Division of Gastroenterology and
   Hepatology
The Johns Hopkins Hospital
Baltimore, Maryland

Edward V. Loftus Jr, MD (Chapter 10)
Professor of Medicine
Chair, Inflammatory Bowel Disease
   Interest Group
Division of Gastroenterology and
   Hepatology
Rochester, Minnesota

Gil Y. Melmed, MD, MS (Chapter 13)
Director, Clinical Trials
Inflammatory Bowel Disease Center
Cedars-Sinai Medical Center
Assistant Clinical Professor of
   Medicine
David Geffen School of Medicine
   at UCLA
Los Angeles, California

*Udayakumar Navaneethan, MD
(Chapter 18)*
Fellow, Digestive Disease Institute
Cleveland Clinic Foundation
Cleveland, Ohio

*Timothy R. Orchard, MA, MD, DM,
FRCP (Chapter 9)*
Consultant Gastroenterologist
St Mary's Hospital
Healthcare NHS Trust
Reader in Gastroenterology
Imperial College
London, United Kingdom

*Sulieman Abdal Raheem, MD
(Chapter 12)*
Fellow, Hepatology
Center for Human Nutrition
Digestive Disease Institute
Cleveland, Ohio

David T. Rubin, MD (Chapter 15)
Associate Professor of Medicine
Co-Director, Inflammatory Bowel
   Disease Center
Program Director, Fellowship in
   Gastroenterology, Hepatology,
   and Nutrition
The University of Chicago Medicine
Chicago, Illinois

David A. Schwartz, MD (Chapter 3)
Director, Inflammatory Bowel
   Disease Center
Associate Professor of Medicine
Vanderbilt University Medical Center
Nashville, Tennessee

Bo Shen, MD (Chapter 18)
Cleveland Clinic
Professor of Medicine
Staff, Digestive Disease Institute
Gastroenterology and Hepatology
Cleveland, Ohio

Miles P. Sparrow, MBBS, FRACP
(Chapter 15)
Consultant Gastroenterologist
The Alfred Hospital
Melbourne, Australia

A. Hillary Steinhart, MD, MSc,
FRCP(C) (Chapter 16)
Head, Combined Division of
  Gastroenterology
Mount Sinai Hospital/University
Toronto, Ontario, Canada

Eva Szigethy, MD, PhD (Chapter 14)
Associate Professor of Psychiatry and
  Pediatrics
Director, Medical Coping Clinic
Children's Hospital of Pittsburgh
Pittsburgh, Pennsylvania

Fernando Velayos, MD, MPH
(Chapter 5)
Associate Professor of Medicine
University of California—
  San Francisco
Center for Crohn's and Colitis
San Francisco, California

David G. Walker, BSc (Hons), MBBS,
MD (Res), MRCP (Chapter 9)
Department of Gastroenterology
  and Hepatology
Imperial College London
United Kingdom

PREFACE

The inflammatory bowel diseases (IBDs), encompassing Crohn's disease and ulcerative colitis, affect more than 1 million Americans, and are often diagnosed at a young age. Treatment of these diseases can be difficult, as patients often develop disease-related complications, which can lead to a decrease in quality of life and work productivity. In addition, recent years have seen not only the introduction of novel therapeutic agents to treat these conditions, but continuing controversies regarding the optimization of clinical outcomes, while minimizing therapy-related adverse events. Physicians need to consider complications due to the natural history of disease, medications, surgery, and general health issues including pregnancy and vaccination, in these complex patients.

Clinical Challenges and Complications of IBD was designed to address the complexities often encountered in the clinical care of patients with IBD. We are thankful to have the expertise of so many nationally and internationally recognized thought leaders as contributors to this book, and we hope that their expertise will be valuable in clarifying the multiple issues that can arise in the care of IBD patients. We believe that gastroenterologists, gastroenterology fellows, nurse practitioners, physician assistants, surgeons, and primary care physicians can all benefit from the management strategies that are emphasized in the book.

The first section deals with the natural history of IBD, including fibrostenotic and penetrating complications, toxic megacolon, dysplasia, and colorectal cancer, and the growing epidemic of infectious complications in IBD patients. Extraintestinal manifestations of IBD are well recognized, and the second section of the book highlights the diagnosis and management of these complications. Many patients with IBD are young people faced with the diagnosis of a significant chronic disease and a high likelihood of eventual surgery. The third section of the book, therefore, details considerations related to this unique patient population, including women's health issues, such as pregnancy, the psychiatric comorbidities associated with IBD, vaccination strategies, and nutritional deficiencies. As mentioned previously, multiple novel medications and treatment algorithms have recently been introduced, and the next section of the book highlights the major adverse events associated with the more commonly used IBD medications. Finally, patients with both ulcerative colitis and Crohn's disease have a significant risk of undergoing surgery during their disease course, which brings with it the possibility of additional complications, as discussed in the final chapter.

In our clinical practice, we care for patients who are simultaneously dealing with one or more of the complications described in this book, and management is never straightforward. Additional factors such as medications, prior or upcoming surgery, and the presence of dysplasia make decision making even more challenging. Although most chapters in this book go into detail regarding the epidemiology and pathophysiology of these conditions, the authors offer practical recommendations in terms of diagnosis and treatment of each complication, which can be easily accessed by the reader. We hope that the clinical pearls in each chapter will help in the day-to-day management of IBD patients and offer a valuable resource for all health professionals involved in their care.

FOREWORD

The treatment of inflammatory bowel diseases (IBD), ulcerative colitis and Crohn's disease, and their complications is a challenge. These idiopathic, chronic immune-mediated inflammatory disorders and their sequelae often have varied clinicopathological courses and unpredictable responses to therapeutic interventions (medical or surgical) such that the concept of "personalized medicine" is both apropos and elusive. Indeed, the evidence base for treatment across the vast array of presentations is quite limited and insufficient to encompass the spectrum of clinical scenarios.

Hence, a compendium of approaches by experts that synthesizes the (limited) evidence and guides by logic and extrapolation the experience of IBD centers is useful to practitioners who will, invariably, encounter diverse and unexpected symptoms and signs of the underlying diseases and/or the medical or surgical interventions.

Drs. Regueiro and Swoger are to be congratulated on their effort to catalog the most common uncommon presentations of IBD and to identify experienced clinicians to synthesize diagnostic and therapeutic options for situations where the evidence is leanest and the risks most perilous. The authors handle both the common manifestations of these uncommon diseases, as well as the uncommon manifestations that will be encountered amidst the spectrum of the ulcerative colitides and the Crohn's diseases. The key points are clearly delineated and the algorithms depict rational, if not completely researched, options. The state of the art of IBD continues to evolve as novel etiopathogenic pathways are elucidated and novel diagnostic strategies and therapies are incorporated into clinical trials and clinical practice. Yet, until the causes are confirmed and long-term approaches are evaluated, the challenges for patients living with, and for physicians attempting to treat IBD, will continue to accrue as the art is gradually translated into science.

Stephen B. Hanauer, MD
Joseph B. Kirsner Professor of Medicine and Clinical Pharmacology
Chief, Section of Gastroenterology, Hepatology, and Nutrition
University of Chicago Medicine
Chicago, Illinois

INTRODUCTION

The aim of this book is to provide a clinically focused, user-friendly approach to the diagnosis, management, and prevention of complications encountered in the care of patients with IBD. Our target audience is not only gastroenterologists who care for IBD patients, but also gastroenterology fellows, nurse practitioners, and physician assistants involved in the care of these often complex patients. We have organized the book to concisely address specific complications related not only to the natural history of IBD, but also to the medical and surgical therapies for these diseases. The main sections of the text are organized as complications related to the natural history of IBD, extraintestinal manifestations of IBD, general health and metabolic complications of IBD, and complications arising from the medical and surgical treatment of IBD. We attempted to create a book that will aid the practitioner in the daily management of IBD patients, and each chapter emphasizes practical knowledge and "clinical pearls." The chapters are organized to promote easy navigation, with sections on epidemiology, etiology and pathophysiology, clinical features, diagnostic evaluation, and management and treatment options. In addition, each chapter includes key clinical points that summarize the main concepts of the text. In addition, we have tried to include concise tables and treatment algorithms, along with representative figures and images to assist clinicians in visually identifying the main pathologies discussed in the text. Caring for patients with Crohn's disease and ulcerative colitis is extremely challenging, and complications, although sometimes rare, present an additional level of complexity. We hope that this book will offer practical information that is both easy to access and clinically relevant to anyone who cares for patients with Crohn's disease and ulcerative colitis.

Section *I*

COMPLICATIONS RELATED TO IBD

Chapter 1

Upper Gastrointestinal Tract Crohn's Disease

Mark Lazarev, MD and Jemilat O. Badamas, MD

CLASSIFICATION AND EPIDEMIOLOGY

Upper gastrointestinal (UGI) Crohn's disease (CD) refers to disease found in the esophagus, stomach, jejunum, or proximal ileum. The original Vienna classification of CD location designated L1 disease as terminal ileal, L2 as colonic, L3 as ileocolonic, and L4 as UGI disease.[1] However, the vast majority of patients with UGI disease also have concurrent distal disease. The Vienna classification was not able to appropriately categorize these patients. More recently, the Montreal Working Party reclassified L4 disease such that it can be separately added to any other established location (Table 1-1).[2] This has improved the ability to more accurately phenotype patients with UGI disease.

Symptomatic UGI disease is rare, reported in only 1% to 5% of CD patients.[3,4] However, UGI disease is much more common than previously thought. Studies have found that upper endoscopy will identify mild macroscopic inflammation in up to 30% to 64% of patients, and microscopic disease has been reported in up to 70% of pediatric patients.[5,6]

Larger population cohort studies have not confirmed a prevalence this high. In a Danish population-based inflammatory bowel disease (IBD) cohort including both adult and pediatric patients, 641 patients with newly diagnosed CD were identified among 3 different time periods, 1962 to 1987, 1991 to 1993, and 2003 to 2004.[7] UGI disease, defined as any disease proximal to the ileum, was identified in 8%, 19%, and 8%, respectively. This observed trend argues against an increased prevalence of UGI disease, even with advances in endoscopy and radiographic imaging. In one of the larger published pediatric cohorts (Pediatric IBD Consortium), Heyman et al collected data on 1370 pediatric IBD patients between 2000 and 2002, 798 of whom had CD.[8] Macroscopic gastroduodenal inflammation was seen in 5% of 0 to 5 year olds, 10% of 6 to 12 year olds, and 13% of 13 to 17 year olds. Thus, prevalence was found to increase slightly with age in the pediatric cohort. A similar UGI prevalence was found in an

Regueiro MD, Swoger JM, eds.
Clinical Challenges and Complications of IBD (pp 3-16).
© 2013 Taylor & Francis Group.

Table 1-1. Montreal Classification of Crohn's Disease	
Age at diagnosis	A1— >17 years old
	A2—17 to 40 years old
	A3— >40 years old
Disease location	L1—Ileal
	L2—Colonic
	L3—Ileocolonic
	L4—Upper gastrointestinal disease*
Disease behavior	B1—Nonpenetrating, nonstricturing
	B2—Stricturing
	B3—Penetrating
	P—Modifier for perianal involvement

*L4 is a modifier applied to L1–L3 disease, when present.
Adapted from Satsangi J, Silverberg MS, Vermeire S, Colombel JF. The Montreal classification of inflammatory bowel disease: controversies, consensus, and implications. *Gut*. 2006;55:749-753.

adult cohort based on the North American IBD genetics consortium.[9] A total of 611 patients with CD were phenotyped to evaluate UGI disease. Disease location was divided into ileal, colonic, ileocolonic, and UGI disease. UGI disease was further subdivided into esophagogastroduodenal (EGD) or jejunal disease. Location of disease was established based on endoscopic reports, radiographic studies, and operative reports. A confirmed endoscopic diagnosis required 10 or more aphthous ulcers to be identified. The presence of histologic disease alone, in this study, was not considered diagnostic. Of the 611 CD patients, 54 (8.8%) had EGD involvement and 57 (9.1%) had jejunal involvement. This study also found racial disparities in the prevalence of UGI CD. The prevalence of EGD disease in Blacks was significantly higher than that in Whites (20% versus 8.5%; $P = 0.003$). However, the prevalence of jejunal involvement was not different between groups.

It has traditionally been thought that UGI disease is more common in children compared to the adult population. This may be a result of detection bias, as pediatric patients are much more likely to undergo routine upper endoscopy, whereas adults only undergo upper endoscopy if they are symptomatic. However, there appears to be evidence to suggest that UGI disease is more common in children. Limbergen et al compared 273 Scottish childhood-onset CD patients with 507 Scottish adult-onset CD patients.[10] With a median follow-up time of 3.7 years from diagnosis in the childhood-onset IBD patients, and 10.3 years from diagnosis in the adult-onset IBD patients, the former group was significantly less likely to have isolated ileal or colonic disease than their adult counterparts. By contrast, childhood-onset patients were far more likely to have "panenteric" or extensive disease (ileocolonic and UGI disease) than adult-onset patients (43.2% versus 3.2%; odds ratio [OR] 23.4) (95% confidence interval [CI] 13.5 to 40.6).

Generally, studies have found esophageal CD to be rare. The prevalence of esophageal disease is approximately 1.8% among adults with CD.[11] Furthermore, isolated esophageal disease is exceedingly rare, mostly described in case reports. Concurrent distal disease involvement is almost always present.

ETIOLOGY: GENETICS OF UPPER GASTROINTESTINAL DISEASE

Few studies have assessed phenotype/genotype correlations of UGI CD. Mutations in NOD2/CARD15 have been associated with the presence of ileal and stricturing disease.[12] Studies of the association of UGI disease with the NOD2 gene have generated mixed results. In a report of 202 mostly White CD patients, 18 were found to have gastroduodenal disease.[13] Of these 18 patients, 10 (56%) were wild type for NOD2, 4 (22%) had 1 gene variant, and 4 (22%) had 2 gene variants. Patients with gastroduodenal CD involvement were more likely to have 2 variants in the NOD2 gene than patients without gastroduodenal involvement (OR 2.7; 95% CI 1.6 to 7.3). Additionally, after controlling for multiple variants including ileal location, homozygosity in the NOD2 L1007P locus was found through multivariable analysis to be independently associated with gastroduodenal involvement. In another study, NOD2/CARD15 variant status was examined in 167 pediatric patients with CD.[14] Carriage of NOD2/CARD15 mutations was present in 50% in patients with jejunal disease, compared to only 18.4% in those without jejunal disease ($P = 0.01$). Notably, there was no difference in carriage rate between patients with or without gastroduodenal disease.

Not all studies, however, have found a definitive link between UGI CD and NOD2 gene expressions. Lesage et al analyzed variants in the NOD2/CARD15 gene among 453 patients with CD.[15] Patients with 2 disease-causing mutations had a younger age of onset, more frequent stricturing phenotype, and less frequent colonic involvement than patients with no mutations. However, there was no difference in UGI tract involvement (total of 23 patients in the entire cohort) between patients who had 2 mutations and patients who had none (20% versus 19%, respectively).

CLINICAL FEATURES AND NATURAL HISTORY

Clinical Features

Typical symptoms of esophageal disease include dysphagia, odynophagia, heartburn, atypical chest pain, and nausea/vomiting.[16] Gastroduodenal disease involvement often mimics symptoms of peptic ulcer disease, including epigastric pain, atypical chest pain, anorexia, and weight loss. Sometimes patients present with symptoms of gastric outlet obstruction, most notably when stricturing disease has developed at the pylorus or in the proximal duodenum. For jejunoileal (JI) disease, Attard et al studied a cohort of 134 pediatric patients from 1996 to 2002.[17]

Twenty-three (17%) of the patients exhibited JI involvement alone, or in combination with colonic disease. The most commonly reported symptoms included abdominal pain (35%), diarrhea (21%), weight loss (18%), and fever (8%). Patients with JI disease had lower mean and standard deviation z-scores for height than patients without JI disease (−0.36 [1.95] versus 0.16 [1.25]; $P = 0.02$). Additionally, patients with JI disease had lower weight and weight-for-height scores.

Natural History

There is evidence that UGI disease may be associated with a predisposition for more aggressive disease. Wolters et al prospectively studied 358 patients with CD from the time of initial diagnosis.[18] Disease phenotype at diagnosis was examined to determine a possible relationship to future recurrence rates. Although only 20 patients (5.6%) had UGI disease, it was found to be a risk factor for future nonsurgical and surgical recurrence. Additionally, UGI disease was the only significant positive predictor for recurrence found in a Cox proportional hazard model ($P < 0.01$). Notably, 19 out of the 20 UGI patients had a nonpenetrating disease phenotype.

Similar findings were reported in a cohort of 132 Chinese patients with CD.[19] Thirty patients (22.7%) were categorized as having L4 disease at diagnosis. Patients with the L4 phenotype were found to have more stricturing (46.7%) and penetrating disease (30.0%) than patients with non-L4 disease (18.6% and 3.9%, respectively; $P < 0.0001$). Over a median follow-up of 5 years, patients with L4 disease were more likely to undergo major surgery (66.7%) than patients without L4 disease (36.3%; $P < 0.0001$). Notably, half of the patients in the L4 group underwent surgery within the first month of diagnosis. In the Cox proportional hazard model, L4 disease independently predicted hospitalization (hazard ratio 2.1, 95% CI 1.3 to 3.5). For major surgery, stricturing and penetrating diseases were found to be independent predictive factors, whereas L2 (colonic disease only) was protective. L4 disease, however, was not found to be an independent predictor for major surgery.

Recently, the National Institute of Diabetes and Digestive and Kidney Diseases IBD genetics consortium presented data on the prevalence and natural history of UGI CD.[20] Of the 1632 CD patients who had been phenotyped, 287 (17.6%) had L4 disease while 1345 did not (82.4%). Of these 287 patients, 137 (47.7%) had EGD involvement, 85 (29.6%) had jejunal involvement, and 65 (22.7%) had both EGD and jejunal involvement. Age at diagnosis was significantly lower for L4 patients compared to non-L4 patients. Notably, patients with jejunal involvement were significantly less likely to have concurrent colonic disease than patients with disease of the esophagus, stomach, or duodenum. In agreement with the findings of Chow et al, patients with L4 disease were more likely to have a stricturing phenotype than patients without L4 disease.[19] However, the results were largely driven by the subgroup of patients with jejunal disease, as patients with EGD disease were no more likely than non-L4 patients to have stricturing disease. There was no difference in the presence of a penetrating phenotype between groups. L4 patients with jejunal disease were also significantly more likely to undergo multiple abdominal surgeries compared to L4 patients with EGD disease. In the multivariable analysis, L4 disease was an independent predictor for stricturing disease (OR 3.3 [2.0 to 5.2]) as well as multiple surgeries (OR 3.5 [1.9 to 6.2]). Ileal involvement and increased disease duration were also independent predictors. L4 disease involving an EGD location was neither a predictor of stricturing disease nor that of multiple surgeries.

In summary, L4 disease appears to be predictive of complicated disease and an increased need for surgery compared to non-L4 disease. There is evidence that jejunal involvement is different from EGD disease, and perhaps should be classified separately. In fact, in the revision of the Montreal Classification for pediatric IBD (termed the *Paris Classification*), L4 disease is divided into L4a (upper disease proximal to the ligament of Treitz) and L4b (upper disease distal to the ligament of Treitz and proximal to the distal one-third ileum).[21]

DIAGNOSTIC EVALUATION

Esophageal Disease

Upper endoscopy is the main diagnostic tool for the assessment of esophageal CD. In a Mayo Clinic study of 20 patients with esophageal CD, 17 (85%) had ulcers, most of which were superficial; 3 patients had deep ulcers.[22] The distal esophagus was most commonly involved, although several patients had mid- or panesophageal involvement. A chronic inflammatory mucosal infiltrate was seen in 75% of patients, while granulomas were not noted on any biopsies.

Gastroduodenal Disease

Generally, upper endoscopy can serve 2 roles in the diagnosis of gastroduodenal CD. First, it is a method of comprehensively staging disease location. Second, it can assist in differentiating CD from ulcerative colitis (UC). However, caution should be used in interpreting results. Several studies have found that the prevalence of inflammation in the esophagus, stomach, and duodenum is comparable in both CD and UC.[23] In the absence of nonsteroidal anti-inflammatory drug (NSAID) use, pronounced *Helicobacter pylori*–negative ulcerations are highly suggestive of CD involvement (Figure 1-1). The presence of granulomas also supports the diagnosis of CD. Importantly, isolated UGI granulomas in the setting of no known IBD diagnosis can be seen in *H pylori* infection, as well as in sarcoidosis. The finding of *H pylori*–negative gastritis is often nonspecific. Findings of focally enhanced gastritis (defined as a periglandular mononuclear or neutrophilic infiltrate around gastric crypts), however, is more suggestive of CD than of UC. In a study of 238 children with UGI biopsies, focal gastritis was seen in 65.1% of CD patients, 20.8% of UC patients, and only 2.3% of controls.[24] Studies have shown a sensitivity of 43% to 52% and a specificity of 79% to 90% for differentiating CD from UC based on the finding of focally enhanced gastritis.[23] Notably, most studies have been performed in the pediatric population, with fewer data available in adult patients. Overall, current recommendations regarding upper endoscopy in pediatric

Figure 1-1. Endoscopic view of gastric CD, with multiple ulcerations (arrow). (Reprinted with permission of Jason M. Swoger, MD, MPH.)

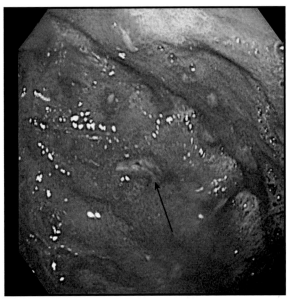

patients are mixed. The value of the procedure in patients with an established diagnosis of CD is questionable. However, for patients in whom the diagnosis is unclear, upper endoscopy can potentially be useful.

Small Bowel Disease

The field of small bowel imaging has been evolving at a dramatic pace. Traditionally, UGI series with small bowel follow-through has been the study of choice in evaluating mucosal detail. Sensitivity can be further enhanced through performance of enteroclysis, in which contrast is delivered via a nasojejunal tube. However, as CD is a transmural process, barium imaging is not ideal in assessing disease activity, nor can it evaluate the presence of extraluminal disease. Additionally, barium studies are significantly user and center dependent, and local expertise is an important factor in the decision of which study to perform. Computed tomography enterography (CTE) was developed in 1992 and uses an oral-based contrast to achieve small bowel distention. This technique has been shown to be very effective and may aid in the differentiation of inflammatory versus fibrostenotic disease (Figure 1-2). More recently, magnetic resonance (MR)–based small bowel imaging has been developed. The performance characteristics of MR enterography (MRE) appear similar to those of CTE.[25] Additionally, there is a strong correlation between findings on MRE and findings at surgery with regard to the detection of inflammation. Important radiographic features described for CTE and MRE, associated with active inflammation, include wall thickening, an increased degree of enhancement, the comb sign (prominent vasa recta), and fistulization.[26] Traditionally, MR imaging has been time consuming; however, sequences are becoming more rapid and can provide as much information as CTE. Additionally, MRE does not subject the patient to ionizing radiation, which is a significant concern given the number of radiographic studies many CD patients undergo over their disease course.

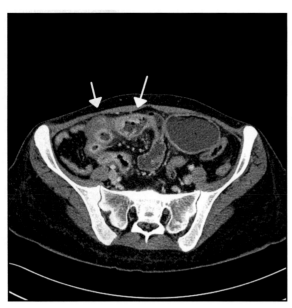

Figure 1-2. CTE showing radiographic signs of proximal small bowel inflammation, including wall thickening and mucosal hyperenhancement (arrows). (Reprinted with permission of David Bruining, MD.)

With regard to small bowel endoscopy, options include small bowel enteroscopy and wireless capsule endoscopy (WCE). WCE allows for the identification of mucosal lesions that may not be visualized with other modalities. Due to the ability to identify subtle mucosal lesions, WCE has a high negative predictive value for the diagnosis of small bowel CD. However, due to the high rate of lesion detection, its positive predictive value is poor. One must be cautioned by nonspecific lesions such as lymphangiectasia, villous denudation, or nodular lymphoid hyperplasia. Additionally, there are no prospectively validated diagnostic criteria for establishing a diagnosis of CD based on WCE alone. Generally, the presence of greater than 3 ulcerations in the absence of NSAID use has been used to confirm a diagnosis of CD (Figure 1-3). Among adults, WCE may be more effective in identifying small bowel mucosal lesions than small bowel follow-through, CTE, or MRE. A recent meta-analysis showed that WCE is superior to small bowel radiography, CTE, or ileocolonoscopy in the evaluation of suspected CD.[27] WCE was also more effective in confirming active small bowel disease in patients with established CD when compared to barium imaging, CTE, or push enteroscopy. Importantly, one must counsel patients about the risk of capsule retention, particularly in those who already have established CD. These patients should have a small bowel imaging study to rule out stricturing disease. Alternatively, a dissolvable patency capsule can be placed prior to capsule placement.

Recommendations for Diagnosis

In summary, multiple radiographic and endoscopic options are available for either the diagnosis of CD or the evaluation of UGI involvement in a patient who already has an established CD diagnosis. Generally, small bowel evaluation with CTE, MRE, or capsule endoscopy is preferred for the initial diagnosis of CD or for the establishment of disease location. The performance of an upper endoscopy should be reserved for adult patients who are symptomatic.

Figure 1-3. Capsule endoscopy view of an aphthous ulceration (arrow) typical of jejunal CD. (Reprinted with permission of Jason M. Swoger, MD, MPH.)

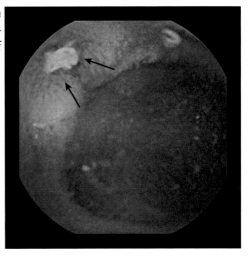

TREATMENT: MEDICAL AND SURGICAL THERAPY

Proton Pump Inhibitors

Proton pump inhibitors (PPIs) are potent suppressants of intragastric acid production and are often recommended in the management of UGI CD to minimize symptoms associated with gastritis. Although PPIs provide symptomatic relief in patients with esophageal or gastric CD, they have little role in controlling mucosal inflammation.[28]

5-Aminosalicylic Acid Drugs

5-aminosalicylic acid (5-ASA) agents have traditionally been used in the treatment of mild-to-moderately active CD. Disulfide bond–dependent 5-ASA preparations, including sulfasalazine, olsalazine, and balsalazide, release their active 5-ASA compound in the distal ileum and colon, thus serving no function in the management of UGI CD. The same applies to pH-dependent mesalamine preparations. Pentasa (mesalamine) is a medication consisting of ethyl cellulose–coated microgranules of mesalamine. Through a moisture-dependent and pH-independent process, Pentasa allows for continuous release of mesalamine throughout the entire GI tract. A meta-analysis examining the efficacy of Pentasa 4 g/d in active CD among three 16-week trials, including a total of 304 patients, showed a mean decrease of 63 points on the Crohn's Disease Activity Index (CDAI) in the Pentasa group compared to a decrease of 45 points in the placebo group.[29] Although this result was statistically significant ($P = 0.04$), its clinical significance is dubious. Notably, UGI disease was not separately examined in these studies.

Glucocorticoids

Corticosteroids are often utilized in patients with mild-to-moderate disease unresponsive to 5-ASA agents, or in patients with moderate-to-severe CD. In one report of 89 patients with duodenal CD, for example, 49 patients were managed medically with prednisone and followed up for 2 to 25 years, with 90% noting good-to-excellent clinical response.[3] Notably, some of the patients were on concomitant medications, including sulfasalazine, H_2 blockers, metronidazole, and azathioprine.

Budesonide is an oral controlled release steroid preparation that specifically targets the distal small bowel and right colon. Because it undergoes extensive first-pass metabolism, it has significantly fewer systemic adverse effects. Budesonide has been shown to be effective for the induction of remission in CD, but its maintenance effect is not sustained beyond 16 weeks.[30] Although its use in UGI CD has not been formally studied, breaking the capsule and ingesting the contents could theoretically lead to proximal small bowel mucosal contact. Overall, there is no evidence that steroids can maintain long-term remission or lead to mucosal healing.

Antibiotics

Antibiotics are unlikely to be a useful tool in the induction or maintenance of remission in UGI CD. Subanalysis of a double-blinded placebo-controlled trial examining the efficacy of metronidazole in CD patients revealed that it is less effective in patients with disease confined to the small bowel compared to patients with disease of the colon or both the colon and small intestine.[31] This was echoed in a study that randomized patients to receive a combination of ciprofloxacin and metronidazole, or placebo. All patients received concomitant budesonide. Again, patients with isolated ileal disease did not exhibit a positive response.[32]

Immunomodulatory Drugs

Immunomodulatory drugs such as azathioprine and 6-mercaptopurine (6-MP) are indicated in patients who are unresponsive to steroids or who require steroid-sparing maintenance therapy. In a study of 148 CD patients treated with 6-MP, all patients with gastric and duodenal disease had either healing or marked improvement of their disease.[33] Another study of 12 patients with UGI disease found that azathioprine therapy allowed for the discontinuation of prednisone in 70% of patients, after 6 months of treatment, with a significant decrease in both CDAI and C-reactive protein levels.[28] Both 6-MP and azathioprine are generally well tolerated; however, possible adverse effects include a hypersensitivity reaction, leukopenia, pancreatitis, hepatotoxicity, an increased risk of infection, nonmelanoma skin cancers, and lymphoma (see Chapter 16).

Biologic Agents

Anti-tumor necrosis factor (TNF) agents such as infliximab, adalimumab, and certolizumab pegol are the mainstays of medical therapy for patients with moderate-to-severe or fistulizing CD, refractory to conventional therapy. Their efficacy in specifically treating UGI CD involvement has not been prospectively studied. However, case studies of patients with severe esophageal, gastric, and duodenal disease have reported a good clinical response to anti-TNF agents.[34-36]

Useful data can also be taken from a CD clinical trial evaluating infliximab in a new long-term treatment regimen, the ACCENT I trial, the largest trial to compare infliximab to placebo.[37] In this study, all patients received a single dose of infliximab at 5 mg/kg; responders (based on CDAI scores) were then randomized to receive maintenance infliximab infusions of 5 or 10 mg/kg or placebo. Forty-three of the 573 (8%) patients included in the study were found to have gastroduodenal disease. Of these 43 patients, the week 2 response rate of 56% was similar to the overall response rate of 58% for the study population. What is not clear from these data is whether or not maintenance therapy was as successful in patients with gastroduodenal disease as in those without gastroduodenal disease. Currently, there remains much to be learned regarding the role of anti-TNF agents in management of UGI CD.

Nutritional Therapy

Corticosteroid therapy has been found to be superior to enteral nutrition therapy for the induction of remission in pediatric patients.[38] Additionally, nutritional therapy, with exclusive enteral therapy has been shown to suppress inflammation and promote bowel healing in patients with CD. Attard et al found that, among 23 patients with JI disease, nutritional therapy was associated with an improvement in height (OR 5.87; $P < 0.03$) compared to patients without jejunoileitis.[17] However, this should not be surprising as JI patients were found to be more stunted at the time of diagnosis. Total parenteral nutrition and complete bowel rest have also been shown to be effective in inducing remission in distal CD; however, high rates of relapse occur with resumption of regular feeding. These effects have not been studied specifically in patients with isolated UGI CD.

Endoscopic Therapy

Stenotic UGI CD lesions may be managed with balloon dilation, although the rate of recurrence is high. Matsui et al described 5 cases of successful dilation of gastroduodenal CD. However, 3 of the 5 patients developed recurrent obstructive symptoms over a period of 4.2 years.[39] Generally, endoscopic dilation should be confined to patients with short, noninflammed, accessible strictures, particularly those at anastomotic sites. Esophageal dilation is one treatment option for esophageal CD. However, this procedure carries a higher risk of perforation due to the presence of esophageal wall inflammation, and thus must be performed with caution.

Surgery

As already mentioned, L4 disease, particularly jejunal disease, is associated with stricturing behavior and the need for one or more surgeries. Additionally, when diffuse jejunoileitis is present, surgical resection is frequently required. Stricturoplasty is the mainstay of surgical therapy in those with extensive small bowel disease. This is a bowel-conserving technique, which minimizes the risk of short bowel syndrome. The most common procedures include the Heineke-Mikulicz technique (for stenoses 7 cm or less) and the Finney technique (for longer strictures) (Figure 1-4). The Michelassi isoperistaltic stricturoplasty is less

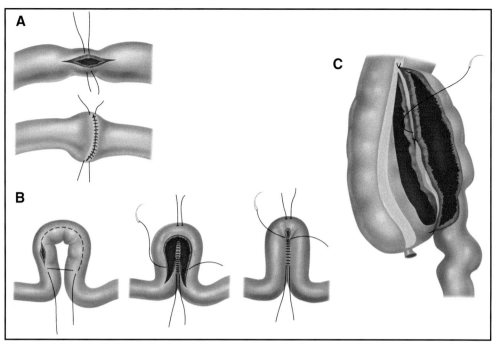

Figure 1-4. Small intestinal stricturoplasty techniques. (A) Heineke-Mikulicz, (B) Finney, (C) Michelassi (isoperistaltic).

frequently used. A study from the Cleveland Clinic examined 123 patients with diffuse jejunoileitis who underwent an index stricturoplasty between 1984 and 1999.[40] Patients required a median of 5 stricturoplasties, and greater than two-thirds of the patients also underwent a synchronous bowel resection. The surgical recurrence rate was 29%, with a median follow-up interval of 6.7 years. This recurrence rate did not differ between patients with diffuse jejunoileitis or with limited small bowel disease who underwent stricturoplasty. Other studies have reported higher rates of recurrence associated with stricturoplasty; one such study found a 52% reoperation rate 4.3 years after an initial stricturoplasty.[41]

In patients with stricturing or fistulizing gastric or duodenal disease, bypass operations (gastrojejunostomy, duodenojejunostomy, and gastroduodenostomy) may be preferred to gastric or duodenal resection due to the increased risk of morbidity associated with bowel resection.[42] Few studies have compared stricturoplasty to bypass surgery. Overall, results have been varied. One study found equal rates of reoperation between stricturoplasty (2/13, 15%) and bypass (2/21, 10%) patients.[43] However, Yamamoto et al reported higher rates of reoperation with stricturoplasty (9/13, 69%) compared to bypass (6/13, 46%) patients.[44] Thus, a definitive recommendation for one approach over the other cannot be made.

CONCLUSION

There are limited data on the effectiveness of medical treatment options specifically aimed at UGI CD. However, there is no reason to believe that the medical treatment for UGI CD should differ from that of more distal disease. Although the evidence is weak, a top-down treatment strategy can be considered in patients with jejunal involvement. As for surgical options, stricturoplasty appears to be the best-studied option and has the advantage of being a bowel-sparing procedure, which helps to decrease long-term complications.

☑ Key Points

- ☑ The diagnosis of UGI CD is not based on clearly delineated guidelines. Generally, a diagnosis is made by gross findings on endoscopy and bowel wall thickening on small bowel imaging (small bowel follow-through, CT, or MRE).

- ☑ UGI CD is common, occurring in up to 64% of patients on a gross macroscopic level. However, symptomatic UGI CD is rare.

- ☑ UGI disease almost always occurs in combination with more distal disease.

- ☑ The genetic basis behind UGI disease is not well understood— NOD2 mutations may be involved.

- ☑ UGI disease appears to be predictive of a more aggressive phenotype. Jejunal disease in particular is linked to a stricturing disease phenotype and the need for multiple resections.

- ☑ Medical therapy has not been well studied for UGI CD. There is no evidence to suggest that the efficacy of medical therapy is any better or worse for patients with or without UGI CD.

- ☑ Stricturoplasty is the mainstay of surgical therapy for those with diffuse obstructive small bowel disease.

REFERENCES

1. Gasche C, Scholmerich J, Brynskov J, et al. A simple classification of Crohn's disease: report of the Working Party for the World Congresses of Gastroenterology, Vienna 1998. *Inflamm Bowel Dis.* 2000;6:8-15.
2. Silverberg MS, Satsangi J, Ahmad T, et al. Toward an integrated clinical, molecular, and serological classification of inflammatory bowel disease: report of a Working Party of the 2005 Montreal World Congress of Gastroenterology. *Can J Gastroenterol.* 2005;19(suppl A):5-36.
3. Nugent FW, Roy MA. Duodenal Crohn's disease: an analysis of 89 cases. *Am J Gastroenterol.* 1989;84:249-254.
4. Tan WC, Allan RN. Diffuse jejunoileitis of Crohn's disease. *Gut.* 1993;34:1374-1378.
5. Lenaerts C, Roy CC, Vaillancourt M, et al. High incidence of upper gastrointestinal tract involvement in children with Crohn's disease. *Pediatrics.* 1989;83:777-781.
6. Sawczenko A, Sandhu BK. Presenting features of inflammatory bowel disease in Great Britain and Ireland. *Arch Dis Child.* 2003;88:995-1000.
7. Jess T, Riis L, Vind I, et al. Changes in clinical characteristics, course, and prognosis of inflammatory bowel disease during the last 5 decades: a population-based study from Copenhagen, Denmark. *Inflamm Bowel Dis.* 2007;13:481-489.
8. Heyman MB, Kirschner B, Gold B, et al. Children with early-onset inflammatory bowel disease (IBD): analysis of a pediatric IBD consortium registry. *J Pediatr.* 2005;146:35-40.

9. Nguyen GC, Torres EA, Reguiero M, et al. Inflammatory bowel disease characteristics among African Americans, Hispanics, and non-Hispanic Whites: characterization of a large North American Cohort. *Am J Gastroenterol*. 2006;101:1012-1023.

10. Limbergen J, Russell RK, Drummond HE, et al. Definition of phenotypic characteristics of childhood-onset inflammatory bowel disease. *Gastroenterology*. 2008;135:1114-1122.

11. Isaacs KL. Crohn's disease of the esophagus. *Curr Treat Options Gastroenterol*. 2007;10:61-70.

12. Abreu MT, Taylor KD, Lin YC, et al. Mutations in NOD2 are associated with fibrostenosing disease in patients with Crohn's disease. *Gastroenterology*. 2002;123:679-688.

13. Mardini HE, Gregory KJ, Nasser M, et al. Gastroduodenal Crohn's disease is associated with NOD2/CARD15 gene polymorphisms, particularly L1007P homozygosity. *Dig Dis Sci*. 2005;50:2316-2322.

14. Russell RK, Drummond HE, Nimmo EE, et al. Genotype-phenotype analysis in childhood-onset Crohn's disease: NOD2/CARD15 variants consistently predict phenotypic characteristics of severe disease. *Inflamm Bowel Dis*. 2005;11:955-964.

15. Lesage S, Habib Z, Cezad J, et al. CARD15/NOD2 mutational analysis and genotype-phenotype correlation in 612 patients with inflammatory bowel disease. *Am J Hum Genet*. 2002;70:845-857.

16. Wagtmans MJ, Hogezand RA, Griffioen G, et al. Crohn's disease of the upper gastrointestinal tract. *Neth J Med*. 1997;50:S2-S7.

17. Attard TM, Horton KM, DeVito K, et al. Pediatric jejunoileitis: a severe Crohn's disease phenotype that requires intensive nutritional management. *Inflamm Bowel Dis*. 2004;10(4):357-360.

18. Wolters FL, Russel MG, Sijbrandij J, et al. Phenotype at diagnosis predicts recurrence rates in Crohn's disease. *Gut*. 2006;55:1124-1130.

19. Chow DK, Sung J, Yu JC, et al. Upper gastrointestinal tract phenotype of Crohn's disease is associated with early surgery and further hospitalization. *Inflamm Bowel Dis*. 2009;15:551-557.

20. Lazarev, M, Hutfless S, Bitton A, et al. Divergence in L4 Crohn's disease: jejunal, not esophagogastroduodenal involvement, is protective of L2 disease location, and a risk for stricturing behavior and multiple abdominal surgeries. Report from the NIDDK-IBDGC Registry. *Gastroenterology*. 2010;138(suppl 1):S105(abstract).

21. Levine A, Griffiths A, Markowitz J, et al. Pediatric modification of the Montreal classification for inflammatory bowel disease. *Inflamm Bowel Dis*. 2011;17:1314-1321.

22. Decker GA, Loftus EV, Pasha TM, et al. Crohn's disease of the esophagus: clinical features and outcomes. *Inflamm Bowel Dis*. 2001;7:113-119.

23. Bousvaros A, Antonioli DA, Colletti RB, et al. Differentiating ulcerative colitis from Crohn's disease in children and young adults: report of a working group of North American Society for Pediatric Gastroenterology, Hepatology and Nutrition and the Crohn's and Colitis Foundation of America. *J Pediatr Gastroenterol Nutr*. 2007;44:653-674.

24. Sharif F, McDermott M, Dillon M, et al. Focally enhanced gastritis in children with Crohn's disease and ulcerative colitis. *Am J Gastroenterol*. 2002;97:1415-1420.

25. Schreyer AG, Hoffstetter P, Daneschnejad M, et al. Comparison of conventional abdominal CT with MR-enterography in patients with active Crohn's disease and acute abdominal pain. *Acad Radiol*. 2010;17:352-357.

26. Zappa M, Stefanescu C, Cazals-Hatem D, et al. Which magnetic resonance imaging findings accurately evaluate inflammation in small bowel Crohn's disease? A retrospective comparison with surgical pathologic analysis. *Inflamm Bowel Dis*. 2011;17:984-993.

27. Dionisio PM, Gurudu SR, Leighton JA, et al. Capsule endoscopy has a significantly higher diagnostic yield in patients with suspected and established small-bowel Crohn's disease: a meta-analysis. *Am J Gastroenterol*. 2010;105:1240-1248.

28. Miehsler W, Puspok A, Oberhuber T, et al. Impact of different therapeutic regimens on the outcome of patients with Crohn's disease of the upper gastrointestinal tract. *Inflamm Bowel Dis*. 2001;7:99-105.

29. Hanauer SB, Stomberg U. Oral Pentasa in the treatment of active Crohn's disease: a meta-analysis of double blind, placebo controlled trials. *Clin Gastro Hepatol*. 2004;2:379-388.

30. Benchimol EI, Seow CH, Otley AR, Steinhart AH. Budesonide for maintenance of remission in Crohn's disease. *Cochrane Database Syst Rev*. 2009;(1):CD002913.

31. Sutherland L, Singleton J, Sessions J, et al. Double blind, placebo controlled trial of metronidazole in Crohn's disease. *Gut*. 1991;32:1071-1075.

32. Steinhart AH, Feagan BG, Wong CJ, et al. Combined budesonide and antibiotic therapy for active Crohn's disease: a randomized controlled trial. *Gastroenterology.* 2002;123:33-40.

33. Korelitz BI, Adler DJ, Mendelsohn RA, Sacknoff AL. Long-term experience with 6-mercaptopurine in the treatment of Crohn's disease. *Am J Gastroenterol.* 1993;88:1198-1205.

34. Heller T, James SP, Drachenberg C, Hernandez C, Darwin PE Treatment of severe esophageal Crohn's disease with infliximab. *Inflamm Bowel Dis.* 1999;5:279-282.

35. Noe JD, Pfefferkon M. Short-term response to adalimumab in childhood inflammatory bowel disease. *Inflamm Bowel Dis.* 2008;14:1683-1687.

36. Firth JJ, Prather C. Unusual gastric Crohn's disease treated with infliximab. A case report. *Am J Gastroenterol.* 2002;97:S190.

37. Hanauer SB, Feagan BG, Lichtenstein GR, et al. Maintenance infliximab for Crohn's disease: the ACCENT I randomized trial. *Lancet.* 2002;359:1541-1549.

38. Lochs H, Steinhardt HJ, Klaus-Wentz B, et al. Comparison of enteral nutrition and drug treatment in active Crohn's disease. Results of the European Cooperative Crohn's Disease Study. IV. *Gastroenterology.* 1991;101:881-888.

39. Matsui T, Hatakeyama S, Ikeda K, Yao T, Takenaka K, Sakurai T. Long-term outcome of endoscopic balloon dilation in obstructive gastroduodenal Crohn's disease. *Endoscopy.* 1997;29:640-645.

40. Dietz DW, Fazio VW, Laureti S, et al. Strictureplasty in diffuse Crohn's jejunoileitis. *Dis Colon Rectum.* 2002;45:764-770.

41. Fearnhead NS, Chowdhury R, Box B. Long-term follow-up of strictureplasty for Crohn's disease. *Br J Surg.* 2006;93:475-482.

42. Murray JJ, Schoetz DJ Jr, Nugent FW, Coller JA, Veidenheimer MC. Surgical management of Crohn's disease involving the duodenum. *Am J Surg.* 1984;147:58-65.

43. Worsey MJ, Hull T, Ryland L, et al. Strictureplasty is an effective option in the operative management of duodenal Crohn's disease. *Dis Colon Rectum.* 1999;42:596-600.

44. Yamamoto T, Allan RN, Keighley RB. Long-term outcome of surgical management for diffuse jejunoileal Crohn's disease. *Surgery.* 2001;129:96-102.

SUGGESTED READINGS

Bousvaros A, Antonioli DA, Colletti RB, et al. Differentiating ulcerative colitis from Crohn disease in children and young adults: report of a working group of North American Society for Pediatric Gastroenterology, Hepatology and Nutrition and the Crohn's and Colitis Foundation of America. *J Pediatr Gastroenterol Nutr.* 2007;44:653-674.

Heyman MB, Kirschner B, Gold B, et al. Children with early-onset inflammatory bowel disease (IBD): analysis of a pediatric IBD consortium registry. *J Pediatr.* 2005;146:35-40.

Lazarev M, Hutfless S, Bitton A, et al. Divergence in L4 Crohn's disease: jejunal, not esophagogastroduodenal involvement, is protective of L2 disease location, and a risk for stricturing behavior and multiple abdominal surgeries. Report from the NIDDK-IBDGC Registry. *Gastroenterology.* 2010;138(suppl 1):S105 (abstract).

Lesage S, Habib Z, Cezad J, et al. CARD15/NOD2 mutational analysis and genotype-phenotype correlation in 612 patients with inflammatory bowel disease. *Am J Hum Genet.* 2002;70:845-857.

Levine A, Griffiths A, Markowitz J, et al. Pediatric modification of the Montreal classification for inflammatory bowel disease. *Inflamm Bowel Dis* 2011;17:1314-1321.

Limbergen J, Russell RK, Drummond HE, et al. Definition of phenotypic characteristics of childhood-onset inflammatory bowel disease. *Gastroenterology.* 2008;135:1114-1122.

Nguyen GC, Torres EA, Reguiero M, et al. Inflammatory bowel disease characteristics among African Americans, Hispanics, and non-Hispanic whites: characterization of a large North American cohort. *Am J Gastroenterol.* 2006;101:1012-1023.

Wolters FL, Russel MG, Sijbrandij J, et al. Phenotype at diagnosis predicts recurrence rates in Crohn's disease. *Gut.* 2006;55:1124-1130.

Chapter 2

Internal Fistula, Abscesses, and Strictures

Evaluation With Novel Radiographic Techniques and Clinical Management

Peter D.R. Higgins, MD, PhD, MSc

EPIDEMIOLOGY

Crohn's disease (CD) is classified into inflammatory (B1, nonpenetrating, nonstricturing), stricturing (B2, stenotic), and penetrating (B3, fistulas and/or abscesses) disease.[1] Although this is the standard Montreal classification, the stricturing and penetrating categories have significant overlap; most fistulas/penetrating complications arise upstream from a stenosis.[2,3] Epidemiologic data on the prevalence of stricturing disease demonstrate a correlation with disease duration, in that, after a decade of disease, approximately one-third of patients with CD will have developed a stricture.[4] Numerous studies have documented a steady progression of patients over time to increasingly complicated disease phenotypes (Figure 2-1).

A 5-year prospective study of a cohort of 646 patients identified a 12% risk for stricture 5 years after diagnosis and an 18% risk 20 years after diagnosis.[5] In a retrospective analysis of 297 patients with CD, the incidence of stricturing disease increased over time, with a 10% rate of stricturing disease at diagnosis, which increased to 30% after 10 years of disease. Over 10 years, 27% of the patients initially characterized as having an inflammatory phenotype had developed stricturing disease.[4] In a recent population-based cohort study, 19% of patients had a stricture or penetrating complication by 90 days after diagnosis, and half of all patients had experienced a complication by 20 years

Regueiro MD, Swoger JM, eds.
Clinical Challenges and Complications of IBD (pp 17-42).

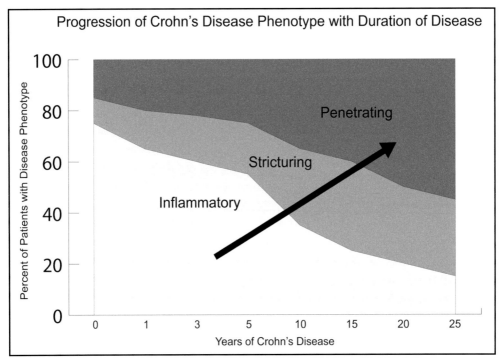

Figure 2-1. Progression of CD over time to complicated phenotypes. CD is largely inflammatory in the majority of patients at diagnosis, but becomes complicated (strictured, fistulizing, or abscess forming) in a majority of patients over time. (Adapted from Cosnes J, Cattan S, Blain A, et al. Long-term evolution of disease behavior of Crohn's disease. *Inflamm Bowel Dis.* 2002;8:244-250.)

of disease.[6] Despite advances in our understanding of CD, and an increased use of immunosuppressants and biologics, the frequency of strictures and the need for surgery for CD have not significantly decreased.[7-10]

Risk Factors for Stricturing Disease and Penetrating Complications

Several studies have identified disease severity, small bowel disease location, and disease duration as important risk factors for stricture development. A prospective cohort study found disease location to be the most important predictor of disease behavior, with stricturing disease being associated with small bowel involvement (ileal or jejunal), absence of colonic involvement, and absence of anal disease.[5] An analysis of the Crohn's Therapy Resource Evaluation and Assessment Tool (TREAT) Registry identified duration of disease, disease severity, ileal disease, and new corticosteroid use as significant predictors of intestinal stricture, stenosis, or obstruction.[11] It is believed that the combination of disease severity and duration (moderate chronic or severe acute inflammation) is a risk factor for stricture development and that inflammation appears necessary for initiating fibrotic stenosis.[12] The Olmsted County cohort study identified upper gastrointestinal or ileal involvement and 5-aminosalicylic acid (5-ASA) use as risk factors for complicated disease.[6]

The role of genes, including NOD2/CARD15, and serologic markers such as anti-*Saccharomyces cerevisiae* antibodies (ASCA) in prognosticating stricture risk remain unclear.[13-15] Although there is consensus that NOD2/CARD15 status is associated with small bowel disease and young age at disease onset, whether or not it is also an independent risk factor for fibrostenosing disease is arguable, as the data are not consistent.[13,15,16] A recent meta-analysis of genetic studies found that the predictive ability of NOD2 heterozygote status for complicated disease was poor, with a sensitivity of 36% and a specificity of 73%, but the presence of 2 NOD2 mutations was a powerful predictor of disease complications, with a specificity of 98%.[17] ASCA serologies are frequently associated with CD, and higher antibody levels have been associated with both fibrostenosing and penetrating CD[18]; however, in a multivariate analysis, ASCA status was not identified as an independent predictor of disease behavior.[15] Other serologic markers including antibodies to the outer membrane porin C of *Escherichia coli* (OmpC), *Pseudomonas fluorescens*–associated sequence I2 (anti-I2), and flagellin CBir1 (anti-CBir1) have been studied and appear to be associated with complicated disease[18,19]; however, their ability to predict future disease behavior remains unclear. Furthermore, no prospective studies have proven that any interventions can change the natural history of patients who have a high risk of fibrostenotic CD.

There is evidence that disease location, duration, 5-ASA use, and degree of inflammation are risk factors for CD complications. The role of potential genetic or serologic markers remains unclear. Other than homozygosity for NOD2 mutations, current laboratory tests do not allow us to confidently predict which patients with CD will develop complications or to act on this information even if it were available.

Abscess Formation

Internal fistulas in CD are almost exclusively found adjacent to luminal strictures, although these strictures may not always be apparent on imaging studies. An epidemiologic estimate of nonperianal fistulas in CD patients in Olmsted County, Minnesota, found a prevalence rate of 12% at 10 years and 24% by 20 years of disease.[20] An unknown fraction of these internal fistulas result in intra-abdominal abscesses in CD, but because case ascertainment is largely limited to patients with symptoms, we do not have an accurate estimate of what proportion of patients with internal fistulas develop abscesses. Asymptomatic patients presenting with internal fistulas are not uncommon, and it appears that steroid or anti-tumor necrosis factor (TNF) use is associated with increased formation and growth of abscesses. However, without prospective imaging of a cohort of patients, we are unable to determine the rate of conversion of stricturing to fistulizing to abscess-forming CD. Intra-abdominal abscesses eventually occur in 10% to 25% of all patients with CD[21] and are more likely after recent steroid use.[22] Abscesses appear to occur as a consequence of deep ulceration and transmural inflammation in combination with locally increased intraluminal pressure (often related to stenotic disease), which drives the initiation of a perforating fistula. When this perforation is contained by adjacent tissues, it becomes an intra-abdominal abscess.

ETIOLOGY AND PATHOGENESIS

Although intestinal narrowing in CD is often described as inflammatory or fibrotic, it is important to state that nearly all chronic strictures have a mix of inflammation and fibrosis and that all strictures with associated penetrating complications have a prominent fibrotic component. Clinical evaluation focuses on whether these strictures are predominantly inflammatory or fibrotic, as this characterization is thought to predict both response to anti-inflammatory therapy and prognosis. Although this characterization is generally believed to be true, there is a paucity of prospective data on any imaging evaluation of fibrosis versus inflammation describing the long-term outcomes of these strictures.

The pathogenesis of fibrotic strictures in CD is poorly understood.[23,24] Chronic inflammation and recurrent episodes of intestinal wound healing are believed to play a central role, but the physiologic pathways, and potential anti-fibrotic therapeutic targets, are not well defined. It remains unclear why some CD patients rapidly develop recurrent strictures, whereas others are rarely affected, although homozygote status for NOD2 mutations is a specific predictor of future complicated disease.[17] Fibrosis is believed to be the result of "excessive wound healing" triggered by severe or chronic inflammation,[12] and inflammatory cells, cytokines, and mesenchymal cells all likely play a role in the ultimate development of fibrosis.[23] Mesenchymal cells including fibroblasts, myofibroblasts, and smooth muscle cells are believed to participate in the fibrogenesis process, as they produce components of the extracellular matrix.[25] An imbalance between extracellular matrix synthesis and degradation may contribute to the accumulation of fibrosis.[24] The stiffness of the matrix may play a role in activating myofibroblasts, and the propagation of fibrosis, once it is initiated by inflammation.[26] The role of specific cytokines continues to be studied. Particular cytokines involved in wound healing, including transforming growth factor-β1 and interleukin-13, appear to be profibrotic.[24] Animal models of intestinal fibrosis have been developed and continue to be studied to improve our understanding of the pathogenesis of stricture formation.[25,27]

A critical and unanswered clinical question is what causes strictures to progress to penetrating complications, which often require invasive management. Retrospective data suggest that the combination of increased intraluminal pressure (within or upstream of a stricture) and a weak bowel wall (from transmural inflammation) is required for penetrating complications to occur. It is commonly believed that deep ulcers are a risk marker for future penetrating disease. Matrix metalloproteinases may be important in the breakdown of extracellular matrix components and the formation of fistulas.[27,28]

CLINICAL PRESENTATION

The initial presentation of strictures and internal penetrating complications can be subtle. Patients with CD frequently develop strictures slowly over time, and often adapt remarkably well to a chronic, slow narrowing of the small intestine. The formation of enteroenteric, enterocolonic, enterovesicular, and enterovaginal fistulas can decompress a dilated segment of bowel, leading to a paradoxical improvement of symptoms. Patient adaptation can hide signs of complicated disease. Concrete questioning should inquire about changes in diet (decreased fiber, small meals), weight loss, bubbles in or the stopping and starting of the urine stream, fecaluria or dysuria, and discharge from the vagina. These questions will occasionally yield important information that patients often fail to volunteer. To add to the diagnostic challenge, initial symptoms can be masked by steroids, anti-TNF therapy, or narcotic medications.

As high-resolution cross-sectional imaging, including computed tomography enterography (CTE) and magnetic resonance enterography (MRE), is being used with increasing frequency in CD, more cases of "silent" strictures and enteric fistulas are being discovered. The ascertainment bias inherent in which patients are undergoing imaging studies makes it difficult to know how common mildly symptomatic penetrating disease or strictures truly are. Identifying "clinically significant" strictures is often dependent on dilation upstream from a stricture, but this approach is likely insensitive for 2 reasons. First, patients with strictures find it difficult to drink enough oral contrast to dilate the small bowel, and second, the decompressive effect of fistulas and abscesses relieves the pressure that causes upstream dilation. Even experienced radiologists will miss up to 17% of strictures that are found at surgery by passing an inflated balloon catheter through the small bowel,[29] and CD patients with no apparent obstructive symptoms can be obstructed by a pill camera at a rate of up to 13%.[30]

When penetrating complications are symptomatic, patients generally present initially with a vague, visceral pain that is difficult to localize. Later focal localization suggests transmural inflammation and peritonitis and is often a sign of bowel perforation upstream of a stricture. When a perforation is contained, an abscess can result, which can produce vague fatigue, malaise, sweats, and fevers, often with an elevated white blood cell count and erythrocyte sedimentation rate (ESR). Unfortunately, this presentation is often masked by the use of steroids, which can diminish all of these symptoms, and often significantly reduce the ESR. However, recurrent fevers and discomfort during steroid tapering should be a worrisome sign. Low-grade fever while on an anti-TNF agent can also be a subtle presentation of an abscess. Both steroids and anti-TNF agents can effectively reduce evidence of inflammation, masking the presence of an abscess, and allowing it to increase in size, until constitutional signs or mass-effect symptoms predominate. Another nonspecific presentation can be the patient report that "food goes right through me," with a large-volume watery diarrhea. Although this is often interpreted as *Clostridium difficile* infection, or rapid motility as a manifestation of postinflammatory irritable bowel syndrome, this can be a sign of either an enlarging fistula or multiple fistulas creating a functional ileal-sigmoid bypass.

A truly complex stricture with multiple fistulas will often form a phlegmon that is palpable and sometimes surprisingly nontender on examination. Rarely, a superficial abscess can be a red, warm, and tender distention of the abdominal wall, which should not be confused with an abdominal wall hernia. More commonly, a deep intra-abdominal or pelvic abscess presents as a vague, difficult to localize discomfort or mild pain, and systemic symptoms can predominate.

CLINICAL AND RADIOGRAPHIC EVALUATION

Patients with complicated CD generally present in 3 forms: clinically silent (detected by imaging for another indication), clinically smoldering, and symptomatically overt presentations. The clinically smoldering patients often require a high level of clinical suspicion to trigger an evaluation. Patients with a past history of penetrating complications, a history of perianal disease, smoking, previous surgery, previous bowel wall thickening on imaging, or subtle obstructive symptoms should be considered high risk. Because patients often adapt to slowly worsening obstruction, direct questioning about appetite, nausea, and vomiting can be helpful. At times, validation of appetite and eating patterns with a spouse or family member can be valuable, as patients can adapt by eating small amounts or largely liquid diets. Asking whether the patient eats like other family members and finding out how his or her eating habits differ from his or her family's can be revealing.

The physical examination is limited in the detection of an abdominal abscess deeper than the abdominal wall. Psoas abscesses present with difficulty in standing up straight and pain on straight leg-raising or on flexion. In most cases, an elevated index of suspicion and an imaging study are required to detect abscesses. A study of which (non-inflammatory bowel disease [IBD]) emergency department patients are most likely to have intra-abdominal abscesses found that anorexia; chills; and elevations in hematocrit, white blood cell count, and platelet count were most predictive.[31] Given the frequency of abscesses, and their often nebulous presentation when symptoms are masked by immune suppressants in CD, the need for accurate diagnosis and intervention is crucial. Maconi et al's prospective study showed that standard oral contrast CT and ultrasound (US) have comparable accuracy in detecting intra-abdominal abscesses, although CT may have a higher specificity and positive predictive value. It is important to note that CT and US can miss up to 17% of intra-abdominal abscesses that are small or located deep within the abdominal cavity, and a single negative imaging test (eg, a middle of the night emergency department scan) in a clinically suspicious setting should not necessarily close off this line of diagnostic thinking.[32]

In addition to CT and US, CTE and MRE have rapidly become popular in diagnosing and monitoring CD. Both of these cross-sectional imaging techniques use negative oral contrast, allowing better visualization of the bowel wall than standard CT. MRE has nearly the resolution of CTE, but due to slower acquisition time, is more susceptible to motion (including peristaltic movement) artifacts. CTE and MRE are helpful for identifying abscesses and fistulas, providing accurate assessment of bowel wall inflammation, and identifying nearby bowel strictures (Figures 2-2 and 2-3). The choice of imaging study should depend in part on local expertise, as CT, US, and MR appear

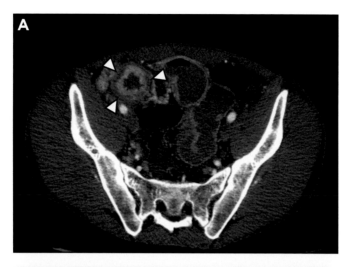

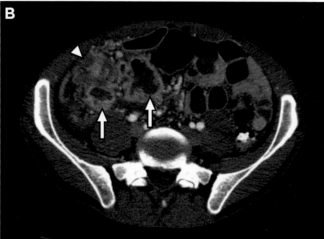

Figure 2-2. Radiographic assessment of intra-abdominal abscesses in a CD patient. Axial images from CTE performed with intravenous and low-density oral contrast. (A) Active inflammatory stricture involving the terminal ileum (arrowheads) is shown, demonstrating increased mucosal enhancement, circumferential bowel wall thickening, and stranding of the surrounding mesenteric fat. (B) Slightly more superior image shows at least 2 adjacent mesenteric fluid collections (arrows) consistent with multiple abscesses.

to be comparable in accuracy, although CT may be the most specific of the 3 modalities for abscess identification.[32,33]

The initial evaluation of suspected complicated disease should include both imaging and laboratory testing. Repeated longitudinal use of imaging tests that have high costs, significant patient inconvenience, and radiation risk should be minimized, and interval follow-up with serologic markers of inflammation can be helpful. Evaluations with a complete blood count, ESR, and

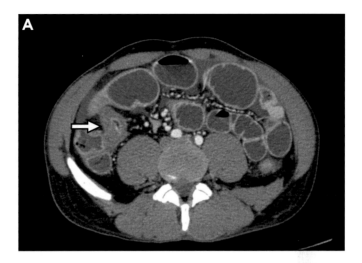

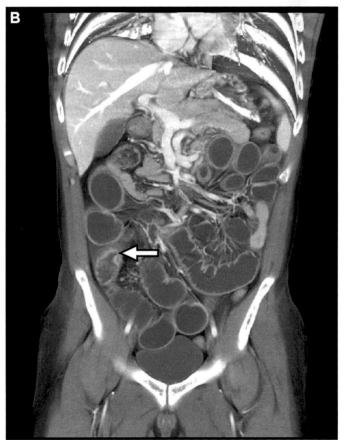

Figure 2-3. Radiographic assessment of small bowel stricturing disease. CTE performed with intravenous and low-density oral contrast. (A and B) Axial and coronal 3-dimentional reformatted images show active inflammatory stricture involving the terminal Ileum (arrow) demonstrating luminal narrowing, increased mucosal enhancement, circumferential bowel wall thickening, and stranding of the surrounding mesenteric fat.

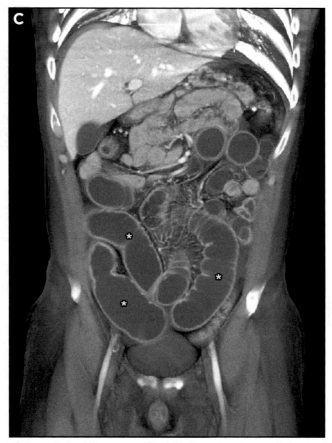

Figure 2-3. (*Continued*). (C) Proximal small bowel loops are dilated (*), consistent with distal small bowel obstruction secondary to the terminal ileal fibrotic stricture.

C-reactive protein (CRP), along with cross-sectional imaging (MRE or CTE), are the initial steps in the evaluation.

Lifetime radiation exposure can be substantial in patients with complicated CD,[34,35] and it is important to identify and discuss this risk with patients, particularly those younger than 50 years. Patients with CD should know how many abdominal CT scans and films they have had in their lives and should feel comfortable questioning the need for more radiation. Preference should be given to MRE over CTE for patients younger than 50, when it is available. Small bowel follow-through can be used to evaluate CD, and occasionally a dynamic study can be useful to evaluate a narrowed segment of small bowel. However, MRE and CTE are more sensitive and add value with extraluminal data.[36]

The critical questions to be addressed by cross-sectional imaging are (1) whether small bowel luminal narrowing is present, (2) the diameter of the lumen, (3) the length of the narrowing, (4) the diameter of the lumen of the proximal small bowel, (5) whether (and how active) inflammation is present in the narrowed segment, and (6) whether penetrating complications (fistulas, abscesses, free air) have already occurred (see Figure 2-2). Internal fistulas most often arise from the ileum, often connecting to the cecum, ileum, sigmoid colon, bladder, vagina, or the abdominal wall. Rarely, gastrocolic or duodenocolic fistulas can occur and are associated with significant nutritional bypass, weight loss, and occasional telltale fecal vomiting.

Assessment of Bowel Strictures

Patients with CD who present with obstructive symptoms, including postprandial abdominal pain, distention, and nausea and vomiting, require evaluation to assess for obstruction. If obstruction or partial obstruction is suspected, it is also important to evaluate the underlying cause, which in CD can be secondary to inflammatory narrowing, fibrotic stricture, combined inflammation and fibrosis, cancer, or adhesive disease from previous surgeries. This characterization is essential to the selection of appropriate treatment. The initial clinical impression does not always correlate with radiographic findings, and imaging can add important information to a physician's assessment.[37] Radiographic imaging including CTE and MRE, which allow for detailed visualization of the small bowel, can be very helpful in this diagnostic evaluation. Clinical indices and laboratory markers are often less informative.[38]

On imaging, prestenotic dilation (luminal widening proximal to the narrowing) is not commonly seen in purely inflammatory stenosis and is suggestive of a fibrotic component (see Figure 2-3).[39] Mucosal enhancement and increased vascularity (comb sign) on CTE or MRE are highly correlated with active inflammation and can be helpful in distinguishing between an inflammatory narrowing and fibrotic stricture.[40,41] These imaging modalities are also helpful in identifying the location, as well as the length of involved bowel, which are important considerations for subsequent management. Historically, small bowel follow-through was the imaging modality of choice for the evaluation of active CD; however, CTE and MRE are better at detecting inflammation, provide more comprehensive imaging, and are today's preferred imaging modalities.[42] When choosing between CT and magnetic resonance imaging (MRI) for the evaluation of small bowel stenosis in Crohn's, consideration should be given to local expertise, patient age, and patient radiation exposure.[43]

US, which is more commonly used in Europe in the evaluation of CD, may also be able to distinguish inflammation from fibrosis.[38] Contrast-enhanced US appears to accurately detect active inflammation in CD, and may provide useful prognostic information on response to anti-inflammatory therapy; however, more studies are needed.[44]

Novel imaging methods are being used in research settings to address the question of whether a given stricture is predominantly fibrotic or predominantly inflammatory. These new approaches include magnetization transfer MRI,[45,46] and ultrasound elasticity imaging.[47] Each approach uses a distinct methodology to assess the presence of fibrosis. Magnetization transfer MRI uses the delayed relaxation of hydrogen atoms attached to macromolecules to detect the presence and concentration of macromolecules, such as actin and collagen, in the bowel wall. Ultrasound elasticity imaging uses mechanical stiffness and the compressibility of the bowel wall to assess for the presence of fibrosis. Both of these methods have been shown to correlate with histologic fibrosis in rodent and human bowels, but need to be prospectively validated in clinical care. Ideally, these approaches would be able to accurately predict whether a given patient is likely to respond to anti-inflammatory therapy or to require mechanical intervention (balloon dilation or surgery) in the following year. Prospective measurement of sensitivity and specificity, with masking of the results for clinicians making the decisions about medical or mechanical intervention, will be needed to demonstrate the clinical value of these novel approaches.

Assessment of Abscesses

The goals of imaging studies for abscess assessment include (1) assessment of the presence of an abscess; (2) determination of whether the abscess location, size, and loculations allow for safe and complete percutaneous drainage; (3) determination of whether there is an adjacent stricture or fistula contributing to the abscess; (4) determination of whether there is adjacent bowel inflammation contributing to the abscess; (5) establishing a baseline for longitudinal assessment of the success of treatment; and (6) establishing the readiness of the patient for immunosuppressive therapy (see Figure 2-2B). Communication with the diagnostic radiologist and the interventional radiology team that performs abscess drainage are important in obtaining all of the essential information from the baseline imaging study and in formulating a plan for evacuation of the infectious material.

The characteristics of the abscess and the nearby bowel can help predict the likelihood of nonoperative success. A complex, loculated abscess, or one that is in a location not amenable to percutaneous drainage, is more likely to require surgical intervention. An adjacent stricture and a wide fistula from the bowel to the abscess are both associated with an increased likelihood of requiring surgery. Finally, active inflammation in the adjacent bowel makes treatment more challenging, as the use of systemic anti-inflammatory therapy, particularly with steroids[22] or anti-TNF-α agents, can contribute to the growth and persistence of an incompletely drained abscess.

Indications for Intervention

When a stricture is identified, the lumen size and length are important in establishing whether it is amenable to endoscopic dilation and whether fluoroscopy will be required. Generally, strictures less than 4 cm in length and more than 5 mm in luminal diameter will respond well to dilation without requiring fluoroscopy.[48-51] Very narrow or angulated short strictures can respond to dilation, but require careful fluoroscopic visualization during the dilation procedure. Whether a particular stricture is "clinically significant" and warrants intervention is largely a matter of clinical judgment. A stricture that is associated with penetrating complications, significant proximal dilation, or occurs in a patient with significant vomiting and/or admissions for partial obstruction is clearly worthy of intervention. The presence of signs of active inflammation, including mucosal enhancement and increased vascularity, indicate the need for medical anti-inflammatory therapy. The presence of penetrating complications, including fistulas and abscesses, is an indication for medical intervention, often followed by a surgical intervention. Short-term management goals are to simultaneously (1) remove and treat purulent fluid collections, (2) control inflammation, and (3) reduce intraluminal pressure from adjacent strictures that contributed to the penetrating complication.

CLINICAL MANAGEMENT OF STRICTURES AND PENETRATING COMPLICATIONS IN CROHN'S DISEASE

General Principles of Management

Patients with CD who have developed strictures and/or penetrating complications often have important comorbidities that impact their disease course. First, many patients have significant weight loss and malnutrition at presentation. The optimization of enteral feeding and supplementation to the greatest extent possible will be important in improving wound healing and in reducing fluid shifts due to hypoalbuminemia. However, timely surgery should not be delayed for optimization of nutrition, as many studies have shown delayed surgery results in worse outcomes, and that no nutritional interventions, including parenteral nutrition, have been shown to improve outcomes.

Next, decisions about anti-inflammatory therapy need to be made. If significant inflammation is seen on imaging, and can be followed with blood markers including ESR and CRP, this inflammation should be treated both to minimize the obstructive effects and to reduce the risk of additional penetrating complications. However, if purulent extraluminal material is present, anti-inflammatory therapy can be problematic. Abscesses appear to increase in size in response to steroid or anti-TNF therapy and require drainage before these therapies can be used. Methotrexate, an immune suppressant medication with antimicrobial properties, can be a good choice in this setting, if the patient is not a fertile female (methotrexate is pregnancy category X).

Several interventions have been evaluated to reduce the flow of intestinal contents through CD fistulas to encourage healing. These include bowel rest with total parenteral nutrition (TPN)[52] and octreotide injections to reduce the volume of pancreatic secretions.[53] These approaches have been reported in case series[54,55] but are rarely successful in the setting of a Crohn's stricture with associated bowel wall inflammation. No prospective randomized studies support their use.

Clinical Management of Strictures

Patients with minimally symptomatic, partially obstructing small bowel strictures may have developed numerous adaptations to their stricture, and careful questioning can often identify these adaptations. Endoscopic dilation can often greatly improve the quality of life in these patients, even when they initially minimize their complaints. These patients are also at risk for small intestinal bacterial overgrowth, with resultant gas, distention, and bloating. Temporary response of these symptoms to a 2-week course of antibiotics directed at gut flora (rifaximin, ciprofloxacin, and metronidazole) is often rapid and significant.

The appropriate treatment of asymptomatic stricture depends on several factors, including the length, diameter, and evidence of significant inflammation. Small bowel strictures tend to progress over time, and watchful waiting, even in patients who respond to conservative measures with nasogastric suction and bowel rest, often fails over time. An aggressive and timely approach to strictures is important, in order to prevent penetrating complications and to perform an elective surgery with minimal resection, when surgery is needed.

Although more aggressive medical management can be successful in the setting of an inflammatory stricture, and may avoid or delay a surgery, it is unlikely to be of benefit if the stricture is largely fibrotic. Evidence of active inflammation, including biomarkers (CRP, ESR) and findings on US, CTE, or MRE, can direct a step up in anti-inflammatory therapy. Titration of medical therapy to reduce inflammation can be immediately helpful in producing increased luminal diameter and symptom relief. Unfortunately, evidence to support a long-term benefit in truly slowing the progression of fibrosis with anti-inflammatory therapy is limited, and prospective evidence is lacking. In fact, numerous case reports and a prospective cohort study, the TREAT database, suggest that anti-inflammatory therapy with either anti-TNF medications or thiopurines has a trend toward association with more stenosis, stricture, and obstruction events.[11] This association may largely be due to disease severity and pre-existing partial obstruction, but at least suggests that these therapies are unlikely to reverse fibrotic stenosis.[11] Infliximab is not contraindicated in the presence of strictures but is clearly most effective when inflammation, rather than mechanical obstruction, is the primary cause of symptoms. Importantly, this medication may be especially effective after the surgical removal of strictures.[56] More striking and statistically significant associations are found between steroid or narcotic use and stenosis, stricture, and obstruction events. Patients with a stricture who are dependent on steroids or narcotics require an intervention before penetrating complications occur, in order to avoid complications including peritonitis and adhesions, which make future surgical interventions more difficult.

If imaging and laboratory testing suggest a narrowing is primarily fibrotic, options including balloon dilation and surgery should be considered. It is important to intervene on strictures and lower intraluminal pressure before penetrating complications occur. Although data are limited and there have been no randomized controlled trials, through-the-scope balloon dilation is considered a safe and effective treatment for short and uncomplicated primary or anastomotic strictures. Although surgical resection has been the traditional treatment for strictures, a course of repeated extensive bowel resections can lead to short bowel syndrome. Therefore, effort should be taken to avoid or limit bowel resection when possible. Short (<5 cm long) strictures without penetrating complications should be considered for balloon dilation.[49] We usually endoscopically dilate over several sessions to gradually increase the diameter by 5-mm increments per session to a goal diameter of 20 mm.

A systematic review of endoscopic dilation in CD identified 13 retrospective studies, in which a total of 353 strictures were dilated in 347 patients. A majority of the strictures were postsurgical, anastomotic strictures. The procedure was technically successful in 86% of patients, and 68% of those patients had avoided surgery by study end (mean follow-up 33 months). Overall, there was a 58% long-term success rate. Surgery was ultimately required in 42% of patients who underwent an attempted dilation. More than one-third of patients remained surgery-free after only one dilation session. The overall mean complication rate was 2%, in which the majority were bowel perforations; however, reported complication rates including bleeding and perforation range from 0% to 18%.[57] Data regarding through-the-scope dilation for primary nonanastomotic strictures are particularly limited (Figure 2-4). Although there is more literature on the dilation of anastomotic strictures, data suggest it is equally safe and effective for the treatment of primary, nonanastomotic strictures.[58] Appropriate stricture selection is important, and endoscopic balloon dilation for short strictures ≤4 cm in length has been associated with the best outcomes.[57] Steroid injection into the stricture after dilation appears to be safe, and it may be a useful adjunct to dilation. However, to date, there are only 3 retrospective studies, the largest of which has 17 patients,[50,59,60] and only a single small randomized controlled trial has been published, which found no benefit to steroid injection.[61]

Although data suggest endoscopic balloon dilation is safe and effective in appropriately selected strictures, there have been no randomized trials comparing different dilation approaches. There are no specific guidelines regarding optimal dilation technique, or timing or re-treatment in CD, and there is wide variation in published clinical practice. Variations exist in the maximum balloon diameter used, whether serial dilations or a single dilation is performed in a session, the duration of balloon insufflation during a dilation session, and the frequency of dilation.[57]

If endoscopic dilation is ineffective, the stricture is long, or penetrating complications are present surgical options should be considered. Retrospective data comparing stricturoplasty versus resection suggest that there is no significant difference in long-term outcomes, but these data are likely subject to selection and ascertainment bias.

Stricturoplasty preserves intestinal length while increasing the diameter of the lumen. This is particularly advantageous for patients with a prior history of repeated resection and those at risk for short bowel syndrome. Stricturoplasty is generally contraindicated in the presence of active perforating disease. Although there are no randomized controlled trials comparing stricturoplasty to resection, stricturoplasty is considered safe and effective, and time

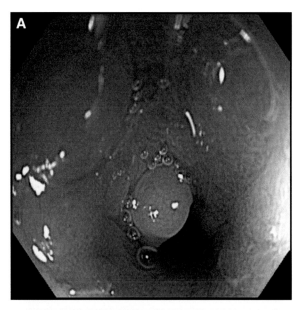

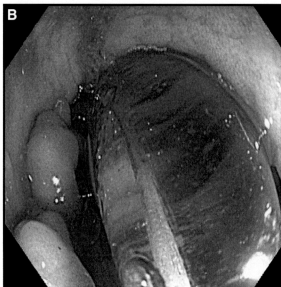

Figure 2-4. Endoscopic dilation of a colonic stricture in a patient with CD. (A) Colonic stenosis compatible with fibrostenotic stricture and (B) Through-the-scope balloon dilation of colonic stricture. (Reprinted with permission of Jason M. Swoger, MD, MPH.)

to recurrence is believed to be comparable to that of resection.[62] Prospective, randomized studies are needed to evaluate the relative benefit of balloon dilation, stricturoplasty, and resection, and to identify whether specific subgroups of patients will derive long-term benefit from a particular approach.

Clinical Management of Internal Fistulas

The presence of an internal fistula identifies a segment of bowel that previously experienced the combination of inflammation (weak bowel wall) and elevated intraluminal pressure. Whether or not a stricture is readily visualized with imaging, it is highly likely that a stricture is present. Clinical symptoms may be reduced by the reduction in intraluminal pressure by the fistula, but patients remain at risk for small intestinal bacterial overgrowth, abscess formation, and eventual complete obstruction. Unfortunately, medical anti-inflammatory therapies, including anti-TNF therapy, are less successful for abdominal fistulas than for perianal disease. In general, these patients should have imaging to identify the location and character of the nearby stricture, rule out an associated abscess, and plan eventual elective surgery. Anti-inflammatory therapy should be optimized and steroid therapy minimized to prepare for eventual surgery and to optimize the healing of the anastomosis and the abdominal wound.

Patients can smolder with abdominal fistulas, strictures, and phlegmons for some years if they are willing to significantly adapt their eating habits to their disordered anatomy. However, these patients generally have increasing numbers of penetrating complications and adhesions over time, making timely elective surgery important in optimizing outcomes. Penetrating complications are, in themselves, an indication for surgery. Endoscopic dilation, while it may improve an obstruction, does not lower the risk of abscess formation. Prospective randomized trial data to guide the timing of surgery do not exist, but a timely elective surgery can dramatically change the eating habits and quality of life of these patients.

Clinical Management of Abdominal Abscesses

There are numerous options in the treatment of intra-abdominal abscesses associated with CD. Unfortunately, most of the available data are from retrospective case series, and no therapies have been evaluated with controlled trials in this patient population. We have to extrapolate largely from the results of case series, with conclusions tempered by the high probability of substantial selection bias in all of the published series. Options include surgical incision and drainage with antibiotics, percutaneous drainage with antibiotics, antibiotic therapy without drainage, combining 1 of these 3 options with anti-inflammatory therapy, and/or combining one of these options with surgical resection of the diseased bowel.

Antibiotic therapy should be chosen to target gram-negative rods and anaerobes, and initial parenteral delivery is generally used to maximize delivery in CD patients, who often have active small bowel inflammation. Ampicillin/sulbactam and piperacillin/tazobactam are often initial choices, although a penicillin allergy may require the use of metronidazole plus either ceftriaxone or levofloxacin. Antibiotic therapy should ideally be commenced prior to the initiation of the drainage procedure. Parenteral antibiotics are generally continued for 1 week, or at least 2 days beyond defervescence and an improvement in the white blood cell count. Antibiotics can then be converted to once daily or oral administration to facilitate outpatient care. Oral antibiotics, which may include a quinolone plus metronidazole, amoxicillin clavulanate, or trimethoprim/sulfamethoxazole plus metronidazole, are generally continued until at least 3 days after the drainage catheter is removed and repeat imaging has confirmed that the cavity has been fully evacuated.

A team approach to defining the optimal route for drainage of all infectious material is helpful. Location of abscesses near vessels can require alternate access routes for percutaneous drainage, and a transgluteal approach to pelvic fluid collections is often needed. Very small collections (<1 cm) may be difficult to access, whereas those 1 to 3 cm can often be effectively drained with an aspiration needle. Those greater than 3 cm in diameter will generally require placement of a 8- to 14-French catheter, followed by irrigation with 10 to 20 mL of sterile normal saline every 6 to 12 hours, depending on the size of the abscess and the thickness of the draining material. Drainage output volume and character should be recorded with each irrigation and monitored for changes.[63-65]

Ideally, catheter output should become steadily less thick and purulent and decrease in volume over the first week. The patient should also defervesce over the first 3 days and have a fall in white blood cell count and ESR with successful drainage. A sudden cessation in output, or a failure to defervesce and demonstrate laboratory parameter improvement, are indications for reimaging, as the catheter may be dislodged or kinked, or incompletely draining a portion of the abscess, which would require repositioning or placement of an additional drainage catheter. A sudden increase in fluid output may occur if a clogged catheter is reopened by irrigation, but this could also indicate a new or enlarging fistulous connection to bowel. A more watery, bilious, or feculent appearance with increased output is an indication for a fistulagram, with contrast injected through the catheter to evaluate for a wide fistula from the abscess to the bowel.

An abscess drainage catheter can be removed after output becomes nonpurulent, decreases to <20 mL/day for 3 consecutive days, and repeat imaging confirms the resolution of the entire abscess. This required an average of 10.5 days (but ranged up to 23 days) in Golfieri et al's series. Initial drainage was successful, without abscess recurrence in 74% of spontaneous Crohn's abscesses in this series. An additional 10% could be successfully treated after recurrence, with a 16% overall failure rate.[63] It is important to emphasize that with large or complex abscesses, recurrence should be expected in 25% to 50%, and can be successfully treated in approximately 40% of cases with a second round of percutaneous drainage.

With high-resolution CT scanners, small abscesses <1 cm in size are more likely to be found and reported than in the past. If these can be aspirated safely, they should be, but these are often detected as part of a cluster of small, undrainable abscesses adjacent to actively inflamed bowel proximal to a stricture. In this setting, therapy with antibiotics alone can be attempted and has been moderately successful in a retrospective series. Kim et al treated 20 Crohn's patients with intra-abdominal abscesses (average size 3.3 cm) with antibiotics alone, when percutaneous drainage was not possible. Eighteen responded initially, and 13 of 20 had no recurrence at 6 months, without percutaneous drainage or surgery.[64]

Patients must be instructed on how to care for and irrigate drainage catheters before outpatient care is begun and need to be able to describe and record their daily abscess catheter output. Monitoring progress toward the resolution of an intra-abdominal abscess requires regular imaging. This can be done with weekly CT scans as per Golfieri et al,[63] but this approach can result in substantial radiation exposure. It is often effective to use US or MRI, or less frequent CT imaging for repeated evaluation, particularly with a complex collection that is likely to require a long treatment course. We typically perform follow-up imaging with US at 2-week intervals, unless there has been a change in catheter output to suggest that the catheter has been displaced or kinked or that a new enteric fistula has formed.

Dietary restriction to enteral formulas or TPN is controversial in the treatment of intra-abdominal Crohn's abscesses, and minimal data are available to support dietary restriction. A few retrospective case series have suggested that TPN in patients kept nothing by mouth (NPO) might be beneficial, but Greenberg et al's randomized controlled trial of TPN while NPO in CD found that this therapy did not significantly improve outcomes either during hospitalization or after 1 year of follow-up.[66] TPN is associated with an increased risk of line infections and bacteremia, which are of particular concern in immunosuppressed IBD patients. Central lines are also associated with an increased incidence of venous thromboembolism, which is further increased in IBD patients with active disease. Given these risks and the substantial costs of TPN, a clear benefit to TPN and bowel rest needs to be demonstrated before this can be routinely recommended for Crohn's patients with intra-abdominal abscess.

Systemic steroid therapy and anti-TNF-α therapy have both been strongly associated with increased skin and soft tissue infections, wound infections, and an increased incidence and growth of abscesses. The risk of infection in association with steroid use is both dose and duration related, with an odds ratio of 6.3 for infection with <20 mg daily prednisone and 18.9 for >40 mg daily.[67] The risk of infection also increases with a cumulative steroid dose of >700 mg. Several studies have shown an increased risk of surgical complications and infection in association with anti-TNF-α therapy; the largest is from the British Society for Rheumatology Biologics Registry. With more than 10,000 patients, and more than 2000 surgeries, they were able to show that anti-TNF-α therapy is associated with skin and soft tissue infections and that the perioperative risk is strongest if anti-TNF-α agents have been administered in the 2 weeks preceding surgery. The risk diminishes if greater than 2 weeks has elapsed since dosing of the anti-TNF-α medication and is reduced further if the anti-TNF-α medication was administered more than 4 weeks prior to surgery.[68,69]

Systemic steroid and anti-TNF-α therapies are usually avoided until complete drainage of the infectious material is confirmed with repeat imaging and catheter removal, or definitive surgery is performed. Some centers will initiate therapy with these agents within 24 to 48 hours after initial drainage is accomplished, if the radiologic team feels that the entire abscess cavity has been accessed and/or an effective drain is in place. This approach can be safe and effective, but requires close monitoring to ensure that the drainage catheter remains in place and does not become clogged or displaced before complete eradication of the access is achieved.

Thiopurines and methotrexate appear to pose substantially less risk of interfering with abscess eradication and can be initiated during abscess drainage, although their onset of action is delayed, and more rapidly acting nonsystemic agents may be needed in combination with one of these immunomodulators. Subcutaneous methotrexate, which is well absorbed and has antibacterial properties similar to trimethoprim, is particularly appealing in patients with purulent complications. Nonsystemic anti-inflammatory therapies can be used immediately, including budesonide for the ileum and right colon and mesalamine enemas for the left colon. In our experience, budesonide can also be used for upper tract inflammation, if the patient opens the capsule and mixes the contents with applesauce, then chews the granules thoroughly before swallowing. This method of administration produces a more rapid release of budesonide but may produce more systemic side effects.

Surgical planning should also affect the choices and timing of anti-inflammatory therapy. Many Crohn's patients with intra-abdominal abscesses will have strictures or large fistulas that will require elective surgery, and at least 10% are likely to fail percutaneous drainage and antibiotic therapy. Ideally, after removal of all infectious material, anti-inflammatory therapy will be used to control bowel inflammation prior to surgery. This will minimize bowel wall friability when creating an ostomy or an anastomosis, reducing the risk of bowel leak and subsequent peritonitis, or the formation of new abscesses. Thiopurines and methotrexate do not appear to significantly increase the risk of infections or complications in the postoperative period, while current systemic steroids and recent (infusion or injection in prior 2 to 4 weeks) anti-TNF-α agents have been associated with worse surgical outcomes. If it is clear that surgery is likely in the near future, and infectious material has been drained, effective control of bowel inflammation should be achieved with immunomodulators and/or biologics, and systemic steroids should be tapered to minimum doses. The scheduling of surgery should be targeted, when possible, for the trough period of anti-TNF-α agent dosing.

Traditionally, intra-abdominal abscesses due to CD have been managed with surgical drainage and systemic antibiotic therapy, coupled with resection of the involved inflamed or fibrotic segment of bowel. Due to concerns about postoperative complications from contamination of the operative field by the abscess, this was often approached with a 2-stage surgical procedure, with initial surgical incision and drainage of the abscess, followed by a delayed bowel resection. This led to attempts to accomplish the first stage, drainage of infectious material, by a percutaneous route, enabling a single-stage surgery, with a primary re-anastomosis. Even if percutaneous drainage is only partially effective, it may provide benefit in reducing the amount of infectious material in the operative field and in buying time to treat and control bowel wall inflammation prior to surgery.

Numerous retrospective studies have reported success rates of percutaneous catheter drainage of Crohn's abscess ranging from 37% to 90%. Surgical therapy, while offering more open access and allowing definitive therapy of the abscess and nearby strictured or fistulizing bowel, can have an abscess recurrence rate comparable to that of percutaneous drainage. Furthermore, surgery is more likely

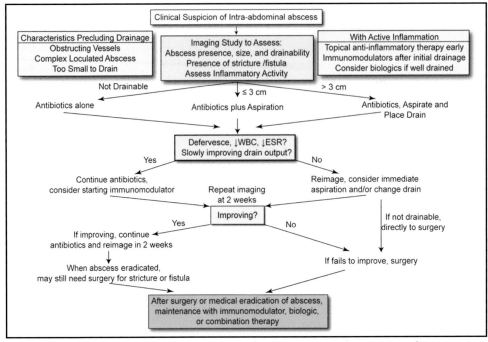

Figure 2-5. Abscess management algorithm. ESR = erythrocyte sedimentation rate; WBC = white blood cell.

than percutaneous drainage to lead to an enterocutaneous fistula. Immediate surgical approaches also often require substantial resection of adjacent bowel, putting patients at risk for future short bowel syndrome. Although percutaneous drainage will fail to prevent recurrence of abscesses in a number of patients, and many patients will require surgery for strictures or fistulas irrespective of the abscess outcome, an initial medical approach has a number of attractive features. Initial antibiotics and attempts at percutaneous drainage are inexpensive and less invasive than surgery; evacuation of infectious material will reduce subsequent perioperative infectious risk; and drainage of infectious material allows subsequent anti-inflammatory therapy, which can make elective Crohn's surgery less complicated and often requires less extensive resection of bowel.

The determination that medical therapy has failed can be difficult when there is partial improvement with antibiotic treatment and percutaneous drainage. In general, if at least 3 weeks of antibiotics and 2 attempts at percutaneous drainage have failed to demonstrate continuing progress on repeated imaging, surgical intervention is indicated. Occasionally, a complex, loculated collection will require multiple percutaneous interventions and drains over 30 to 60 days. However, if the abscess has not improved in the interval since the previous imaging, despite continuing effective drainage, maximum medical benefit has been achieved,[64] and surgery should be planned. An algorithm for the management of intra-abdominal abscesses in CD is presented in Figure 2-5.

A history of an intra-abdominal abscess implies severe transmural inflammation and a contained perforation and is a powerful prognostic factor for a future of complicated CD requiring highly effective postoperative medical therapy. These patients should not rely on maintenance therapy with antibiotics, mesalamine, herbal therapies, or modified diets. Evidence from randomized controlled trials suggests that patients who have required surgical resection derive endoscopic and clinical benefit from 3 months of metronidazole and long-term azathioprine. Regueiro et al's data suggest that initiation of infliximab is also very beneficial in preventing the recurrence of mucosal ulceration.[56] Further, the Study of Biologic and Immunomodulator Naïve in Crohn's Disease (SONIC) trial data show that, in the subset of patients with active inflammation early in the disease course, combination therapy with azathioprine and infliximab is superior to biologic monotherapy.

At a minimum, these patients should receive 3 months of antibiotics and be started or continued on an immunomodulator (azathioprine 2.5 mg/kg/day or 6-mercaptopurine 1.5 mg/kg/day). Methotrexate may have similar benefits, but there are limited data available in patients who have had intra-abdominal abscesses. Many of these patients will have risk factors for recurrence that merit serious discussion of use of biologic or combination therapy. A full discussion with the patient should make it clear that these patients are at high risk for future complications, and should contrast the potential benefits of combination therapy with azathioprine and infliximab with the potential for long-term harm from recurrence of intra-abdominal abscesses, perforation, peritonitis, and chronic bowel adhesions.

☑ Key Points

- ☑ Internal penetrating complications appear to arise from a combination of high intraluminal pressure (in or upstream of strictures) and transmural inflammation.

- ☑ Symptoms of penetrating complications may be difficult to detect because intraluminal pressure is reduced and/or they are masked by steroids or anti-TNF therapy.

- ☑ Initial evaluation requires imaging, which is usually cross-sectional, unless focal signs direct US evaluation.

- ☑ Percutaneous drainage of abscesses, antibiotic therapy, and reduction/withdrawal of systemic steroids and anti-TNF therapy are first-line therapy for abscesses.

- ☑ Short strictures (<5 cm) can be effectively endoscopically dilated.

- ☑ Strictures with associated penetrating complications are often best treated with reduction of infectious and inflammatory burden, followed by elective surgery.

References

1. Satsangi J, Silverberg MS, Vermeire S, Colombel JF. The Montreal classification of inflammatory bowel disease: controversies, consensus, and implications. *Gut.* 2006;55:749-753.

2. Kelly JK, Preshaw RM. Origin of fistulas in Crohn's disease. *J Clin Gastroenterol.* 1989;11: 193-196.

3. Oberhuber G, Stangl PC, Vogelsang H, Schober E, Herbst F, Gasche C. Significant association of strictures and internal fistula formation in Crohn's disease. *Virchows Arch.* 2000;437:293-297.

4. Louis E, Collard A, Oger AF, Degroote E, El Yafi FAN, Belaiche J. Behaviour of Crohn's disease according to the Vienna classification: changing pattern over the course of the disease. *Gut.* 2001;49:777-782.

5. Cosnes J, Cattan S, Blain A, et al. Long-term evolution of disease behavior of Crohn's disease. *Inflamm Bowel Dis.* 2002;8:244-250.

6. Thia KT, Sandborn WJ, Harmsen WS, Zinsmeister AR, Loftus EV Jr. Risk factors associated with progression to intestinal complications of Crohn's disease in a population-based cohort. *Gastroenterology.* 2010;139:1147-1155.

7. Jones DW, Finlayson SR. Trends in surgery for Crohn's disease in the era of infliximab. *Ann Surg.* 2010;252:307-312.

8. Cosnes J, Nion-Larmurier I, Beaugerie L, Afchain P, Tiret E, Gendre JP. Impact of the increasing use of immunosuppressants in Crohn's disease on the need for intestinal surgery. *Gut.* 2005;54:237-241.

9. Poritz LS, Rowe WA, Koltun WA. Remicade does not abolish the need for surgery in fistulizing Crohn's disease. *Dis Colon Rectum.* 2002;45:771-775.

10. Cannom RR, Kaiser AM, Ault GT, Beart RW Jr, Etzioni DA. Inflammatory bowel disease in the United States from 1998 to 2005: has infliximab affected surgical rates? *Am Surg.* 2009;75:976-980.

11. Lichtenstein GR, Olson A, Travers S, et al. Factors associated with the development of intestinal strictures or obstructions in patients with Crohn's disease. *Am J Gastroenterol.* 2006;101:1030-1038.

12. Rieder F, Brenmoehl J, Leeb S, et al. Wound healing and fibrosis in intestinal disease. *Gut.* 2007;56:130-139.

13. Abreu MT, Taylor KD, Lin YC, et al. Mutations in NOD2 are associated with fibrostenosing disease in patients with Crohn's disease. *Gastroenterology.* 2002;123:679-688.

14. Lesage S, Zouali H, Cezard JP, et al. CARD15/NOD2 mutational analysis and genotype-phenotype correlation in 612 patients with inflammatory bowel disease. *Am J Hum Genet.* 2002;70:845-857.

15. Louis E, Michel V, Hugot JP, et al. Early development of stricturing or penetrating pattern in Crohn's disease is influenced by disease location, number of flares, and smoking but not by NOD2/CARD15 genotype. *Gut.* 2003;52:552-557.

16. Vermeire S, Vermeire S. NOD2/CARD15: relevance in clinical practice. *Best Pract Res Clin Gastroenterol.* 2004;18:569-575.

17. Adler J, Rangwalla S, Higgins PDR. The prognostic power of NOD2 genotype for complicated Crohn's disease: a meta-analysis. *Am J Gastroenterol.* 2011;106:699-712.

18. Targan SR, Landers CJ, Yang H, et al. Antibodies to CBir1 flagellin define a unique response that is associated independently with complicated Crohn's disease. *Gastroenterology.* 2005;128:2020-2028.

19. Mow WS, Vasiliauskas EA, Lin YC, et al. Association of antibody responses to microbial antigens and complications of small bowel Crohn's disease. *Gastroenterology.* 2004;126:414-424.

20. Schwartz DA, Loftus EV, Jr, Tremaine WJ, et al. The natural history of fistulizing Crohn's disease in Olmsted County, Minnesota. *Gastroenterology.* 2002;122:875-880.

21. Yamaguchi A, Matsui T, Sakurai T, et al. The clinical characteristics and outcome of intraabdominal abscess in Crohn's disease. *J Gastroenterol.* 2004;39:441-448.

22. Agrawal A, Durrani S, Leiper K, Ellis A, Morris AI, Rhodes JM. Effect of systemic corti-costeroid therapy on risk for intra-abdominal or pelvic abscess in non-operated Crohn's disease. *Clin Gastroenterol Hepatol*. 2005;3:1215-1220.

23. Powell DW, Mifflin RC, Valentich JD, Crowe SE, Saada JI, West AB. Myofibroblasts. II. Intestinal subepithelial myofibroblasts. *Am J Physiol*. 1999;277:C183-C201.

24. Powell DW, Mifflin RC, Valentich JD, Crowe SE, Saada JI, West AB. Myofibroblasts. I. Paracrine cells important in health and disease. *Am J Physiol*. 1999;277:C1-C9.

25. Burke JP, Mulsow JJ, O'Keane C, et al. Fibrogenesis in Crohn's disease. *Am J Gastroenterol*. 2007;102:439-448.

26. Blanco LP, Johnson LA, Sauder KL, et al. Increased matrix stiffness induces a fibrogenic phenotype in human colonic mesenchymal cells. *Gastroenterology*. 2010;138(suppl 1):S752 (abstract).

27. Di Sabatino A, Jackson CL, Pickard KM, et al. Transforming growth factor beta signalling and matrix metalloproteinases in the mucosa overlying Crohn's disease strictures. *Gut*. 2009;58:777-789.

28. Kirkegaard T, Hansen A, Bruun E, Brynskov J. Expression and localisation of matrix metalloproteinases and their natural inhibitors in fistulae of patients with Crohn's disease. *Gut*. 2004;53:701-709.

29. Vogel J, da Luz Moreira A, Baker M, et al. CT enterography for Crohn's disease: accurate preoperative diagnostic imaging. *Dis Colon Rectum*. 2007;50:1761-1769.

30. Cheifetz AS, Kornbluth AA, Legnani P, et al. The risk of retention of the capsule endoscope in patients with known or suspected Crohn's disease. *Am J Gastroenterol*. 2006;101:2218-2222.

31. Freed KS, Lo JY, Baker JA, et al. Predictive model for the diagnosis of intraabdominal abscess. *Acad Radiol*. 1998;5:473-479.

32. Maconi G, Sampietro GM, Parente F, et al. Contrast radiology, computed tomography and ultrasonography in detecting internal fistulas and intra-abdominal abscesses in Crohn's disease: a prospective comparative study. *Am J Gastroenterol*. 2003;98:1545-1555.

33. Maconi G, Parente F, Bollani S, Cesana B, Bianchi Porro G. Abdominal ultrasound in the assessment of extent and activity of Crohn's disease: clinical significance and implication of bowel wall thickening. *Am J Gastroenterol*. 1996;91:1604-1609.

34. Brenner DJ, Hall EJ. Computed tomography—an increasing source of radiation exposure. *N Engl J Med*. 2007;357:2277-2284.

35. Peloquin JM, Pardi DS, Sandborn WJ, et al. Diagnostic ionizing radiation exposure in a population-based cohort of patients with inflammatory bowel disease. *Am J Gastroenterol*. 2008;103:2015-2022.

36. Solem CA, Loftus EV Jr, Fletcher JG, et al. Small-bowel imaging in Crohn's disease: a prospective, blinded, 4-way comparison trial. *Gastrointest Endosc*. 2008;68:255-266.

37. Higgins PD, Caoili E, Zimmermann M, et al. Computed tomographic enterography adds information to clinical management in small bowel Crohn's disease. *Inflamm Bowel Dis*. 2007;13:262-268.

38. Maconi G, Carsana L, Fociani P, et al. Small bowel stenosis in Crohn's disease: clinical, biochemical and ultrasonographic evaluation of histological features. *Aliment Pharmacol Ther*. 2003;18:749-756.

39. Sorrentino D, Sorrentino D. Role of biologics and other therapies in stricturing Crohn's disease: what have we learnt so far? *Digestion*. 2008;77:38-47.

40. Bodily KD, Fletcher JG, Solem CA, et al. Crohn disease: mural attenuation and thickness at contrast-enhanced CT enterography—correlation with endoscopic and histologic findings of inflammation. *Radiology*. 2006;238:505-516.

41. Koh DM, Miao Y, Chinn RJ, et al. MR imaging evaluation of the activity of Crohn's disease. *AJR Am J Roentgenol*. 2001;177:1325-1332.

42. Lee SS, Kim AY, Yang SK, et al. Crohn disease of the small bowel: comparison of CT enterography, MR enterography, and small-bowel follow-through as diagnostic techniques. *Radiology*. 2009;251:751-761.

43. Brenner DJ, Hall EJ, Brenner DJ, Hall EJ. Computed tomography—an increasing source of radiation exposure. *N Engl J Med*. 2007;357:2277-2284.

44. Migaleddu V, Quaia E, Scano D, et al. Inflammatory activity in Crohn disease: ultrasound findings. *Abdom Imaging.* 2008;33:589-597.

45. Adler J, Schmiedlin-Ren P, Higgins P, Verrot T, Zimmermann E. Magnetization transfer MRI for quantitative assessment of intestinal fibrosis in Crohn's disease. *Inflamm Bowel Dis.* 2007;13:648-649.

46. Adler J, Swanson SD, Schmiedlin-Ren P, et al. Magnetization transfer helps detect intestinal fibrosis in an animal model of Crohn disease. *Radiology.* 2011;259:127-135.

47. Kim K, Johnson LA, Jia C, et al. Noninvasive ultrasound elasticity imaging (UEI) of Crohn's disease: animal model. *Ultrasound Med Biol.* 2008;34:902-912.

48. Van Assche G. Intramural steroid injection and endoscopic dilation for Crohn's disease. *Clin Gastroenterol Hepatol.* 2007;5:1027-1028.

49. Van Assche G, Vermeire S, Rutgeerts P. Endoscopic therapy of strictures in Crohn's disease. *Inflamm Bowel Dis.* 2007;13:356-358.

50. Singh VV, Draganov P, Valentine J, Singh VV, Draganov P, Valentine J. Efficacy and safety of endoscopic balloon dilation of symptomatic upper and lower gastrointestinal Crohn's disease strictures. *J Clin Gastroenterol.* 2005;39:284-290.

51. Saunders BP, Brown GJ, Lemann M, Rutgeerts P. Balloon dilation of ileocolonic strictures in Crohn's disease. *Endoscopy.* 2004;36:1001-1007.

52. Evans JP, Steinhart AH, Cohen Z, McLeod RS. Home total parenteral nutrition: an alternative to early surgery for complicated inflammatory bowel disease. *J Gastrointest Surg.* 2003;7:562-566.

53. Lavy A, Yasin K. Octreotide for enterocutaneous fistulas of Crohn's disease. *Can J Gastroenterol.* 2003;17:555-558.

54. Ostro MJ, Greenberg GR, Jeejeebhoy KN. Total parenteral nutrition and complete bowel rest in the management of Crohn's disease. *JPEN J Parenter Enteral Nutr.* 1985;9:280-287.

55. Schraut WH, Block GE. Enterovesical fistula complicating Crohn's ileocolitis. *Am J Gastroenterol.* 1984;79:186-190.

56. Regueiro M, Schraut W, Baidoo L, et al. Infliximab prevents Crohn's disease recurrence after ileal resection. *Gastroenterology.* 2009;136:441-450.

57. Hassan C, Zullo A, De Francesco V, et al. Systematic review: endoscopic dilatation in Crohn's disease. *Aliment Pharmacol Ther.* 2007;26:1457-1464.

58. Atrjeja A, Dwivedi S, Lashner B, Vargo JJI, Shen B. Short and long-term outcomes of endoscopic stricture dilation for primary and anastomotic strictures in patients with Crohn's disease. *Gastroenterology.* 2010;138:S528-S529.

59. Brooker JC, Beckett CG, Saunders BP, et al. Long-acting steroid injection after endoscopic dilation of anastomotic Crohn's strictures may improve the outcome: a retrospective case series. *Endoscopy.* 2003;35:333-337.

60. Ramboer C, Verhamme M, Dhondt E, et al. Endoscopic treatment of stenosis in recurrent Crohn's disease with balloon dilation combined with local corticosteroid injection. *Gastrointest Endosc.* 1995;42:252-255.

61. East JE, Brooker JC, Rutter MD, Saunders BP. A pilot study of intrastricture steroid versus placebo injection after balloon dilatation of Crohn's strictures. *Clin Gastroenterol Hepatol.* 2007;5:1065-1069.

62. Yamamoto T, Fazio VW, Tekkis PP, Yamamoto T, Fazio VW, Tekkis PP. Safety and efficacy of strictureplasty for Crohn's disease: a systematic review and meta-analysis. *Dis Colon Rectum.* 2007;50:1968-1986.

63. Golfieri R, Cappelli A, Giampalma E, et al. CT-guided percutaneous pelvic abscess drainage in Crohn's disease. *Tech Coloproctol.* 2006;10:99-105.

64. Kim DH, Cheon JH, Moon CM, et al. Clinical efficacy of nonsurgical treatment of Crohn's disease-related intraabdominal abscess. *Korean J Gastroenterol.* 2009;53:29-35.

65. Gutierrez A, Lee H, Sands BE. Outcome of surgical versus percutaneous drainage of abdominal and pelvic abscesses in Crohn's disease. *Am J Gastroenterol.* 2006;101:2283-2289.

66. Greenberg GR, Fleming CR, Jeejeebhoy KN, Rosenberg IH, Sales D, Tremaine WJ. Controlled trial of bowel rest and nutritional support in the management of Crohn's disease. *Gut.* 1988;29:1309-1315.

67. Aberra FN, Lewis JD, Hass D, Rombeau JL, Osborne B, Lichtenstein GR. Corticosteroids and immunomodulators: postoperative infectious complication risk in inflammatory bowel disease patients. *Gastroenterology.* 2003;125:320-327.

68. Dixon WG, Symmons DP, Lunt M, Watson KD, Hyrich KL, Silman AJ. Serious infection following anti-tumor necrosis factor alpha therapy in patients with rheumatoid arthritis: lessons from interpreting data from observational studies. *Arthritis Rheum.* 2007;56:2896-2904.

69. Dixon WG, Watson K, Lunt M, Hyrich KL, Silman AJ, Symmons DP. Rates of serious infection, including site-specific and bacterial intracellular infection, in rheumatoid arthritis patients receiving anti-tumor necrosis factor therapy: results from the British Society for Rheumatology Biologics Register. *Arthritis Rheum.* 2006;54:2368-2376.

SUGGESTED READINGS

Agrawal A, Durrani S, Leiper K, Ellis A, Morris AI, Rhodes JM. Effect of systemic corticosteroid therapy on risk for intra-abdominal or pelvic abscess in non-operated Crohn's disease. *Clin Gastroenterol Hepatol.* 2005;3:1215-1220.

Cannom RR, Kaiser AM, Ault GT, Beart RW Jr, Etzioni DA. Inflammatory bowel disease in the United States from 1998 to 2005: has infliximab affected surgical rates? *Am Surg.* 2009;75:976-980.

Cosnes J, Cattan S, Blain A, et al. Long-term evolution of disease behavior of Crohn's disease. *Inflamm Bowel Dis.* 2002;8:244-250.

Lichtenstein GR, Olson A, Travers S, et al. Factors associated with the development of intestinal strictures or obstructions in patients with Crohn's disease. *Am J Gastroenterol.* 2006; 101:1030-1038.

Oberhuber G, Stangl PC, Vogelsang H, Schober E, Herbst F, Gasche C. Significant association of strictures and internal fistula formation in Crohn's disease. *Virchows Arch.* 2000;437:293-297.

Chapter 3

Perianal Disease and Perianal Fistulizing Disease in Crohn's Disease

Leyla J. Ghazi, MD and David A. Schwartz, MD

NONFISTULIZING PERIANAL DISEASE

Perianal Crohn's disease (CD) can be categorized as fistulizing and nonfistulizing. Nonfistulizing disease includes skin tags or anal canal abnormalities such as stenosis, fissures, and ulcers. The Cardiff anatomical classification (later modified by Hughes) categorizes nonfistulizing perianal disease as ulceration (U) or stricture (S), and grades these according to severity, location, and reversibility (ie, presence of fissure, ulcer, stricture). The American Gastroenterological Association (AGA) identifies each type of lesion separately (ie, ulceration, stricture, skin tags) and includes cancer.[1]

Anal Fissures

Fissures are longitudinal cuts in the anal canal that typically start at the anal verge and extend to the dentate line. The prevalence of anal fissures in CD is 21% to 35%.[1] In this setting, fissures are commonly eccentric, rather than arising at the midline posterior position of the anus as is common in idiopathic fissures (>90%). Therefore, fissures that are found outside of midline, are multiple, or do not heal should alert the physician to an alternative diagnosis such as CD, infection, or neoplasm. The etiology of anal fissures is unknown, but low blood flow may be one cause.[2] These lesions can be asymptomatic; however, typical symptoms include pain, burning, and/or bleeding upon defecation. The first line of treatment should be medical management. Treatment of symptomatic fissures includes soaking in sitz bath to relax the sphincter, stool softeners if there is associated constipation, or topical ointments. A widely used topical preparation is 0.2% to 0.4% nitroglycerin ointment.

Regueiro MD, Swoger JM, eds.
Clinical Challenges and Complications of IBD (pp 43-60).
© 2013 Taylor & Francis Group.

Randomized trials and systematic reviews have reported marginal results. One study showed induction of healing in one-third of patients at 6 months.[3] Intolerance to the drug, including headache and flushing, requires slow dosage escalation (from once to 3 times daily) and has limited its widespread use. Calcium channel blockers have also been used for their effect on relaxing the internal anal sphincter. Topical 2% diltiazem and 0.2% nifedipine have proven efficacious in a number of studies, with healing rates as high as 50% to 95%, and have demonstrated even better results after the addition of lidocaine ointment.[4] Although botulinum toxin A has gained popularity for the treatment of chronic anal fissures, its utility in Crohn's perianal disease has not been investigated. In patients with persistent fissures without proctitis, Fleshner et al found that 7 of 8 (88%) patients healed after sphincterotomy. Surgery should be avoided if there is evidence of associated proctitis.[5]

Skin Tags

Skin tags are found in 40% to 70% of patients with CD[6,7] and can vary in shape and size. Skin tags may arise secondary to lymphatic obstruction or may be associated with recurrent fissures and fistulas.[1] Though often asymptomatic, soft, and mobile, they may become inflamed, painful, or firm during a CD flare. Skin tags are benign processes, and a majority persist for as long as a decade.[8] In general, surgical intervention should be reserved for persistent symptoms or hygiene purposes, due to difficulty with wound healing in these patients.

Anal Ulcer

Five to 10% of patients with CD present with deep or large, cavitating anorectal ulcers.[1] Symptoms include discharge, bleeding, pruritis, and anorectal pain. Pain is the most common symptom and is often unremitting, with dyschezia being reported in up to 35% of patients.[8] Associated proctitis is present in 75% to 96% of patients.[9] Local treatment with topical metronidazole, tacrolimus, and intralesional methylprednisolone has been studied in small case series, with moderate success.[1] A retrospective review of patients with CD anal ulcerations showed a 43% early and a 72% long-term response to infliximab induction and maintenance therapy, respectively, supporting the use of anti-tumor necrosis factor (anti-TNF) agents for this indication.[10]

Strictures

A CD stricture is believed to occur as a consequence of chronic inflammation or fistulization in either the anus (34%) or the rectum (50%). These strictures can be short or long and result in functional symptoms such as obstipation, perianal pain, overflow diarrhea, or incontinence. Severe stenosis can cause subacute obstruction. Classifying a stricture as either inflammatory or fibrostenotic significantly impacts management. Inflammatory strictures have the potential for response to medical therapy. However, a fibrostenotic stricture may require manual or surgical intervention. Medical therapy using immunomodulators and anti-TNF can be used to treat inflammatory strictures and luminal disease. Commonly, anal dilation with a single finger or balloon is done to break the fibrous band of tissue that makes up the stricture. This should be done gently and under anesthesia, as there is a risk of perforation. The presence of luminal disease, namely proctitis, along with an anal canal stricture (occurs in 43%) has been associated with need for proctectomy.[11]

FISTULIZING PERIANAL DISEASE

Epidemiology

Perianal involvement is a common and devastating complication of CD. Patients typically suffer from sequela such as persistent purulent drainage, vaginal or rectal pain, and incontinence. The course is one of frequent relapses and long episodes of actively draining fistulas. In referral centers, the frequency of perianal fistulas in CD ranges from 17% to 43%.[12] Two population-based studies have estimated the cumulative incidence of perianal fistulas in patients with CD to be 21% to 23%.[12,13] In the Olmsted County, Minnesota, population, perianal disease was present at or before time of diagnosis in 45% of cases. The remaining 55% were found at median of 4.8 years (8 days to 18.7 years) following diagnosis. The distribution of CD fistulas include 54% perianal and 9% rectovaginal, with the remainder being internal or enterocutaneous.[12] Luminal disease is typically present; however, approximately 5% of individuals will have isolated perianal disease. The risk of developing CD perianal fistulas increases when the disease involves the distal bowel. Rectal involvement occurs in 92% of cases, while only 10% to 15% of patients have ileocolonic or small bowel disease.[13] Rectal sparing is associated with a better prognosis.

A majority of patients with fistulizing CD will undergo operative intervention during their disease course. Natural history studies have found that 71% of patients with perianal fistulas require an operation; major operations, such as proctectomy and diverting ileostomy, are required in 32% of patients.[12] Available medical therapies have not appeared to thwart the progression of disease. Introduction of anti-TNF therapy has been the most promising and effective therapeutic option to date, although its effect on the natural history of the disease remains to be determined.

Etiology and Pathophysiology

Knowledge of perianal anatomy is fundamental in order to better understand and accurately classify perianal fistulas. The normal anal canal comprises the internal and external anal sphincters, intersphincteric space, anorectal musculature, and the dentate line (Figure 3-1). The external anal sphincter is formed from the downward extension of skeletal muscle from the puborectalis. The internal anal sphincter is an extension of the continuous band of circular smooth muscle of the rectum.[14] The dentate, or pectinate line, lies in the mid-portion of the internal anal sphincter, adjacent to the

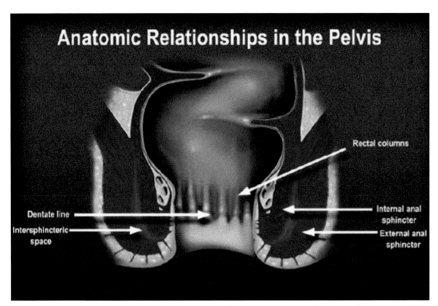

Figure 3-1. Schematic diagram of anatomic relationships in the perianal region.

venous plexus. It separates the squamous epithelium of the anus and columnar epithelium of the rectum. Anal glands exist at the base of many anal crypts present at the level of the dentate line; these may be an important source for the development of perianal fistulas.

Classification of perianal anatomy is essential for optimizing the care of patients with fistulizing CD and for facilitating communication between gastroenterologists and surgeons. Fistulas are divided into high and low; those that originate below the dentate line are considered to be low fistulas, whereas those above the dentate line are considered to be high fistulas.[15] Alternatively, a more precise system is the Parks classification of perianal fistulas. Using the external sphincter as a central point of reference, it categorizes 5 types of fistulas: superficial, intersphincteric, transsphincteric, suprasphincteric, and extrasphincteric (Figure 3-2).[16,17] Although it is the most accurate method of describing fistula anatomy, it has several limitations, including the failure to identify other perianal manifestations, such as skin tags or anal strictures. In addition, clinically important abscesses and/or tracts leading to other structures, such as the vagina or bladder, are not part of this scheme. The AGA has proposed an alternative approach to the classification of perianal fistulas that may be more clinically relevant, namely dividing the fistulas into 2 categories: simple and complex (Figure 3-3).[18] Simple fistulas are those that are considered superficial, intersphincteric, or low transsphincteric; have a single opening; and are not associated with an abscess or tract to another organ. Complex fistulas involve more of the anal sphincters (ie, supra-, extra-, or transsphincteric), have multiple openings, cross the midline (horseshoe fistula), are associated with an abscess, and/or involve the bladder or vagina (AGA). In other words, complex fistulas have features that make them less likely to heal completely (ie, connection to the vagina) and/or involve a significant portion of the external

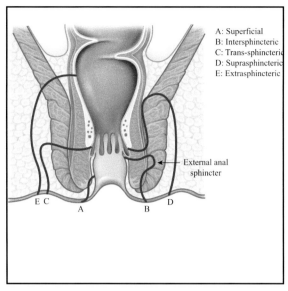

Figure 3-2. The Parks classification. (A) A superficial fistula tracks below both the internal anal sphincter and external anal sphincter complexes. (B) An intersphincteric fistula tracks between the internal anal sphincter and the external anal sphincter in the intersphincteric space. (C) A transsphincteric fistula tracks from the intersphincteric space through the external anal sphincter. (D) A suprasphincteric fistula leaves the intersphincteric space over the top of the puborectalis and penetrates the levator muscle before tracking down to the skin. (E) An extrasphincteric fistula tracks outside of the external anal sphincter and penetrates the levator muscle into the rectum.

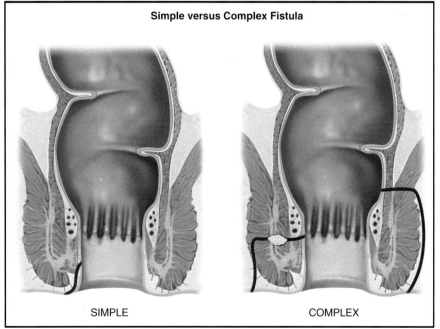

Figure 3-3. AGA classification of perianal fistulas. (Reprinted and published with permission from AGA Position Statement 2003.)

sphincter; these may result in an increased risk of incontinence with aggressive surgical intervention. The AGA system is the preferred method for the classification of perianal fistulas given its ease of application and clinical relevance.

The pathogenesis of perianal CD is not clear, although 2 main mechanisms have been proposed. One hypothesis is that perianal fistulas begin as deep penetrating ulcers in the anus or rectum that extend over time as feces are forced into them with the pressure of defecation.[19] Alternatively, fistulas may form as a result of infection or abscess of the anal glands that exist at the base of the anal crypts. The affected glands can then penetrate into the intersphincteric space, forming tracts to the skin or through the external anal sphincter.[15] The etiology of extrasphincteric fistula formation is less clear, but surgical trauma has been implicated (ie, probing).[20,21]

Clinical Features

The acute presentation of perianal CD may include rectal pain, fevers suggesting an abscess, and/or significant perianal drainage if an active fistula is present. Drainage of perianal abscesses typically relieves the severity of the pain; however, the patient may continue to suffer from persistent perianal drainage, odor, and disfiguring scars. The drainage may be purulent or serosanguinous and vary in amount. The presence of rectovaginal or rectovesicular fistulas can lead to frequent vaginal and urinary tract infections. Overall, the presence of perianal fistulizing disease has a negative impact on the quality of life of patients with CD.[22] Medical therapy with infliximab has been shown to improve quality of life of patients with active CD and fistulizing disease, increasing their ability to work and decreasing feelings of fatigue, depression, and anger.[23,24] The ultimate, yet challenging, goal in treating perianal CD is complete and sustained closure of all fistulas, without the sequelae of abscesses or internal fistula (ie, rectovaginal or rectovesicular) formation. This ultimately aims to avoid the need for invasive surgery and improves the patient's quality of life.

Diagnostic Evaluation

Accurate diagnosis of perianal fistulas is of paramount importance prior to institution of medical or surgical therapy. Patients with suspected perianal CD should undergo a comprehensive diagnostic evaluation to classify fistula anatomy, identify perianal abscesses, and determine whether or not the rectum is actively inflamed or stenotic. This evaluation includes visualization of the perianal region, endoscopy, and endoscopic ultrasound (EUS) or pelvic magnetic resonance imaging (MRI). Objective measures of fistula activity exist. The Fistula Drainage Assessment Measure, based upon the examiner's understanding of fistula anatomy, classifies fistulas as improved (ie, decrease from baseline in number of open draining fistulas by ≥50%) and in remission (ie, closure of all fistulas). A fistula is considered to be open if purulent material can be expressed with the application of gentle pressure to the tract.[25] The term *closed* is appropriate, but misleading and clinically incorrect as imaging studies with EUS or MRI have demonstrated persistent fistula activity for several months after the fistula stops draining.[26] The perianal equivalent to the Crohn's Disease Activity Index, and a more exhaustive measure of perianal symptoms caused by CD, is the Perianal Disease Activity Index (PDAI). This validated index measures fistulas according to 5 categories including discharge, pain, restriction of sexual activity (ie, none to unable), type of perianal disease (ie, skin tags to anal sphincter ulceration), and degree of induration.[27] Higher scores indicate more severe or active disease. The PDAI has been validated as a secondary outcome measure in several trials assessing the efficacy of antibiotics, azathioprine, and anti-TNF therapy.[25,28,29]

There are several imaging techniques used for the identification and classification of CD perianal fistulas. Fistulography involves the injection of the contrast into an open fistula tract; it can be painful and has a theoretical risk of septic spread of infected feculent material. Overall, it has low accuracy because it cannot visualize the anal sphincters. Cross-sectional imaging with computed tomography scan has a mediocre (24% to 60%) accuracy rate secondary to its poor spatial resolution in the pelvis. Attenuation values for the sphincters, levator ani, fibrotic fistulous tracks, and active fistulas are similar, making it difficult to characterize these structures accurately. Conversely, unenhanced T_1-weighted MRI images of the pelvis provide an excellent anatomic overview of the sphincter complex, levator plate, and the ischiorectal fossae. Fistulous tracts, inflammation, and abscesses, however, appear as areas of low-to-intermediate signal intensity and may not be distinguished from normal structures such as the sphincters and levator ani muscles. Alternatively, dynamic contrast-enhanced MRI gives additional information regarding disease activity.[30]

Rectal EUS is also an effective modality to identify fistula tracts and abscesses, assess the degree of active inflammation surrounding a fistula tract, and guide medical and surgical therapy.[26,31] Prospective blinded studies comparing MRI, EUS, and examination under anesthesia (EUA) have demonstrated comparably high accuracy in patients with suspected perianal CD fistulas (EUS 91%, MRI 87%, and EUA 91%). An accuracy of 100% was achieved when MRI or EUS was combined with EUA.[32]

Treatment

Treatment of perianal fistulas consists of medical or surgical therapy, and frequently requires a combination of both treatment modalities. The ultimate goal of therapy is the abolition of existing draining abscesses, followed by the permanent closure or fibrosis of any active perianal fistulas. Identification of the type of fistula and the degree of rectal or luminal inflammation can guide the therapeutic algorithm.

Antibiotics

The efficacy of antibiotics in treating perianal CD has mainly been studied in small case series. Metronidazole and ciprofloxacin are commonly used and appear to provide clinical benefit. However, precise therapeutic guidelines have not been established to date. Long-term tolerability of antibiotic treatment may be poor due to side effects. Common adverse effects with metronidazole include metallic taste, nausea, and peripheral neuropathy. Ciprofloxacin can cause nausea, diarrhea, rash, and rarely tendon rupture. One small randomized, double-blind, placebo-controlled trial comparing the 2 antibiotics (metronidazole and ciprofloxacin) to placebo for treating perianal CD suggested that remission and response may be better with ciprofloxacin.[33]

Immunomodulators

6-mercaptopurine (6-MP) and azathioprine have been used for the treatment of active inflammatory CD in several studies. However, these studies were not designed to test the efficacy of these agents in perianal CD. A meta-analysis of trials looking at fistula response (defined as complete healing or decreased discharge) as a secondary endpoint found that a greater proportion of patients on immunomodulator therapy responded in comparison to placebo (54% versus 21%, odds ratio [OR] 4.44).[34] The early use of antibiotics (ciprofloxacin or metronidazole) in combination with immunomodulator therapy has also been associated with better medium-term response, especially in patients with simple fistulas.[29] This study showed that those patients who were maintained on azathioprine after antibiotics were discontinued had a higher response rate at week 20 compared to those who were not bridged to azathioprine (48% versus 15%; $P = 0.03$).

Small uncontrolled case series and retrospective chart reviews have reported on the effectiveness of methotrexate for the treatment of perianal disease.[35,36] Most patients had at least partial response; however, the lack of controlled studies and short-term efficacy do not support the use of methotrexate for perianal disease as a first-line agent. Consideration should be given to its use for patients intolerant to 6-MP/azathioprine or in lieu of surgical intervention for medically refractory disease.

Tacrolimus

A randomized placebo-controlled study found higher rates of fistula improvement in patients treated for 10 weeks with tacrolimus (0.2 mg/kg/day) versus placebo.[37] However, complete fistula closure was rare, with only 10% of those patients randomized to tacrolimus having complete cessation of drainage in all fistulas. These and other results have not demonstrated high complete fistula closure rates with tacrolimus.[38] A small pilot study of medically refractory fistulizing CD using tacrolimus (0.05 mg/kg every 12 hours) found a greater proportion of partial responders (50%) and fewer complete responders (40%) within 6 to 24 months of follow-up.[39] Currently, given these results, tacrolimus is reserved for patients who have not responded to anti-TNF antibody treatment. Larger randomized trials are needed to identify the subpopulation that may potentially benefit from this alternative therapy in refractory patients. Adverse effects include headache, paresthesias, tremors, insomnia, and renal insufficiency. Additionally, there is a need for close monitoring of drug levels and serum creatinine when using tacrolimus.

Cyclosporine

Cyclosporine has not been studied in a randomized, double-blinded, placebo-controlled trial with the primary endpoint of fistula closure. Open-label data have shown improvement in fistula drainage, but results are tempered by high relapse rates and a substantial side effect profile. The advent of anti-TNF agents has limited its use.[40,41]

Tumor Necrosis Factor Antagonists

Biologic therapies currently available for the treatment of CD include infliximab (a chimeric monoclonal antibody to TNF-α), adalimumab (a fully human immunoglobulin IgG1 anti-TNF-α monoclonal antibody), and certolizumab pegol (a humanized anti-TNF Fab' monoclonal antibody fragment linked to polyethylene glycol). Each of these agents has been shown to be effective in the induction and maintenance of remission of CD. Two double-blind placebo-controlled trials have specifically evaluated the efficacy of infliximab for the treatment of fistulizing CD. These studies demonstrated that infliximab is effective at reducing fistula drainage (5 mg/kg at 0, 2, and 6 weeks) and maintaining cessation of fistula drainage with regular dosing (5 mg/kg every 8 weeks).[25,42] Results showed a 68% response rate in the infliximab (5 mg/kg)-treated group, compared to a 26% placebo response rate ($P = 0.002$). Furthermore, there was a 55% fistula "closure rate" compared to a 13% rate in the placebo group ($P = 0.001$). At 54 weeks, a significantly greater proportion of the infliximab-treated group (36%) maintained complete fistula closure than with placebo (19%, $P = 0.009$).

The efficacy of adalimumab in fistula healing was assessed in the CHARM (CD trial of the Fully Human Antibody Adalimumab for Remission Maintenance) trial. Fistula healing was a secondary endpoint in this trial and was achieved in 33% of patients at 56 weeks (combined 40 mg weekly and every other week versus 13% placebo, $P = 0.016$). In addition, early closure at 26 weeks was predictive of a durable response. Follow-up data of patients with fistulas at baseline in CHARM also revealed durable fistula closure rates at 2 years of 60%.[43,44] Similarly, fistula healing has been examined as a secondary endpoint in the certolizumab maintenance trials (PRECISE—Pegylated Antibody Fragment Evaluation in Crohn's Disease Safety and Efficacy). PRECISE and PRECISE 2 were underpowered to assess the efficacy of certolizumab in fistula closure; however, the latter did show a high rate of short-term fistula closure in those that had a response in the open-label induction portion of the study (67% at week 26).

The efficacy of the different anti-TNF therapies for fistula healing has not been studied in head-to-head trials. However, medical therapy with anti-TNF in conjunction with surgical intervention with EUA and seton placement has been examined in a retrospective study. Patients with fistulizing perianal disease who had a EUA with seton placement prior to receiving infliximab had a 100% response versus 82% in the infliximab-alone group. Response was defined as a complete closure and cessation of drainage from the fistula.

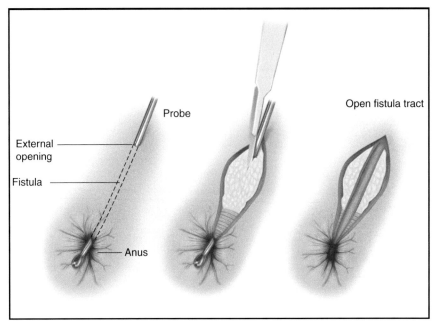

Figure 3-4. Schematic of surgical fistulotomy. (Reprinted with permission from Schwartz Schwartz DA, Wiersema MJ, Dudiak KM, et al. A comparison of endoscopic ultrasound, magnetic resonance imaging, and exam under anesthesia for evaluation of Crohn's perianal fistulas. *Gastroenterology.* 2001;121:1064-1072.)

Durable treatment outcomes (lower recurrence rates and longer time to recurrence) were seen in the combination therapy group (44% versus 79%, 13.5 versus 3.6 months).[45]

Surgical Options

The reported incidence of surgery for perianal CD is from 25% to 30% to as high as 71% in those with perianal fistulizing disease.[12,46] The surgical options include, but are not limited to, EUA with seton placement, fistulotomy, advancement flaps, fibrin glue or fistula plugs, diverting ileostomy, and proctectomy. In fact, the rate of proctectomy in the era prior to the introduction of anti-TNF therapy was 14% based upon a 20-year review of patients with perianal CD.[47] In general, the goal of surgical intervention in patients with complex fistulas is to evacuate the perianal sepsis that is present and to control fistula healing to prevent abscess formation, which helps to maximize the effectiveness of subsequent medical therapy. Drainage of active abscesses should take place prior to the initiation of medical therapy to avoid further pelvic septic complications. The surgical approach can include local incision and drainage, catheter placement, or seton placement for abscesses directly associated with a fistula tract.

For patients with simple or superficial fistulas and no active proctitis, fistulotomy is a reasonable option (Figure 3-4). This involves the fistula tract being surgically incised open to allow it to heal. Active proctitis is a relative contraindication to fistulotomy, as it is associated with poor outcomes in this setting. The dilemma arises in the treatment of deeper, transsphincteric and

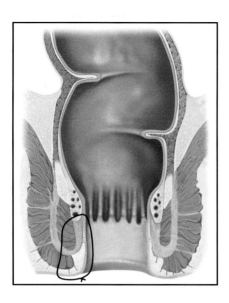

Figure 3-5. Schematic of seton. (Reprinted with permission from Schwartz DA, Wiersema MJ, Dudiak KM, et al. A comparison of endoscopic ultrasound, magnetic resonance imaging, and exam under anesthesia for evaluation of Crohn's perianal fistulas. *Gastroenterology*. 2001;121:1064-1072.)

extrasphincteric or rectovaginal fistulas (RVFs) due to the risk of sphincter compromise and subsequent fecal incontinence. Therefore, the main objective for the surgical therapy of CD perianal fistulas includes (1) the successful elimination of current and recurrent disease and (2) the preservation of sphincter function.

The control of perianal fistula healing is generally done through the placement of a noncutting or draining seton (Figure 3-5). A vessel loop or suture is typically threaded through a fistula tract and is tied outside of the anal canal. This allows the fistula to continue to drain while there is active inflammation, reducing the risk of abscess formation. It has been shown that combination therapy with both a medical and surgical approach results in the most successful outcomes for these patients.[45,48] There is a theoretical risk of abscess formation with premature closure of the cutaneous opening of the fistula on medical therapy alone. In the infliximab trials evaluating patients with perianal disease, the rate of abscess formation was 11% to 15%.[25,42] For this reason, surgical intervention to maintain a patent drainage tract is recommended prior to starting anti-TNF therapy. Most commonly, EUA with seton placement or fistulotomy is performed prior to the initiation of medical therapy. Imaging with MRI of the pelvis or EUS can then be obtained to confirm fistula healing and closure. The seton can be removed if the fistula tract becomes inactive or stay in place if healing has not occurred.

Other less commonly used surgical options for refractory fistulas include endorectal advancement flap, fibrin glue injection, or placement of a fistula plug. The advancement flap procedures involve the oversewing of a mucosal flap onto the internal opening of the fistula tract. The flap prevents fecal material and bacteria from entering the fistulous tract, permitting it to heal. Dissection of the sphincter fibers is not required, thereby minimizing functional disturbance.[49] Although overall success rates for the closure of anorectal and RVFs vary (29% to 95%), CD and obstetrical fistulas appear to have the highest failure rates.[50] Recurrence rates for CD fistulas are as high as 50% within 2 years or less of postoperative follow-up. Prior incision and drainage of abscess or seton placement seems to be associated with greater EAF success rates (73% in one study). A systematic review of the literature from 1978 to 2008 revealed a 12% incontinence rate in the CD subpopulation (range 0% to 35% overall).[51]

Fibrin glue injection involves injection of the fistula with a biodegradable glue. The fistula plug involves fixing of a porcine-derived plug in the anal fistula. The presence of active inflammation or abscess is associated with a decreased chance of success for these procedures. The use of fibrin glue takes advantage of the activation of thrombin to form a fibrin clot, which mechanically seals the fistula tract from the inside out and allows it to heal naturally. The process of wound healing including fibroblast growth and collagen formation has been estimated to occur in 1 to 2 weeks.[52] Most reports using fibrin glue are relatively small, rarely randomized, and infrequently reported on CD patients exclusively, and certainly not with the uniformity of fistula and patient characterization observed in a multicenter randomized trial. The overall closure rates for both cryptoglandular and CD fistulas are highly variable. A recent open-label randomized trial looking at actively draining complex and simple CD perianal fistulas found fibrin glue plugs were significantly effective in 38% of patients (versus 16% in observation group). Patients with complex fistulas appear to have less benefit, as do those with RVFs. The study was limited by its small sample size and the exclusion of patients with prior anti-TNF therapy (within 3 months).[53] Combined therapy with seton placement and fibrin glue has been proposed for the treatment of complex perianal fistulas in the literature with an estimated closure rate of 50% by 1 year.[52] A phase III clinical trial is currently investigating the benefit of combining expanded adipose-derived stem cells and fibrin glue for the treatment of complex fistulas associated with CD or of cryptoglandular origin. The published phase II trial has shown promising results at 1 year (71% adipose-derived stem cells with glue versus 16% fibrin glue alone, $P < 0.001$).[54]

RVFs in women can be especially devastating and require special attention. Up to 10% of women with CD will develop an RVF.[55] Patients commonly describe dyspareunia, chronic feculent or malodorous vaginal discharge, or passage of flatus. In comparison to other perianal fistula, Crohn's-related RVF has higher recurrence rates, ranging from 25% to 50%. Steroids and smoking have been associated with higher treatment failure, and immunomodulators with successful healing.[56] Patients with Crohn's RVF may require on average more surgical procedures to achieve healing,[57] with a 29% to 54% first attempt failure. Patients with minor symptoms may be able to avoid surgery. Those with extensive anorectal disease, on the other hand, may be poor surgical candidates for primary reparative surgery. Operative interventions such as endorectal advancement flap, fistulotomy, transperineal repair, fibrin glue injection, and collagen plug insertion have been used with variable and overall poor outcomes.[58]

Fecal diversion or proctocolectomy is typically reserved for patients with severe rectal and/or perianal disease refractory to medical and surgical treatment. In a 20-year review of patients with perianal CD prior to the introduction of infliximab, the rate of proctectomy was 14%.[47] Reported proctectomy rates for RVFs are 34% to 53%.[58] In practice, some patients may not benefit from diversion and may continue to have symptoms despite aggressive medical therapy. Those in remission after surgery have a high risk of recurrence once the fecal stream is restored. There are currently no parameters that can identify patients who may have more successful outcomes.[59] Limited data are available for the use of hyperbaric oxygen for perianal CD fistulas. Small case reports suggest its benefit for severe, medically refractory disease; however, the method is plagued by potential complications (oxygen toxicity, middle ear or sinus trauma), unknown effect on complete healing, and the drawback of treatment frequency.[60]

Overall, there are very few randomized controlled trials comparing the various modalities of surgery for fistula-in-ano. A Cochrane systematic review of 10 studies of simple, noninflammatory bowel disease–related fistulas showed no difference between the various techniques in regards to recurrence rates.[61] It is clear that combination of medical and surgical therapy is paramount to achieve the greatest long-term success in the treatment of CD perianal fistulas.

Management

The presence of fistulizing disease is one of the predictors of poor outcome in patients with CD (Figure 3-6).[62] When counseling patients about the treatment of perianal CD, many advocate the top-down approach, treatment with an anti-TNF agent and a concomitant immunomodulator. Early response rates (cessation of drainage and EUS inactivity) of 86% and maintenance of response rates of 76% (median 68 weeks) have been shown in retrospective case series using combination medical therapy, along with seton placement and image guidance.[26] Fifty-two percent of patients had complete fistula healing by EUS at a median of 21 weeks. A subsequent study looking at patients with complex fistulas treated with combination medical therapy, antibiotics, and pre-emptive seton placement found similar results (80% cessation of drainage at 54 weeks). EUS-guided inactivity occurred at 18 weeks.[31] Similarly, a study from Ng et al looked at 34 CD patients with perianal fistulas, followed with serial MRIs during treatment. Those patients with inadequate fistula response on MRI at the midway point of the study (week 22) had their medical therapy increased. This resulted in 3 of the 4 initial nonresponders achieving either fistula remission or response at week 52.[63]

The recommended strategy of utilizing combination medical (top-down therapy) and surgical therapy with image guidance is based upon available guidelines put forth by the AGA, the European Crohn's and Colitis Organization, and randomized controlled trials. First, the perianal anatomy should be well defined with physical examination and imaging using either pelvic MRI or EUS. If a simple fistula is found without evidence of luminal disease (namely proctitis), then a combination of antibiotics, immunosuppressive therapy (6-MP/azathioprine), or anti-TNF (if intolerant to immunomodulators) should be initiated. If there is no response within approximately 3 months,

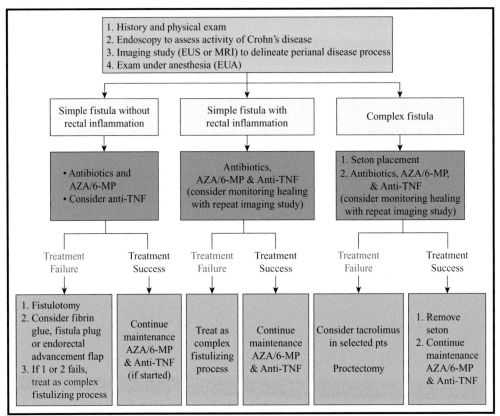

Figure 3-6. Algorithm for the management of perianal fistulizing disease. EUS = endoscopic ultrasound; MRI = magnetic resonance imaging; AZA = azathioprine; 6-MP = 6-mercaptopurine; TNF = tumor necrosis factor.

then the fistula should be treated as complex. The presence of proctitis reduces the chance of fistula healing and limits surgical options; therefore, consideration should be given to starting anti-TNF therapy early. If a complex fistula is found, such as high (extra-, trans-, or suprasphincteric) or low (trans- or intersphincteric), or there is an associated abscess, then a surgical consult for EUA should be obtained with the goal of seton placement.[64] All abscesses should be drained promptly, and antibiotics (ciprofloxacin and/or metronidazole) should be initiated. Anti-TNF therapy, preferably in combination with immunomodulator (6-MP 1 to 1.5 mg/kg/azathioprine 2 to 2.5 mg/kg), if tolerated, is recommended. Seton removal should only be considered after confirmation of fistula inactivity by EUS or MRI. Setons should not be removed if there is persistent purulent drainage or if imaging suggests ongoing fistula activity. For refractory cases, a discussion of alternative surgical approaches such as fibrin plug, advancement flap, or fecal diversion should take place.

☑Key Points

☑ Perianal CD is a common manifestation of CD, with long-term devastating sequelae if not adequately treated.

☑ Knowledge of the perianal anatomy and recognition of fistulizing and nonfistulizing perianal lesions is paramount in developing a treatment plan.

☑ The management of perianal CD involves a multidisciplinary approach, including diagnostic imaging with MRI or EUS, surgical drainage of abscesses, EUA with seton placement, and timely initiation of medical therapy.

☑ Combination therapy with immunomodulators (6-MP/azathioprine) and anti-TNF agents has proven to be successful in the induction and maintenance of fistula closure.

☑ Alternative medical (ie, cyclosporine, tacrolimus, methotrexate) and surgical therapies (ie, fibrin glue, fistulotomy, fecal diversion) exist for those patients refractory to the more conventional approach.

REFERENCES

1. Bouguen G, Siproudhis L, Bretagne J, et al. Nonfistulizing perianal Crohn's disease: clinical features, epidemiology, and treatment. *Inflamm Bowel Dis.* 2010;16(8):1431-1442.
2. Hull TL. Diseases of the anorectum. In: Feldman M, Friedman LS, Brandt LJ, eds. *Sleisenger and Fordtran's Gastrointestinal and Liver Diseases.* 8th ed. Philadelphia, PA: Saunders Elsevier; 2006:2834-2854.
3. Richard CS, Gregoire R, Plewes EA, et al. Internal sphincterotomy is superior to topical nitroglycerin in the treatment of chronic anal fissure: results of a randomized, controlled trial by the Canadian Colorectal Surgical Trials Group. *Dis Colon Rectum.* 2000;43:1048.
4. Dhawan S, Chopra S. Nonsurgical approaches for the treatment of anal fissures. *Am J Gastroenterol.* 2007;102:1312-1321.
5. Fleshner PR, Schoetz DJ, Roberts PL. Anal fissure in Crohn's disease: a plea for aggressive management. *Dis Colon Rectum.* 1995;38(11):1137-1143.
6. Keighley MR, Allan RN. Current status and influence of operation on perianal Crohn's disease. *Int J Colorectal Dis.* 1986;1(2):104-107.
7. Buchmann P, Keighley MR, Allan RN, et al. Natural history of perianal Crohn's disease. Ten year follow-up: a plea for conservatism. *Am J Surg.* 1980;140(5):642-644.
8. Lewis RT, Maron DJ. Anorectal Crohn's disease. *Surg Clin North Am.* 2010;90(1):83-97.
9. Siproudhis L, Mortaji A, Mary JY, et al. Anal lesions: any significant prognosis in Crohn's disease? *Eur J Gastroenterol Hepatol.* 1997;9(3):239-243.
10. Bouguen G, Trouilloud I, Siproudhis L, et al. Long-term outcome of non-fistulizing (ulceration, stricture) perianal Crohn's disease in patients treated with infliximab. *Aliment Pharmacol Ther.* 2009;30:749-756.
11. Fields S, Rosainz L, Korelitz BI, et al. Rectal strictures in Crohn's disease and coexisting perirectal complications. *Inflamm Bowel Dis.* 2008;14:29-31.

12. Schwartz DA, Loftus EV Jr, Tremaine WJ, et al. The natural history of fistulizing Crohn's disease in Olmsted County, Minnesota. *Gastroenterology.* 2002;122(4):875-880.

13. Hellers G, Bergstrand O, Ewerth S, et al. Occurrence and outcome after primary treatment of anal fistulae in Crohn's disease. *Gut.* 1980;21(6):525-527.

14. Bannister L, Martin MB, Peter LM et al, eds. Alimentary system. In: *Gray's Anatomy.* Vol. 38. New York, NY: Churchill Livingstone; 1995:1683-1812.

15. Goligher J. Fistulas-in-ano. In: Goligher J, ed. *Surgery of the Anus, Rectum, and Colon.* 5th ed. London, England: Bailliere Tindall; 1984:178-220.

16. Parks A. The pathogenesis and treatment of fistula-in-ano. *Br Med J.* 1961;1:463-469.

17. Parks AG, Gordon PH, Hardcastle JD. A classification of fistula-in-ano. *Br J Surg.* 1976;63(1):1-12.

18. American Gastroenterological Association. American Gastroenterological Association medical position statement: perianal Crohn's disease. *Gastroenterology.* 2003;125(5): 1503-1507.

19. Hughes L. Surgical pathology and management of anorectal Crohn's disease. *J R Soc Med.* 1978;71:644-651.

20. Hawley PR. Anorectal fistula. *Clin Gastroenterol.* 1975;4(3):635-649.

21. Vasilevsky C, Stein B. Fistula-in-ano. In: Wexner S, Vernava A, eds. *Clinical Decision Making in Colorectal Surgery.* New York, NY: Igaku-Shoin; 1995:137-141.

22. Shen B, Fazio VW, Remzi FH, et al. Clinical features and quality of life in patients with different phenotypes of Crohn's disease of the ileal pouch. *Dis Colon Rectum.* 2007;50(9):1450-1459.

23. Lichtenstein GR, Bala M, Chenglong H, et al. Infliximab improves quality of life in patients with Crohn's disease. *Inflamm Bowel Dis.* 2002;8:237-243.

24. Cadahia V, Garcia-Carbonero S, Vivas S, et al. Infliximab improves quality of life in the short-term in patients with fistulizing Crohn's disease in clinical practice. *Rev Esp Enferm Dig (Madrid).* 2004;96(6):369-378.

25. Present DH, Rutgeerts P, Targan S, et al. Infliximab for the treatment of fistulas in patients with Crohn's disease. *N Engl J Med.* 1999;340(18):1398-1405.

26. Schwartz DA, White CM, Wise PE, et al. Use of endoscopic ultrasound to guide combination medical and surgical therapy for patients with perianal fistulas. *Inflamm Bowel Dis.* 2005;11:727-732.

27. Irvine EJ. Usual therapy improves perianal Crohn's disease as measured by a new disease activity index. McMaster IBD Study Group. *J Clin Gastroenterol.* 1995;20(1):27-32.

28. Farrell RJ, Shah SA, Lodhavia PJ, et al. Clinical experience with infliximab in 100 patients with Crohn's disease. *Am J Gastroenterol.* 2000;95(12):3490-3497.

29. Dejaco C, Harrer M, Waldhoer T, et al. Antibiotics and azathioprine for the treatment of perianal fistulas in Crohn's disease. *Aliment Pharmacol Ther.* 2003;18(11-12):1113-1120.

30. Horsthuis K, Lavini C, Bipat S, et al. Perianal Crohn's disease: evaluation of dynamic contrast-enhanced MR imaging as an indicator of disease activity. *Radiology.* 2009;251(2): 380-387.

31. Spradlin NM, Wise PE, Herline AJ, et al. A randomized prospective trial of endoscopic ultrasound to guide combination medical and surgical treatment for Crohn's perianal fistulas. *Am J Gastroenterol.* 2008;103:2527-2535.

32. Schwartz DA, Wiersema MJ, Dudiak KM, et al. A comparison of endoscopic ultrasound, magnetic resonance imaging, and exam under anesthesia for evaluation of Crohn's perianal fistulas. *Gastroenterology.* 2001;121:1064-1072.

33. Thia KT, Mahadevan U, Feagan BG, et al. Ciprofloxacin or metronidazole for the treatment of perianal fistulas in patients with Crohn's disease: a randomized, double-blind, placebo-controlled pilot study. *Inflamm Bowel Dis.* 2009;15:17-24.

34. Pearson DC, May GR, Fick GH, et al. Azathioprine and 6-mercaptopurine in Crohn's disease. A meta-analysis. *Ann Intern Med.* 1995;123:132-142.

35. Schroder O, Blumenstein I, Schulte-Bockholt A, et al. Combining infliximab and methotrexate in fistulizing Crohn's disease resistant or intolerant to azathioprine. *Aliment Pharmacol Ther.* 2004;19(3):295-301.

36. Mahadevan U, Marion JF, Present DH. Fistula response to methotrexate in Crohn's disease: a case series. *Aliment Pharmacol Ther.* 2003;18(10):1003-1008.

37. Sandborn WJ, Feagan BG, Hanauer SB, et al. A review of activity indices and efficacy endpoints for clinical trials of medical therapy in adults with Crohn's disease. *Gastroenterology.* 2002;122:512-530.

38. González Lama Y, Abreu LE, Vera MI, et al. Long-term oral tacrolimus in refractory to infliximab fistulizing Crohn's disease: comments from Spanish experience. *Gastroenterology.* 2004;126(3):942-943.

39. Gonzalez Lama Y, Abreu LE, Vera MI. Long-term oral tacrolimus in refractory to infliximab fistulizing Crohn's disease: a pilot study. *Inflamm Bowel Dis.* 2005;11:8-15.

40. Lichtiger S. Cyclosporine therapy in inflammatory bowel disease: open-label experience. *Mt. Sinai J Med.* 1990;57:315-319.

41. Hanauer SB, Smith MB. Rapid closure of Crohn's disease fistulas with continuous intravenous cyclosporine A. *Am J Gastroenterol.* 1993;88:646-649.

42. Sands BE, Anderson FH, Bernstein CN, et al. Infliximab maintenance therapy for fistulizing Crohn's disease. *N Engl J Med.* 2004;350:876.

43. Colombel JF, Sandborn WJ, Rutgeerts P, et al. Adalimumab for the maintenance of clinical response and remission in patients with Crohn's disease: the CHARM trial. *Gastroenterology.* 2007;132(1):52-65.

44. Panacionne R, Colombel JF, Sandborn WJ, et al. Adalimumab sustains clinical remission and overall clinical benefit after 2 years of therapy for Crohn's disease. *Aliment Pharmacol Ther.* 2010;31(12):1296-1309.

45. Regueiro M, Mardini H. Treatment of perianal fistulizing Crohn's disease with infliximab alone or as an adjunct to exam under anesthesia with seton placement. *Inflamm Bowel Dis.* 2003;9:98-103.

46. Fichera A, Michelassi F. Surgical treatment of Crohn's disease. *J Gastrointest Surg.* 2007; 11:791-803.

47. Williamson PR, Hellinger MD, Larach SW, et al. Twenty-year review of the surgical management of perianal Crohn's disease. *Dis Colon Rectum.* 1995;38:389-392.

48. Topstad DR, Panaccione R, Heine JA, et al. Combined seton placement, infliximab infusion, and maintenance immunosuppressives improve healing rate in fistulizing anorectal Crohn's disease: a single center experience. *Dis Colon Rectum.* 2003;46:577-583.

49. Hyman N. End anal advancement flap repair for complex perianal fistulas. *Am J Surg.* 1999;178:337-340.

50. Sonora T, Hull T, Piedmont MR, Fazio VW. Outcomes of primary repair of anorectal and rectovaginal fistulas using the endorectal advancement flap. *Dis Colon Rectum.* 2002;45(12):1622-1628.

51. Sultana A, Kaiser AM. Endorectal advancement flap for cryptoglandular or Crohn's fistula-in-ano. *Dis Colon Rectum.* 2010;53(4):486-495.

52. De Parades V, Safe Far H, Seaton EJ, et al. Seton drainage and fibrin glue injection for complex anal fistulas. *Colorectal Dis.* 2009;12:459-463.

53. Grimed JC, Munoz-Bong N, Siproudhis L, et al. Fibrin glue is effective healing perianal fistulas in patients with Crohn's disease. *Gastroenterology.* 2010;138:2275-2281.

54. Garcia-Olmos D, Herreros D, Pascual I, et al. Expanded adipose-derived stem cells for the treatment of complex perianal fistula: a phase II clinical trial. *Dis Colon Rectum.* 2009; 52:79-86.

55. Radcliffe AG, Ritchie JK, Hawley PR, et al. Innovational and rectovaginal fistulas in Crohn's disease. *Dis Colon Rectum.* 1988;31:94-99.

56. El-Gaza G, Hull T, Minnelli E, et al. Analysis of function and predictors of failure in women undergoing repair of Crohn's related rectovaginal fistula. *J Gastrointest Surg.* 2010;14:824-829.

57. Pinto RA, Peterson TV, Shaky S, et al. Are there predictors of outcome following rectovaginal fistula repair. *Dis Colon Rectum.* 2010;53(9):1240-1247.

58. Gartner WB, Madoff RD, Spencer MP, et al. Results of combined medical and surgical treatment of rectovaginal fistula in Crohn's disease. *Colorectal Dis.* 2011;13(6)678-683.

59. Yamamoto T, Allan RN, Keighley MR. Effect of fecal diversion alone on perianal Crohn's disease. *World J Surg.* 2000;24(10):1258-1262.
60. Boyer CM, Brandt LJ. Hyperbaric oxygen therapy for perianal Crohn's disease. *Am J Gastroenterol.* 1999;94(2):318-321.
61. Jacob TJ, Pea Kath B, Keighley MR. Surgical intervention for anorectal fistula. *Cochrane Database Syst Rev.* 2010;(5):CD006319.
62. Beau Erie L, Seasick P, Nion-Lamurier I, et al. Predictors of Crohn's disease. *Gastroenterology.* 2006;130(3):650-656.
63. Ng SC, Plamondon, S, Gupta A, et al. Prospective evaluation of anti-tumor necrosis factor therapy guided by magnetic resonance imaging for Crohn's perineal fistulas. *Am J Gastroenterol.* 2009;104(12):2973-2986.
64. Siemanowski B, Regueiro M. Management of perianal fistula in Crohn's disease. *Inflamm Bowel Dis.* 2008;14:S266-S268.

SUGGESTED READINGS

Present DH, Rutgeerts P, Targan S, et al. Infliximab for the treatment of fistulas in patients with Crohn's disease. *N Engl J Med.* 1999;340(18):1398-1405.

Schwartz DA, Loftus EV Jr, Tremaine WJ, et al. The natural history of fistulizing Crohn's disease in Olmsted County, Minnesota. *Gastroenterology.* 2002;122(4):875-880.

Schwartz DA, Wiersema MJ, Dudiak KM, et al. A comparison of endoscopic ultrasound, magnetic resonance imaging, and exam under anesthesia for evaluation of Crohn's perianal fistulas. *Gastroenterology.* 2001;121:1064-1072.

Chapter 4

Toxic Ulcerative Colitis and Megacolon

Garret Cullen, MD and Adam S. Cheifetz, MD

Ulcerative colitis (UC) is a chronic inflammatory disease characterized by acute flares of activity between periods of remission. Approximately 15% of patients with UC will develop an acute severe flare over the lifetime of their disease.[1] Ten percent of patients with UC develop an acute severe flare as their initial presentation of the disease.[2,3] Confirmation of the diagnosis on admission is essential and includes a good history, physical examination, laboratory markers, and imaging of the abdomen (to rule out megacolon), as well as exclusion of *Clostridium difficile* and cytomegalovirus (CMV) infections. Narcotics and antidiarrheals should be avoided as they may potentially precipitate megacolon. Patients are also at increased risk for thromboembolic disease and should be given prophylaxis against this complication.

Intravenous (IV) corticosteroids are the first line of therapy for acute severe colitis but up to 30% will fail to respond. Scoring systems that allow prediction of steroid failure are helpful and should be calculated on admission and at day 3. Patients failing IV steroids have the option of medical "rescue" therapy or surgery, and these options should be reviewed with the patient and surgeon by day 3 of hospitalization, if there has been no response.

Cyclosporine offers excellent short-term efficacy (70% to 80%), and long-term efficacy is improved with bridging to thiopurine agents (6-mercaptopurine or azathioprine).

Infliximab has been used in the setting of severe UC, although data supporting its efficacy, particularly long term, are lacking. It appears to be effective in patients with less severe disease. The choice of rescue therapy will depend on whether there has been prior failure of thiopurine therapy because cyclosporine is typically used as a bridge to long-term thiopurine maintenance therapy. Surgery is curative, but one must take into account the morbidity, surgical risks, and long-term functional outcomes. The risks and benefits of all options must be discussed openly and honestly with the patient in a team

Regueiro MD, Swoger JM, eds.
Clinical Challenges and Complications of IBD (pp 61-80).
© 2013 Taylor & Francis Group.

Table 4-1. American College of Gastroenterology Clinical Practice Guidelines: Definitions of Severity of Acute Ulcerative Colitis

SEVERE	FULMINANT
>6 BM per day with:	>10 BM per day with:
• Fever	• Continuous bleeding
• Tachycardia	• Systemic toxicity
• Anemia	• Abdominal tenderness and distention
• ↑ESR	• Anemia requiring transfusion
	• Colonic dilatation on x-ray
BM = bowel movements; ESR = erythrocyte sedimentation rate	

approach involving the gastroenterologist and surgeon, both of whom should be involved in the patient's care from the time of admission.

EPIDEMIOLOGY

Severe flares of UC, which typically require hospitalization, are defined by Truelove and Witts criteria as greater than 6 bloody stools per day plus one of the following: temperature >100°F, pulse >90 bpm, hemoglobin <10.5 g/dL, or erythrocyte sedimentation rate (ESR) >30 mm/h.[4] The term *toxic UC* has been used interchangeably with acute severe colitis. Many gastroenterologists and colorectal surgeons reserve the term toxic UC to refer to a patient who has acute severe UC that is likely to require immediate colectomy. The term *fulminant colitis* is often used as well but can be differentiated based on definitions from the American College of Gastroenterology's Clinical Practice guidelines (Table 4-1).[5] Megacolon refers to the appearance of a dilated colon (≥6 cm) on plain radiograph of the abdomen (Figure 4-1).[6] If this is accompanied by signs of systemic toxicity (tachycardia, fever, hypotension), the patient has a toxic megacolon, which typically requires urgent surgical management (Figure 4-2). Toxic megacolon in the setting of UC was first described in 1950.[7] The lifetime incidence of toxic megacolon in UC is 1% to 2.5%.[8] Italian data have suggested that as many as 17% of admissions for acute severe UC are complicated by toxic megacolon.[9] However, the same group subsequently published prospective data indicating an incidence of 7.9% of UC hospital admissions, which seems closer to what is seen in clinical practice.[10]

Prior to the introduction of corticosteroid therapy, acute severe UC had a mortality rate of approximately 25%.[11] One of the earlier studies of corticosteroids in the setting of toxic megacolon showed a 90% mortality rate in those given supportive therapy without steroids.[12] Those treated with steroids

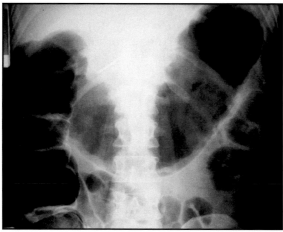

Figure 4-1. Plain radiograph showing gross dilation of the transverse and ascending colon consistent with megacolon.

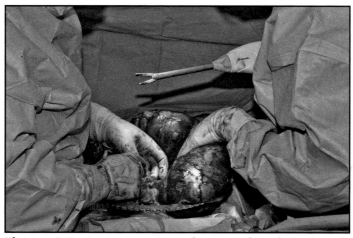

Figure 4-2. Intraoperative photograph of a grossly distended colon removed for acute severe UC. (Reprinted with permission of V. Poylin, MD.)

had a 34% mortality rate, mostly due to delays in surgery.[12] Corticosteroids decreased the mortality in severe UC from 25% to 7%, and improvements in intensive care and surgical techniques have improved mortality even further. Kaplan et al, however, have shown that this condition is still associated with morbidity and mortality, with increased mortality in those undergoing emergency rather than elective colectomy.[13]

ETIOLOGY AND PATHOPHYSIOLOGY

It is not uncommon for a patient with UC to present with a severe flare requiring hospitalization. Just as importantly, approximately 10%

of patients with UC will initially present with an acute severe episode requiring hospitalization. It is particularly important in the latter scenario to confirm the diagnosis of UC and rule out other potential causes of colitis, particularly infection, as there are a number of diseases that can present in a similar fashion to UC or trigger an exacerbation of UC (see Diagnostic Evaluation below). Toxic megacolon can have a variety of causes that must be considered in the absence of a preceding diagnosis of inflammatory bowel disease (IBD). They include pseudo-obstruction (Ogilvie syndrome), ischemia, pseudomembranous colitis (typically caused by *difficile* infection), and a number of other enteric infections (*Shigella, Salmonella, Campylobacter*).[14]

The mechanisms leading to the development of megacolon in the setting of UC are poorly understood, although there is some evidence implicating impaired smooth muscle contraction[15] and inhibition of the gastrocolic reflex[16] in response to a number of mediators, including nitric oxide,[17] vasoactive intestinal polypeptide, and substance P.[18] The severity of disease is also a factor that differentiates a typical severe flare from toxic megacolon; inflammation rarely extends beyond the submucosa in UC, but in cases of toxic megacolon, it can spread to the muscular layers of the bowel wall.[19]

CLINICAL FEATURES

The symptoms of an acute severe flare of UC are bloody diarrhea, abdominal pain, or cramping associated with signs of systemic toxicity. Abdominal distention and features of systemic sepsis are seen in the case of toxic dilation. Symptoms may evolve after admission, and it is important to monitor the following clinical parameters regularly: frequency of bowel movements, rectal bleeding, and abdominal tenderness. Additionally, the patient's pulse, blood pressure, and temperature should be monitored closely, as these are often the first signs of toxicity. As the majority of patients have received high doses of oral steroids prior to admission, it is important to realize that steroids can often mask signs of infection, toxicity, and even perforation. It is imperative to ask about potential triggers such as nonsteroidal anti-inflammatory drugs (NSAIDs) and risk factors for infection, such as travel and recent antibiotic use. Alternative diagnoses such as CMV, *C difficile*, and enteric bacterial infection need to be considered.

DIAGNOSTIC EVALUATION

Due to the possibility of negative outcomes, patients with severe UC need to be evaluated and monitored closely. In addition to following the clinical features and vital signs as described above, serial abdominal examinations should be performed. Laboratory markers such as white blood count, hematocrit (HCT), platelets, electrolytes, and renal function should be checked. Additionally, inflammatory markers (ESR and C-reactive protein

[CRP]), albumin, and liver function tests should be obtained. There are good data to suggest that CRP, in particular, is a good predictor of steroid failure and need for surgery.[20] Serum potassium and sodium may be affected by corticosteroid therapy. Serum magnesium and cholesterol have an important bearing on cyclosporine therapy and should be measured prior to initiation of this medication. Plain abdominal radiographs are important in monitoring for the development of a toxic megacolon and should be performed according to the patient's clinical condition. Abdominal computed tomography (CT) does not need to be routinely performed but should be considered in the event of fever or increasing abdominal pain (to rule out perforation), and may also give information regarding the extent of disease.

Despite the rush to start treatment, it is important to confirm the diagnosis and rule out potential complicating issues such as infection. Stool samples should be sent to rule out enteric infection including *C difficile*.[21] If the level of suspicion is high (eg, prior history or recent antibiotic use), 3 samples should be sent for *C difficile*, to improve sensitivity. The presence of *C difficile* in the setting of acute UC is associated with increased risk of colectomy and worse long-term clinical outcomes.[22] If the *C difficile* toxin is isolated, the patient should be treated with oral vancomycin. In addition, a flexible sigmoidoscopy with biopsies should be performed to confirm the diagnosis of UC and also to exclude CMV infection. There is some evidence that full colonoscopy can precipitate toxic dilation in the setting of acute UC, so endoscopy should be limited to the left colon, without preparation and using minimal insufflation.[23,24]

CMV warrants special attention, as it can cause diagnostic confusion and affects decisions regarding immunosuppression in acute severe UC. CMV can cause an acute colitis and may also trigger relapse in UC.[25] It is important to note that CMV *infection* refers to the presence of CMV antigens or antibodies in the circulation, whereas CMV *disease* implies tissue damage and clinical symptoms.[26] CMV infection (IgG seropositivity) is common, with prevalence ranging from 35% to 80% in the United States.[27,28] The identification of the virus in the colon (by hematoxylin and eosin staining, immunohistochemistry, or polymerase chain reaction) is the most important factor in establishing the diagnosis of CMV colitis.

MANAGEMENT

The aim in treating a patient with acute severe UC is to induce remission and improve quality of life. This should be accomplished by a team approach with the gastroenterologist, experienced colorectal surgeon, and patient. In most instances this can be accomplished by using medical therapy in order to avoid surgery. For optimal management, patients should be admitted to the hospital for work-up, treatment, and close observation. They should be monitored intensively, at least daily, with close communication between the gastroenterologist and colorectal surgeon.

Patients presenting with toxic megacolon due to UC are typically best managed with early surgery. However, there may be cases in which patients have colonic dilation without overt toxicity, where the gastroenterologist may try a short course of medical therapy. Surgery is absolutely indicated in cases of perforation, uncontrollable bleeding, progressive colonic dilation, and toxic dilation with impending colonic perforation. Thankfully, the majority of cases of acute severe UC do not present with toxic megacolon, and there is a window during which medical therapy may be instituted in an attempt to prevent, or at least delay, surgery.

Although medical therapy is focused on immunosuppressive therapy to induce remission, attention should be paid to a myriad of associated factors during the management of the hospitalized patient with UC:

◊ Fluid balance and electrolytes must be monitored carefully and corrected appropriately. Corticosteroids may induce potassium wasting and sodium retention.

◊ The HCT should be checked at least daily, and the patient should be transfused if it falls below 30%.[29,30]

◊ Patients with acute severe UC are at increased risk for thromboembolic disease, and deep vein thrombosis prophylaxis is very important.[31]

◊ A number of medications can potentially increase the risk of a toxic megacolon and should be avoided.[32,33] These include anticholinergic agents, antidiarrheals, and opiates. Additionally, NSAIDs may exacerbate a flare and should not be used.

◊ Finally, attention should be paid to nutrition. Patients should be weighed on admission and seen by a nutritionist with calorie supplementation and/or supplemental feeding instituted where necessary. There is no evidence to support the use of either bowel rest or total parenteral nutrition in acute UC.[34,35]

MEDICAL THERAPY

Aminosalicylates

There are no data to support the use of 5-aminosalicylates in acute severe UC. Most experts recommend that these drugs should not be started during an acute flare and some will discontinue them because of the small risk of acute intolerance (paradoxical response), which can mimic acute colitis (approximately 3%).[36]

Antibiotics

There is little evidence and no randomized controlled trials to show that IV antibiotics are helpful in acute severe UC.[37,38] Despite the paucity of data, many gastroenterologists use agents such as ciprofloxacin and metronidazole, although we do not routinely recommend this practice. Empiric antibiotics should be considered when there is a strong suspicion for an infectious cause of colitis and are indicated in cases where the illness is complicated by toxic megacolon or bowel perforation.

Corticosteroids

Corticosteroids are the mainstay of treatment for severe UC. Prior to the introduction of corticosteroid therapy, acute severe UC had a mortality rate of approximately 25%. The initial trial of corticosteroids in acute severe UC was performed by Truelove and Witts in 1955.[11] Since this study, corticosteroids have remained first-line therapy for this condition. A recent meta-analysis of all trials from 1974 to 2006 showed that the overall response rate to steroids in this setting was 67%.[39] One of the earlier studies of corticosteroids in the setting of toxic megacolon showed a 90% mortality rate in those given supportive therapy without steroids.[12] Those treated with steroids had a 34% mortality, mostly due to delays in surgery.[12] Corticosteroids decreased the mortality in severe UC from 25% to 7%, and improvements in intensive care unit care and surgical techniques have improved mortality even further. Although this reinforces the need for surgery in toxic megacolon, it also highlights the effectiveness of steroids in severe UC.

In general, for acute severe colitis, a daily IV dose of hydrocortisone 300 mg or methylprednisolone 60 mg is appropriate, and there are no data to support use of higher doses.[39,40] It is important to monitor electrolytes during IV steroid therapy. To date, there is no evidence that continuous infusions confer any advantage over bolus dosing.[39,40]

Despite their effectiveness, approximately 30% of those hospitalized for acute UC do not respond to IV steroid therapy after 5 to 7 days and are thus labeled as *steroid refractory*.[39] Early identification of these patients is critical. A variety of factors and models have been identified with the aim of predicting steroid-refractory disease. In the initial study by Truelove and Witts, those with a first-time presentation responded best to steroids.[4] Response is typically measured through a combination of clinical (number of stools, improved stool consistency, reduced bleeding, and abdominal pain) and biochemical (Hb/HCT, CRP, ESR, albumin) parameters. A number of prospective studies have attempted to identify the key factors associated with the need for colectomy. In a simple-to-use model, Travis et al described an 85% colectomy rate in those with >8 stools/day, or with 3 to 8 stools/day and a CRP >45 mg/L by day 3 of IV steroid therapy.[20] This is known as the Oxford index. Other authors have identified albumin levels, colonic dilation, and the need for blood transfusion as predictors of colectomy.[41,42] Recognition of these parameters is important, as there are data to suggest adverse outcomes for those who undergo surgery after a period of prolonged medical therapy.[43] Patients who clearly respond or fail to respond within the first 3 days are often easier to manage, as the course of action is clear. Those with a partial response present the greatest challenge. The options in this situation are to continue steroids for a further 3 to 4 days or to proceed to early use of rescue medical therapy.

SECOND-LINE OR RESCUE MEDICAL THERAPY

As mentioned previously, one-third of patients with acute severe UC will not respond to IV corticosteroids. The current medical options for these patients are cyclosporine or infliximab. We will review the data supporting the use of cyclosporine and infliximab and compare the effectiveness of these medical therapies to the long-term outcomes for surgery.

Cyclosporine

Cyclosporine is a calcineurin inhibitor that has been used extensively in solid organ transplantation since the early 1980s. In 1994, Lichtiger et al performed a randomized, placebo-controlled trial of IV cyclosporine (4 mg/kg) in patients with acute severe UC not responding to corticosteroid treatment.[44] The results were dramatic, with 9 of 11 patients in the active treatment arm responding, compared to none of those who received placebo. The study was prematurely terminated because of these results, and the 5 placebo patients who crossed over to active drug also responded.[44] There are data supporting the use of IV cyclosporine as an alternative to IV corticosteroids, with comparable efficacy.[45] Furthermore, there have been a number of uncontrolled studies of cyclosporine for acute severe UC with an overall short-term response rate of 64% to 86%.[46,47] Cyclosporine is typically given as a continuous infusion with levels drawn on days 2 to 3, aiming for between 250 and 350 ng/mL. There are some data supporting similar efficacy and reduced neurotoxicity with oral microemulsion cyclosporine.[48] Although there are some retrospective data showing a shorter time to relapse and surgery in the IV compared to the oral cyclosporine group, this has not been replicated in a prospective study, and the IV route is preferred.

Despite its efficacy, cyclosporine has not become widely utilized. The major issue limiting the use of cyclosporine by many physicians is likely its perceived safety profile. Data from Mount Sinai in New York suggest a mortality rate of 1.8% associated with its use in UC (Table 4-2).[49] Common adverse events include tremor, hypertension, renal dysfunction, and seizures.[49] The risk of serious infection was 5% in the Mount Sinai data, but these patients had also been on high-dose corticosteroids prior to initiation of cyclosporine, which may have played a role.

A potential strategy for reducing adverse events associated with cyclosporine is to use a lower dose. The dose of 4 mg/kg, used by Lichtiger et al in the initial trial, was compared to 2 mg/kg in a Dutch study and did not show any difference in the day 8 response rates.[50] In this small study, there were no significant differences in side effects, apart from a trend toward hypertension with the higher dose. Although no clear benefit was proven and further investigation is warranted, the hope is that the use of lower doses and plasma levels may help minimize side effects.

There are other strategies that may help to improve the safety of cyclosporine. Hypocholesterolemia and hypomagnesemia have been associated with a lower

Table 4-2. Summary of the Major and Minor Adverse Events Associated With Cyclosporine Therapy in Ulcerative Colitis
MAJOR ADVERSE EVENTS
• Seizure
• Opportunistic infection
• Nephrotoxicity
• Hyperkalemia
• Anaphylaxis
MINOR ADVERSE EVENTS
• Nausea/vomiting
• Headache
• Tremor/paresthesia
• Gingival hypertrophy
• Elevated liver blood tests
• Hypertension
• Hypertrichosis

seizure threshold and should be monitored closely and repleted both before and during treatment. Total cholesterol levels less than 120 mg/dL have been associated with an increased risk of seizures,[51] thought to be due to increased binding of cyclosporine to low-density lipoprotein, facilitating astrocyte delivery via low-density lipoprotein receptors.[52] Many institute prophylaxis against *Pneumocystis* pneumonia in these patients due to the use of multiple immunosuppressants.

Choosing the appropriate candidate for cyclosporine therapy is important. Cyclosporine should be avoided in those patients with active infection, uncontrolled hypertension, or underlying renal dysfunction and should be used with caution in older patients with multiple comorbidities.

Apart from toxicity, the other concern with the use of cyclosporine is whether it remains efficacious over the long term. Several groups have examined long-term outcomes with cyclosporine. Studies have demonstrated disappointing colectomy rates at 7 years of between 58% and 88%, lending support to the idea that few patients will avoid surgery in the long run.[53] Others have demonstrated colectomy rates of 20% at 1 year and 30% at 5.5 years among cyclosporine responders.[54] Several studies confirm better outcomes for those patients who transitioned to an immunomodulator (azathioprine/mercaptopurine).[53] In one study, 80% of cyclosporine responders who were transitioned to mercaptopurine avoided colectomy at 5.5 years.[54] Further data from New York demonstrated very similar results.[55] Thus, oral cyclosporine should not be intended as a long-term therapy, rather as a bridge to therapy with one of the thiopurine drugs. The exception is for those patients who have already been taking a thiopurine at an appropriate dose (preferably confirmed by measurement of metabolite levels) and for an appropriate length of time prior to admission. These patients should be considered to have failed thiopurine therapy, and cyclosporine is not a valid long-term option in these cases because there is no maintenance treatment to which cyclosporine will serve as a bridge. Data from Belgium confirmed this, with 77% of those taking azathioprine on admission undergoing colectomy compared to 35% of those who started it after demonstrating an initial response to cyclosporine.[53]

Those patients who have a clinical response to cyclosporine can be switched to oral cyclosporine while steroids are tapered down. The aim is to discontinue prednisone by 6 to 12 weeks and the cyclosporine at approximately 3 to 6 months. The thiopurine should be started at a weight-appropriate dose, although the exact timing of instituting this therapy is unclear. It is important to remember that the risk of infection is significantly increased (odds ratio 14.5[56]) in those on 3 or more immunosuppressant drugs. In such situations, cotrimoxazole is recommended as *Pneumocystis* pneumonia prophylaxis while the patient is on corticosteroids, cyclosporine, and a thiopurine simultaneously.

The use of cyclosporine in the management of acute severe UC is generally safe and effective when administered by experienced gastroenterologists. Cyclosporine should be seen as an excellent rescue treatment, inducing remission in up to 80% with severe disease. Proponents of cyclosporine argue that the long-term data reflect the efficacy of maintenance therapy with thiopurines, rather than the cyclosporine, and that cyclosporine should only be used as a bridge to further immunomodulation with a thiopurine.

Anti-Tumor Necrosis Factor Antibodies

Monoclonal antibodies against tumor necrosis factor (TNF) are increasingly being used in the setting of acute severe UC. Infliximab was initially licensed for use in Crohn's disease but, following the publication of the Active UC Trials 1 and 2, it was approved for use in moderate to severe UC.[57] Importantly, these studies included nonhospitalized patients, with only 217 of 700 described as steroid refractory, who are not representative of the patients under discussion here. Despite these limitations, and a paucity of data, infliximab is increasingly used as a rescue therapy for patients with IV steroid-refractory acute severe UC. A number of small randomized trials have studied infliximab in hospitalized patients. An initial trial recruited patients with severe UC, refractory to 5 days of IV steroids, and demonstrated a 50% (4 of 8) response to infliximab compared to no (0 of 3) response to placebo.[58] A subsequent study of 43 patients with steroid-refractory disease showed no benefit of 2 infusions of infliximab 14 days apart compared to placebo.[59] This study excluded subjects with the most severe disease (those who were likely to require urgent colectomy). A Scandinavian multicenter trial of 45 subjects, also excluding those at risk of colectomy, showed a reduction in the 3-month colectomy rate in those who received a single dose of infliximab (29% [7 of 24] versus 67% [14 of 21] for placebo).[60]

The long-term follow-up data for infliximab in acute severe UC are limited. Studies are difficult to interpret because they have been inconsistent with their use of either immunomodulators or maintenance anti-TNF therapy following an initial response. Follow-up from the Jarnerot study showed a 2-year colectomy rate of 46% for infliximab versus 76% for placebo.[60] Thirteen of 24 in the infliximab group were transitioned to azathioprine, and only one patient continued maintenance infliximab. Other studies have suggested 1- to 2-year colectomy rates between 30% and 53%.[61,62] Using a 3-dose induction regimen followed by 8 weekly infusions may well yield more favorable long-term outcomes, but further studies are needed.

Similar to cyclosporine, infliximab is associated with a number of serious side effects. Serious and opportunistic infections, particularly tuberculosis, are a concern, as are more rare side effects such as lymphoma and demyelination. Infusion reactions may be an issue, particularly if 1 or 2 doses are being used, rather than scheduled maintenance treatment. Additionally, there has been some debate regarding postoperative complications in patients who have received infliximab. Studies from the United Kingdom and Italy, in addition to the Jarnerot study from Scandinavia, have all shown no increase in postoperative complications over placebo.[60-62] However, there are data to suggest an increase in complications following ileal pouch-anal anastomosis (IPAA) in those who had previous infliximab.[63] These data are complicated by the fact that the patients have also been on high-dose corticosteroids in addition to infliximab, and it is difficult to separate the effects of these treatments on postsurgical complications. Data from the Crohn's Therapy Resource Evaluation and Assessment Tool registry have previously shown that corticosteroids are the main drug of concern with regard to the risk of serious infection or death.[64]

Cyclosporine Versus Infliximab

The decision between using infliximab and cyclosporine in the setting of severe, steroid-refractory UC is a difficult one for the clinician and will remain so until results are available from an ongoing head-to-head trial. Unfortunately, for the moment, the decision is based largely on physician preference and comfort level. If one compares these medical options, the data would appear to indicate that cyclosporine is the more efficacious agent (particularly in those patients with more severe disease) with response rates in the region of 80%. However, cyclosporine use is typically limited to experienced tertiary referral centers. For those patients without a contraindication, and who have not failed treatment with azathioprine/mercaptopurine, cyclosporine should be considered the drug of choice. Infliximab is the preferred option in patients who have failed or are intolerant to thiopurine therapy. It may also be considered in those with less severe disease or indeterminate colitis. Conversely, there may be patients in whom there are specific concerns regarding infliximab, such as previous exposure to tuberculosis or impaired left ventricular function. Although there are no data to suggest cyclosporine is safer in this setting, its shorter half-life is attractive.

Sequential therapy using either cyclosporine or infliximab to "rescue" those who have failed one agent is not currently recommended. Data from Mount Sinai showed low rates (33% to 40%) of remission, and a 16% risk of serious infection, with one death due to sepsis.[65] In a French study, 65 of 86 patients used cyclosporine first, and 62% of those who received both agents avoided short-term colectomy. However, remission rates were below 30%, and the 3-year colectomy rate was 63%.[66] Fourteen patients developed serious infections and one died (postcolectomy pulmonary embolus). A Spanish group reported outcomes for 16 patients treated initially with cyclosporine and then infliximab. The short-term colectomy rate was 30%, and the medication was well tolerated.[67] Based on these data, one must balance the colectomy rate versus the risk of significant toxicity associated with consecutive therapy.

NEW AND ALTERNATIVE MEDICAL THERAPIES

Given the limitations of the current medical therapies for steroid-refractory severe UC, it is not surprising that new drug discovery is an active area of research. Tacrolimus, like cyclosporine, is a calcineurin inhibitor used extensively in the post-transplant setting. There has been one randomized controlled trial that included some subjects with acute severe UC. Nine of 16 patients had a partial response, compared to 2 of 11 on placebo, but the results did not reach significance (possibly due to type 2 error).[68] There have been case series showing results similar to cyclosporine, but a randomized controlled trial with sufficient numbers of the right type of subject is needed to elucidate its role. Basiliximab (Simulect) is a monoclonal antibody to the IL-2 receptor of T cells that has been used in the treatment of post-transplant organ rejection. A pilot study using a single infusion of this agent in acute severe UC resulted in 90% (9/10) remission at 8 weeks, but the result was not sustained, and a follow-up study reported 4 out of 7 requiring colectomy by 24 weeks.[69,70] Visilizumab (Nuvion) is a humanized IgG$_2$ monoclonal antibody to the CD3 receptor on activated T cells. An initial, open-label study resulted in remission in 41% of 32 subjects with severe steroid-refractory UC.[71] Forty-five percent did not require either salvage therapy or colectomy by 1 year. Unfortunately, phase III trials were stopped due to safety concerns and lack of efficacy. Vedolizumab (MLN002) is a humanized antibody to the $\alpha4\beta7$ integrin that has demonstrated efficacy in the induction and maintenance of remission of UC but has not yet been studied in hospitalized, steroid-refractory UC.[72]

SURGICAL MANAGEMENT

As opposed to medical therapy, surgical resection provides a definitive method of treating UC. Despite the risk of significant perioperative complications, and long-term outcomes that are not what most patients would consider "normal," surgery decreases mortality, improves quality of life, and is often delayed for too long. Surgery is clearly indicated in patients with progressive colonic dilation, toxic dilation, severe hemorrhage, or colonic perforation. However, the majority of colectomies performed in acute severe colitis are in those patients with disease refractory to medical therapy. Surgery remains an excellent treatment for UC, as it effectively cures the condition and removes the colorectal cancer risk. However, the timing of surgery is critical. There are data to demonstrate that both short- and long-term postoperative mortality are increased in the setting of acute severe UC. Kaplan et al showed increased mortality in those undergoing emergency rather than elective colectomy.[13] These data showed that those operated on within 5 days of admission for a UC flare had better outcomes than those who waited 6 or more days (odds ratio of 2 for in-hospital mortality). Both advanced age and low hospital volumes also had a negative impact on postoperative mortality in this study.

Prior to the introduction of IPAA surgery, the operation of choice was a total proctocolectomy with a permanent ileostomy. A majority of patients with severe steroid-refractory UC now undergo an abdominal colectomy with end-ileostomy and oversew of the rectum (Hartmann), with a plan to create an ileal pouch at a later date. The advantage of this procedure in the acutely ill patient is that it avoids intestinal anastomosis and pelvic dissection and, more recently, can be performed using laparoscopic techniques. Laparoscopic surgery in this setting offers the advantages of reduced length of stay and faster recovery compared to open procedures.[73] The IPAA can be performed when the patient has recovered from his or her acute flare and, importantly, is no longer on corticosteroids. This also means that the pouch operation can be performed by a surgeon with the relevant expertise, rather than by whoever is "on call" at the time of the colectomy. In some patients with less severe disease, the initial surgery is a total proctocolectomy and IPAA formation, with a protective diverting ileostomy.

Although surgery is considered a cure for colitis, and improves quality of life, it is associated with a number of limitations and morbidities. Additionally, patients with IPAAs do not have what many would consider normal bowel function. Patients may pass up to 6 to 9 bowel movements over 24 hours. Mean daytime frequency is 5.7 movements at the first year.[74] Pouch surgery is associated with a significant reduction in female fertility.[75] Pouchitis, an inflammatory condition affecting the pouch, occurs in 50% of patients in the 10 years after surgery,[76] with chronic pouchitis developing in 15%.[77] Additionally, a number of patients with a preoperative diagnosis of UC develop Crohn's disease of the pouch. There are also functional disorders of the pouch (irritable pouch syndrome) as well as the rare potential for dysplasia and possibly cancer in the remaining rectal mucosa.[78] Despite these limitations, pouch surgery is a major advance for patients with UC, and offers substantially improved health-related quality of life and excellent functional outcomes (see Chapter 19).[74]

The choice between rescue medical therapy and surgery can be a difficult one and should involve open discussion between the patient, gastroenterologist, and colorectal surgeon. Patients should be given information on surgery

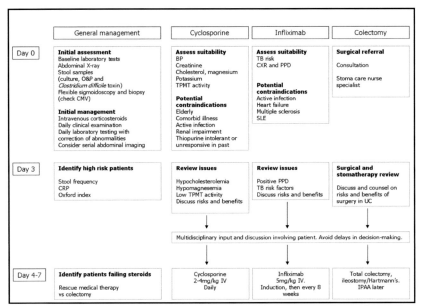

General management	Cyclosporine	Infliximab	Colectomy

Day 0

Initial assessment
Baseline laboratory tests
Abdominal X-ray
Stool samples
(culture, O&P and
Clostridium difficile toxin)
Flexible sigmoidoscopy and biopsy
(check CMV)

Initial management
Intravenous corticosteroids
Daily clinical examination
Daily laboratory testing with
correction of abnormalities
Consider serial abdominal imaging

Assess suitability
BP
Creatinine
Cholesterol, magnesium
Potassium
TPMT activity

**Potential
contraindications**
Elderly
Comorbid illness
Active infection
Renal impairment
Thiopurine intolerant or
unresponsive in past

Assess suitability
TB risk
CXR and PPD

**Potential
contraindications**
Active infection
Heart failure
Multiple sclerosis
SLE

Surgical referral
Consultation
Stoma care nurse
specialist

Day 3

Identify high risk patients
Stool frequency
CRP
Oxford index

Review issues
Hypocholesterolemia
Hypomagnesemia
Low TPMT activity
Discuss risks and benefits

Review issues
Positive PPD
TB risk factors
Discuss risks and benefits

**Surgical and
stomatherapy review**
Discuss and counsel on
risks and benefits of
surgery in UC

Multidisciplinary input and discussion involving patient. Avoid delays in decision-making.

Day 4-7

Identify patients failing steroids
Rescue medical therapy
vs colectomy

Cyclosporine
2-4mg/kg IV
Daily

Infliximab
5mg/kg IV.
Induction, then every 8
weeks

Total colectomy,
ileostomy/Hartmann's.
IPAA later

Figure 4-3. Treatment protocol for acute severe UC based on day of admission to hospital. BP = blood pressure; CMV = cytomegalovirus; CRP = C-reactive protein; CXR = chest x-ray; IPAA = ileal pouch-anal anastomosis; IV = intravenous; O&P = ova and parasites; PPD = purified protein derivative; SLE = systemic lupus erythematosus; TB = tuberculosis; TPMT = thiopurine methyltransferase; UC = ulcerative colitis.

early in their admission rather than at the last minute. Patients should understand the pros and cons of each potential therapy. Many patients will initially opt for medical therapy, but need to understand the success rates, risks, and long-term expectations. Although surgery may seem like a big step for patients, particularly those who are newly diagnosed, it offers a chance to cure the disease, avoid long-term immunomodulators, and eliminate the colorectal cancer risk. Regardless of the decision made, it is crucial that the options are discussed early, so when early escalation of therapy is indicated, it can be done with minimal delay. An algorithm for the treatment of acute severe UC, including general management principles, as well as medical therapy and surgical planning, is presented in Figure 4-3.

CONCLUSION

Acute severe UC will affect 15% of patients with UC during the lifetime of their disease. This condition is a medical emergency requiring close monitoring. It is important to confirm the diagnosis and rule out infections that may mimic or exacerbate acute UC, particularly *C difficile* and CMV.

The management of acute severe UC is complex and requires input and experience from both the gastroenterologist and colorectal surgeon. Timing is the critical issue, and early planning will yield benefits. Patients should know about all available treatment options and should particularly discuss surgery. IV corticosteroids are a mainstay of therapy for severe UC, but 30% of patients will not respond and will require either second-line medical therapy or surgery. Options for rescue medical therapy include cyclosporine and infliximab. At the current time, published data support the use of cyclosporine in this setting. However, it should only be used by those with experience and is best avoided in those who have failed thiopurine therapy. Infliximab may not be as effective in patients with fulminant disease, but may be suitable for those with a flare of moderate severity or in those who have failed thiopurines. The results of a direct head-to-head comparison between cyclosporine and infliximab in acute severe UC will be interesting, but the long-term data may be the most important factor influencing practice.

Colectomy is the definitive treatment for acute severe UC, but patients need to be aware of the long-term risks and benefits of IPAA. It is important to involve the surgical team at the time of admission so that all therapeutic options can be discussed in a balanced manner, allowing patients to make informed decisions regarding their care.

☑ Key Points

☑ Acute severe UC is a medical emergency requiring hospitalization and joint management by an experienced gastroenterologist and colorectal surgeon.

☑ Patients must be monitored carefully for signs of toxicity, bearing in mind that steroid treatment may mask signs of infection and toxicity.

☑ Potential causative or contributory factors such as C difficile or CMV infection should be ruled out at the time of admission.

☑ IV corticosteroids remain the most effective medical treatment, but 30% will not respond and will require rescue medical therapy or surgery.

☑ Timing is the key to successful management of these patients: recognize treatment failure early and move to the next step in the therapeutic algorithm.

☑ For those who fail therapy with corticosteroids, consideration should be given to rescue therapy with cyclosporine, infliximab, or surgery.

REFERENCES

1. Edwards FC, Truelove SC. The course and prognosis of ulcerative colitis. *Gut*. 1963;4:299-315.
2. Farmer RG, Easley KA, Rankin GB. Clinical patterns, natural history, and progression of ulcerative colitis. A long-term follow-up of 1116 patients. *Dig Dis Sci*. 1993;38:1137-1146.
3. Solberg IC, Lygren I, Jahnsen J, et al. Clinical course during the first 10 years of ulcerative colitis: results from a population-based inception cohort (IBSEN Study). *Scand J Gastroenterol*. 2009;44:431-440.
4. Truelove SC, Witts LJ. Cortisone in ulcerative colitis: preliminary report on a therapeutic trial. *Br Med J*. 1954;2:375-378.
5. Kornbluth A, Sachar DB. Ulcerative colitis practice guidelines in adults: American College of Gastroenterology, Practice Parameters Committee. *Am J Gastroenterol*. 2010;105:501-523.
6. Sheth SG, LaMont JT. Toxic megacolon. *Lancet*. 1998;351:509-513.
7. Marshak RH, Lester LJ. Megacolon a complication of ulcerative colitis. *Gastroenterology*. 1950;16:768-772.
8. Greenstein AJ, Sachar DB, Gibas A, et al. Outcome of toxic dilatation in ulcerative and Crohn's colitis. *J Clin Gastroenterol*. 1985;7:137-143.
9. Caprilli R, Latella G, Vernia P, Frieri G. Multiple organ dysfunction in ulcerative colitis. *Am J Gastroenterol*. 2000;95:1258-1262.
10. Latella G, Vernia P, Viscido A, et al. GI distension in severe ulcerative colitis. *Am J Gastroenterol*. 2002;97:1169-1175.
11. Truelove SC, Witts LJ. Cortisone in ulcerative colitis: final report on a therapeutic trial. *Br Med J*. 1955;2:1041-1048.
12. Jalan KN, Sircus W, Card WI, et al. An experience of ulcerative colitis. I. Toxic dilation in 55 cases. *Gastroenterology*. 1969;57:68-82.
13. Kaplan GG, McCarthy EP, Ayanian JZ, Korzenik J, Hodin R, Sands BE. Impact of hospital volume on postoperative morbidity and mortality following a colectomy for ulcerative colitis. *Gastroenterology*. 2008;134:680-687.
14. Gan SI, Beck PL. A new look at toxic megacolon: an update and review of incidence, etiology, pathogenesis, and management. *Am J Gastroenterol*. 2003;98:2363-2371.
15. Snape WJ Jr, Williams R, Hyman PE. Defect in colonic smooth muscle contraction in patients with ulcerative colitis. *Am J Physiol*. 1991;261:G987-G991.
16. Snape WJ Jr, Matarazzo SA, Cohen S. Abnormal gastrocolonic response in patients with ulcerative colitis. *Gut*. 1980;21:392-396.
17. Tomita R, Tanjoh K. Role of nitric oxide in the colon of patients with ulcerative colitis. *World J Surg*. 1998;22:88-91.
18. Snape WJ Jr, Kao HW. Role of inflammatory mediators in colonic smooth muscle function in ulcerative colitis. *Dig Dis Sci*. 1988;33:65S-70S.
19. Buckell NA, Williams GT, Bartram CI, Lennard-Jones JE. Depth of ulceration in acute colitis: correlation with outcome and clinical and radiologic features. *Gastroenterology*. 1980;79:19-25.
20. Travis SP, Farrant JM, Ricketts C, et al. Predicting outcome in severe ulcerative colitis. *Gut*. 1996;38:905-910.
21. Nguyen GC, Kaplan GG, Harris ML, Brant SR. A national survey of the prevalence and impact of *Clostridium difficile* infection among hospitalized inflammatory bowel disease patients. *Am J Gastroenterol*. 2008;103:1443-1450.
22. Jodorkovsky D, Young Y, Abreu MT. Clinical outcomes of patients with ulcerative colitis and co-existing *Clostridium difficile* infection. *Dig Dis Sci*. 2010;55:415-420.
23. Marshak RH. Letter: more on colonoscopy in inflammatory bowel disease. *Gastroenterology*. 1976;70:147.
24. Norland CC, Kirsner JB. Toxic dilatation of colon (toxic megacolon): etiology, treatment and prognosis in 42 patients. *Medicine (Baltimore)*. 1969;48:229-250.
25. Maher MM, Nassar MI. Acute cytomegalovirus infection is a risk factor in refractory and complicated inflammatory bowel disease. *Dig Dis Sci*. 2009;54:2456-2462.

26. Ayre K Warren B, Jeffrey K, Travis S. The role of CMV in steroid-resistant ulcerative colitis: a systematic review. *J Crohns Colitis*. 2009;3:141-148.

27. Staras SA, Dollard SC, Radford KW, Flanders WD, Pass RF, Cannon MJ. Seroprevalence of cytomegalovirus infection in the United States, 1988-1994. *Clin Infect Dis*. 2006;43:1143-1151.

28. Zhang LJ, Hanff P, Rutherford C, Churchill WH, Crumpacker CS. Detection of human cytomegalovirus DNA, RNA, and antibody in normal donor blood. *J Infect Dis*. 1995;171:1002-1006.

29. Garcia-Erce JA, Gomollon F, Munoz M. Blood transfusion for the treatment of acute anaemia in inflammatory bowel disease and other digestive diseases. *World J Gastroenterol*. 2009;15:4686-4694.

30. Gasche C, Berstad A, Befrits R, et al. Guidelines on the diagnosis and management of iron deficiency and anemia in inflammatory bowel diseases. *Inflamm Bowel Dis*. 2007;13:1545-1553.

31. Nguyen GC, Sam J. Rising prevalence of venous thromboembolism and its impact on mortality among hospitalized inflammatory bowel disease patients. *Am J Gastroenterol*. 2008;103:2272-2280.

32. Kornbluth A, Sachar DB. Ulcerative colitis practice guidelines in adults (update): American College of Gastroenterology, Practice Parameters Committee. *Am J Gastroenterol*. 2004;99:1371-1385.

33. Carter MJ, Lobo AJ, Travis SP. Guidelines for the management of inflammatory bowel disease in adults. *Gut*. 2004;53(suppl 5):V1-V16.

34. McIntyre PB, Powell-Tuck J, Wood SR, et al. Controlled trial of bowel rest in the treatment of severe acute colitis. *Gut*. 1986;27:481-485.

35. Dickinson RJ, Ashton MG, Axon AT, Smith RC, Yeung CK, Hill GL. Controlled trial of intravenous hyperalimentation and total bowel rest as an adjunct to the routine therapy of acute colitis. *Gastroenterology*. 1980;79:1199-1204.

36. Loftus EV Jr, Kane SV, Bjorkman D. Systematic review: short-term adverse effects of 5-aminosalicylic acid agents in the treatment of ulcerative colitis. *Aliment Pharmacol Ther*. 2004;19:179-189.

37. Mantzaris GJ, Petraki K, Archavlis E, et al. A prospective randomized controlled trial of intravenous ciprofloxacin as an adjunct to corticosteroids in acute, severe ulcerative colitis. *Scand J Gastroenterol*. 2001;36:971-974.

38. Chapman RW, Selby WS, Jewell DP. Controlled trial of intravenous metronidazole as an adjunct to corticosteroids in severe ulcerative colitis. *Gut*. 1986;27:1210-1212.

39. Turner D, Walsh CM, Steinhart AH, Griffiths AM. Response to corticosteroids in severe ulcerative colitis: a systematic review of the literature and a meta-regression. *Clin Gastroenterol Hepatol*. 2007;5:103-110.

40. Rosenberg W, Ireland A, Jewell DP. High-dose methylprednisolone in the treatment of active ulcerative colitis. *J Clin Gastroenterol*. 1990;12:40-41.

41. Ho GT, Mowat C, Goddard CJ, et al. Predicting the outcome of severe ulcerative colitis: development of a novel risk score to aid early selection of patients for second-line medical therapy or surgery. *Aliment Pharmacol Ther*. 2004;19:1079-1087.

42. Ananthakrishnan AN, McGinley EL, Binion DG, Saeian K. Simple score to identify colectomy risk in ulcerative colitis hospitalizations. *Inflamm Bowel Dis*. 2010;16:1532-1540.

43. Randall J, Singh B, Warren BF, Travis SP, Mortensen NJ, George BD. Delayed surgery for acute severe colitis is associated with increased risk of postoperative complications. *Br J Surg*. 2010;97:404-409.

44. Lichtiger S, Present DH, Kornbluth A, et al. Cyclosporine in severe ulcerative colitis refractory to steroid therapy. *Engl J Med*. 1994;330:1841-1845.

45. D'Haens G, Lemmens L, Geboes K, et al. Intravenous cyclosporine versus intravenous corticosteroids as single therapy for severe attacks of ulcerative colitis. *Gastroenterology*. 2001;120:1323-1329.

46. Shibolet O, Regushevskaya E, Brezis M, Soares-Weiser K. Cyclosporine A for induction of remission in severe ulcerative colitis. *Cochrane Database Syst Rev*. 2005:CD004277.

47. Durai D, Hawthorne AB. Review article: how and when to use ciclosporin in ulcerative colitis. *Aliment Pharmacol Ther.* 2005;22:907-916.

48. Campbell S, Travis S, Jewell D. Ciclosporin use in acute ulcerative colitis: a long-term experience. *Eur J Gastroenterol Hepatol.* 2005;17:79-84.

49. Sternthal MB, Murphy SJ, George J, Kornbluth A, Lichtiger S, Present DH. Adverse events associated with the use of cyclosporine in patients with inflammatory bowel disease. *Am J Gastroenterol.* 2008;103:937-943.

50. Van Assche G, D'Haens G, Noman M, et al. Randomized, double-blind comparison of 4mg/kg versus 2mg/kg intravenous cyclosporine in severe ulcerative colitis. *Gastroenterology.* 2003;125:1025-1031.

51. de Groen PC, Aksamit AJ, Rakela J, Forbes GS, Krom RA. Central nervous system toxicity after liver transplantation. The role of cyclosporine and cholesterol. *N Engl J Med.* 1987;317:861-866.

52. de Groen PC. Cyclosporine, low-density lipoprotein, and cholesterol. *Mayo Clin Proc.* 1988;63:1012-1021.

53. Moskovitz DN, Van Assche G, Maenhout B, et al. Incidence of colectomy during long-term follow-up after cyclosporine-induced remission of severe ulcerative colitis. *Clin Gastroenterol Hepatol.* 2006;4:760-765.

54. Cohen RD, Stein R, Hanauer SB. Intravenous cyclosporin in ulcerative colitis: a five-year experience. *Am J Gastroenterol.* 1999;94:1587-1592.

55. Cheifetz AS, Stern J, Garud S, et al. Cyclosporine is safe and effective in patients with severe ulcerative colitis. *J Clin Gastroenterol.* 2011;45:107-112.

56. Toruner M, Loftus EV Jr, Harmsen WS, et al. Risk factors for opportunistic infections in patients with inflammatory bowel disease. *Gastroenterology.* 2008;134:929-936.

57. Rutgeerts P, Sandborn WJ, Feagan BG, et al. Infliximab for induction and maintenance therapy for ulcerative colitis. *N Engl J Med.* 2005;353:2462-2476.

58. Sands BE, Tremaine WJ, Sandborn WJ, et al. Infliximab in the treatment of severe, steroid-refractory ulcerative colitis: a pilot study. *Inflamm Bowel Dis.* 2001;7:83-88.

59. Probert CS, Hearing SD, Schreiber S, et al. Infliximab in moderately severe glucocorticoid resistant ulcerative colitis: a randomised controlled trial. *Gut.* 2003;52:998-1002.

60. Jarnerot G, Hertervig E, Friis-Liby I, et al. Infliximab as rescue therapy in severe to moderately severe ulcerative colitis: a randomized, placebo-controlled study. *Gastroenterology.* 2005;128:1805-1811.

61. Kohn A, Daperno M, Armuzzi A, et al. Infliximab in severe ulcerative colitis: short-term results of different infusion regimens and long-term follow-up. *Aliment Pharmacol Ther.* 2007;26:747-756.

62. Jakobovits SL, Jewell DP, Travis SP. Infliximab for the treatment of ulcerative colitis: outcomes in Oxford from 2000 to 2006. *Aliment Pharmacol Ther.* 2007;25:1055-1060.

63. Selvasekar CR, Cima RR, Larson DW, et al. Effect of infliximab on short-term complications in patients undergoing operation for chronic ulcerative colitis. *J Am Coll Surg.* 2007;204:956-962.

64. Lichtenstein GR, Feagan BG, Cohen RD, et al. Serious infections and mortality in association with therapies for Crohn's disease: TREAT registry. *Clin Gastroenterol Hepatol.* 2006;4:621-630.

65. Maser EA, Deconda D, Lichtiger S, Ullman T, Present DH, Kornbluth A. Cyclosporine and infliximab as rescue therapy for each other in patients with steroid-refractory ulcerative colitis. *Clin Gastroenterol Hepatol.* 2008;6:1112-1116.

66. Leblanc SAM, Seksik P, Flourie B, et al. Successive treatment with cyclosporine and infliximab in severe ulcerative colitis (UC). *Gastroenterology.* 2009;136:A-88.

67. Manosa M, Lopez San Roman A, Garcia-Planella E, et al. Infliximab rescue therapy after cyclosporin failure in steroid-refractory ulcerative colitis. *Digestion.* 2009;80:30-35.

68. Ogata H, Matsui T, Nakamura M, et al. A randomised dose finding study of oral tacrolimus (FK506) therapy in refractory ulcerative colitis. *Gut.* 2006;55:1255-1262.

69. Creed TJ, Norman MR, Probert CS, et al. Basiliximab (anti-CD25) in combination with steroids may be an effective new treatment for steroid-resistant ulcerative colitis. *Aliment Pharmacol Ther.* 2003;18:65-75.

70. Creed TJ, Probert CS, Norman MN, et al. Basiliximab for the treatment of steroid-resistant ulcerative colitis: further experience in moderate and severe disease. *Aliment Pharmacol Ther*. 2006;23:1435-1442.

71. Plevy S, Salzberg B, Van Assche G, et al. A phase I study of visilizumab, a humanized anti-CD3 monoclonal antibody, in severe steroid-refractory ulcerative colitis. *Gastroenterology*. 2007;133:1414-1422.

72. Feagan BG, Greenberg GR, Wild G, et al. Treatment of ulcerative colitis with a humanized antibody to the alpha4beta7 integrin. *N Engl J Med*. 2005;352:2499-2507.

73. Marceau C, Alves A, Ouaissi M, Bouhnik Y, Valleur P, Panis Y. Laparoscopic subtotal colectomy for acute or severe colitis complicating inflammatory bowel disease: a case-matched study in 88 patients. *Surgery*. 2007;141:640-644.

74. Hahnloser D, Pemberton JH, Wolff BG, Larson DR, Crownhart BS, Dozois RR. Results at up to 20 years after ileal pouch-anal anastomosis for chronic ulcerative colitis. *Br J Surg*. 2007;94:333-340.

75. Waljee A, Waljee J, Morris AM, Higgins PD. Threefold increased risk of infertility: a meta-analysis of infertility after ileal pouch anal anastomosis in ulcerative colitis. *Gut*. 2006;55:1575-1580.

76. Meagher AP, Farouk R, Dozois RR, Kelly KA, Pemberton JH. J ileal pouch-anal anastomosis for chronic ulcerative colitis: complications and long-term outcome in 1310 patients. *Br J Surg*. 1998;85:800-803.

77. Shen B, Remzi FH, Lavery IC, Lashner BA, Fazio VW. A proposed classification of ileal pouch disorders and associated complications after restorative proctocolectomy. *Clin Gastroenterol Hepatol*. 2008;6:145-158.

78. Kariv R, Remzi FH, Lian L, et al. Preoperative colorectal neoplasia increases risk for pouch neoplasia in patients with restorative proctocolectomy. *Gastroenterology*. 2010;139:806-812.

SUGGESTED READINGS

Hart AL, Ng SC. Review article: the optimal medical management of acute severe ulcerative colitis. *Aliment Pharm Ther*. 2010;32:615-627.

Lichtiger S, Halfvarson J, Jarnerot G, Becker J, Stucchi AF, Cohen D. Current controversies: treatment of choice for acute severe steroid-refractory ulcerative colitis. *Inflamm Bowel Dis*. 2009;15(1):141-151.

Dysplasia and Colorectal Cancer

Fernando Velayos, MD, MPH

Colorectal cancer (CRC) is a feared complication of inflammatory bowel disease (IBD). This chapter reviews the most important risk factors for its development, as well as potential strategies for reducing these risks.

EPIDEMIOLOGY

The cumulative probability of developing CRC is significantly higher among persons with IBD than in the general population.[1,2] IBD is the third highest risk condition for CRC after 2 genetic syndromes: familial adenomatous polyposis syndrome and hereditary nonpolyposis CRC.[3] Data from a comprehensive meta-analysis suggest that the probability of CRC in IBD is 2% after 10 years of disease, 8% after 20 years, and 18% after 30 years.[4,5] In comparison, the cumulative lifetime probability of developing CRC for the general population in the United States is approximately 5%.[4,5]

Described in terms of relative risk, IBD increases the risk of CRC 5- to 6-fold relative to the general population. The risk is similar in ulcerative colitis (UC) and Crohn's disease (CD) affecting the colon.[5] Notably, CD isolated exclusively to small bowel alone does not confer an increased risk.[5] These data emphasize the important link between chronic inflammation of the colon and colon cancer. They also support historical observations that the risk of developing CRC increases as a greater proportion of the colon is involved by inflammation.[1]

Interestingly, not all populations of IBD patients have an increased risk of CRC. In a Danish population-based cohort, the risk was 0.4% after 10 years, 1.1% after 20 years, and 2.1% after 30 years of disease.[6] These probabilities are comparable to those of an American population-based cohort where the cumulative probability of developing CRC was 0% at 5 years, 0.4% at 15 years, and 2.0% at 25 years after a chronic UC diagnosis.[7] Also notable is that high-risk

Regueiro MD, Swoger JM, eds.
Clinical Challenges and Complications of IBD (pp 81-100).
© 2013 Taylor & Francis Group.

Table 5-1. Risk Factors for Colorectal Cancer in Inflammatory Bowel Disease

Duration of disease
Extent of colonic inflammation
Primary sclerosing cholangitis
Family history of colorectal cancer
Smoking
Inflammatory pseudopolyps
Backwash ileitis
Young age at diagnosis

populations may be experiencing a reduction in cancer risk and mortality over time. A UK surveillance colonoscopy cohort reported a reduction in cancer risk over the last 30 years (1970 to 2000) and quantified the risk as a 2.5% at 20 years, 7.6% at 30 years, and 10.8% after 40 years of disease.[8] A cohort in Sweden found a still elevated but declining trend in CRC incidence and mortality over a 35-year time period (1960 to 2004).[9]

It is not known why the risk of CRC is lower in certain populations than others, or if the risk of CRC and mortality from CRC is declining in all populations. However, these promising data suggest that the risk of CRC in IBD is modifiable. Greater rates of proctocolectomy for medical treatment failures, better rates of surveillance colonoscopy with resultant proctocolectomy for dysplasia, and finally, greater use of maintenance anti-inflammatory therapy in the form of 5-aminosalicylic acid (5-ASA) could all be important factors that reduce the risk of CRC in a given population of IBD patients.[10,11]

Unfortunately, the most important risk factors in IBD-related CRC, namely duration and anatomic extent of colonic inflammation, are not modifiable (Table 5-1).[1] Other important nonmodifiable risk factors include a concomitant diagnosis of primary sclerosing cholangitis (PSC) and a family history of CRC.[12,13] PSC increases the relative risk of CRC 4.8-fold. Family history of CRC increases the risk of CRC 2.5-fold, whereas a family history of CRC at age <50 increases the relative risk even more, to 9.2.[12,13]

Additional epidemiologic risk factors for CRC in IBD have been described; however, their clinical role remains to be determined. Smoking reduces the risk of CRC in chronic UC by 50%[14,15] but increases the risk of CRC in CD 4-fold,[16] perhaps reflecting the different effect smoking has on inflammation in each condition. The presence of pseudopolyps (inflammatory polyps) also increases the risk of CRC 2.5-fold,[15,17] perhaps either as a historical marker of more severe inflammation or because these inflammatory polyps may obscure true polyps. Other described risk factors include backwash ileitis[18] and young age at diagnosis.[1]

ETIOLOGY AND PATHOPHYSIOLOGY

Colorectal adenocarcinoma develops after the accumulation of key mutations. In IBD, chronic inflammation of the colon is hypothesized to be the key etiologic factor in the pathogenesis of CRC, causing increased oxidative stress; promoting repeated cycles of injury, regeneration, and repair; and finally, accelerating the accumulation of key mutations.[19] Over time, sufficient genetic mutations accumulate to result in dysplasia, defined as an unequivocal neoplastic change in the colon without invasion.[20] With accumulation of additional mutations, dysplasia progresses into invasive CRC.

The mutations that lead to the development of CRC in IBD are similar to that in sporadic CRC; however, the order and frequency in which they occur differ.[21] For example, alteration of the tumor suppressor gene p53 is an early event in the development of colitis-related colon cancer, but a late event in sporadic CRC.[22] Function of the p53 gene prevents the clonal expansion of cells that contain damaged DNA, which prevents damaged cells from progressing through the cell cycle. This protective role is inhibited by mutations caused by reactive oxygen species, suggesting a link between these common byproducts of inflammation seen in IBD and cancer.[20] Although the mutations involved in the pathogenesis of colitis-related colon cancer have been well described,[19] as of today, there are no reliable and clinically available biomarkers to predict future cancer or dysplasia risk.

Although it is intuitive that chronic inflammation is a key etiologic factor in the pathogenesis of IBD-related CRC, it is only recently that severity of inflammation, presumably a modifiable biologic risk factor, has been linked to CRC risk. When defined by frequency of symptomatic exacerbations, severity of inflammation has not been a consistent risk factor in studies.[14,23] However, when defined by degree of histologic inflammation at surveillance colonoscopy, greater histologic inflammation has been found to be a consistent risk factor for colorectal neoplasia in 3 studies.[17,24,25] Rutter and colleagues compared the endoscopic and histologic specimens of 68 UC patients enrolled in their surveillance program who developed CRC compared to 136 controls who did not. They rated endoscopic and histologic inflammation using a self-derived 5-point score. They found a highly significant correlation between increasing colonoscopic (odds ratio [OR] 2.5, $P = 0.001$) and histologic (OR 5.1, $P < 0.001$) inflammation scores and risk of colorectal neoplasia.[17] Ullman and colleagues studied a cohort of 418 patients who underwent colonoscopic surveillance and rated colonoscopic inflammation on a 4-point system using a validated scoring system.[26] Seventy four patients developed neoplasia, and again, greater severity of histologic inflammation at surveillance colonoscopy correlated with risk of developing neoplasia (HR 2.4, $P = 0.03$). Finally, Rubin and colleagues assessed inflammation in 146 cases and matched controls and also demonstrated that severity of inflammation was an independent risk factor for the development of CRC (OR 2.8, $P = 0.006$).[24]

Thus, emerging epidemiologic data suggest that chronic inflammation at surveillance colonoscopy, in theory reflecting the amount of background inflammation when the disease is in remission, is an important (and novel) etiologic risk factor for the development of CRC. Unless this risk factor cannot be modified, these data also suggest that reduction of background inflammation, perhaps via chronic use of medications aimed at keeping IBD in remission, could also be an important (and novel) therapeutic strategy for reducing CRC risk.[11,15,27]

CLINICAL FEATURES

There are several clinical features that distinguish IBD-related CRC from CRC in the general population[28]: (1) CRC occurs at a younger age; (2) many cases are not preceded by visible adenomatous polyps; (3) the rate of progression of dysplasia to cancer is more rapid than the progression of adenomas to cancer in the non-IBD population; (4) there is a greater presence of a generalized field effect in which all colitic mucosa is at risk for malignancy because of molecular and genetic changes associated with chronic inflammation; and finally (5) occult cancer, cancer found incidentally at colectomy when only dysplasia was detected at the preceding colonoscopy, is common. Occult cancer is present in 19% of IBD patients with flat low-grade dysplasia (LGD) who undergo immediate colectomy, in 42% with high-grade dysplasia (HGD), and in 43% of patients with a dysplasia-associated lesions or mass (DALM).[29]

It is unclear whether poorer cancer prognosis is a clinical feature of CRC occurring in the setting of IBD. Older series showed patients with CRC and IBD had a worse prognosis than patients without IBD because CRC was diagnosed at a more advanced cancer stage. A recent study from the Mayo Clinic showed that cancer stage at diagnosis (and hence prognosis) for IBD patients is comparable to that of non-IBD patients.[30] In contrast, a Danish population study showed that IBD itself was a risk factor for worse prognosis even when matching for stage.[31] A Japanese population study also showed a poorer signature for UC–CRC compared to sporadic CRC. However, on further analysis, the difference in survival was driven by a difference in survival in stage III cancers (node positive); survival was similar in limited (stage I/II) and widely metastatic (stage IV) stages.[32] Additional studies are needed to help clarify these discrepancies regarding whether IBD-related CRC has a poorer prognosis.

DIAGNOSTIC EVALUATION

Many patients and their physicians choose to follow a diagnostic program of screening and surveillance colonoscopy, with a goal of detecting dysplasia and other early neoplastic lesions at a curable stage.[33] The rationale for undergoing surveillance colonoscopy is based on the premise that determining which patients are likely to progress to cancer in the near term can be reliably predicted by the presence or absence of histologic dysplasia on colonoscopy.

In all patients, CRC develops from a dysplastic precursor lesion (Figure 5-1). Dysplasia is often categorized as either flat (endoscopically not visible and

Type	Pit pattern	Definition	Usual histopatho-logical findings
Type I	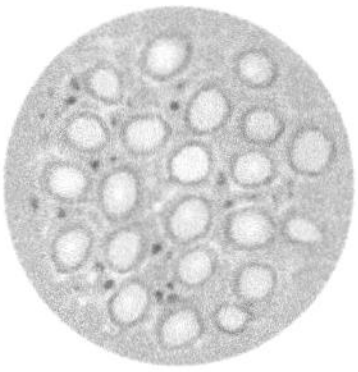	round pits	normal
Type II	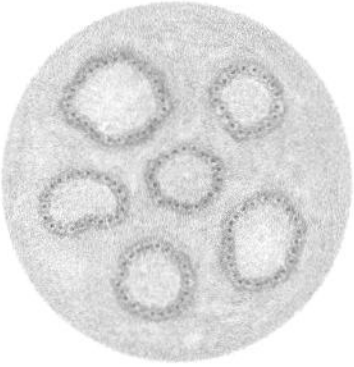	asteroid or papillary pits	hyperplastic
Type IIIS	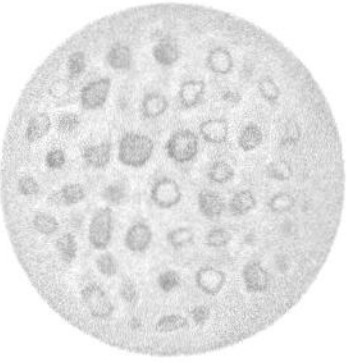	small tubular or roundish pits	intramucosal andenocarcinoma (28.3%) adenoma (73%) (depressed lesion)
Type IIIL	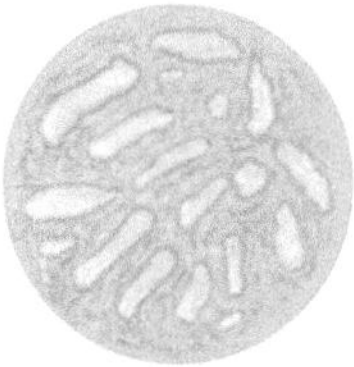	large tubular or roundish pits	adenoma (86.7%) (protruded lesion)
Type IV	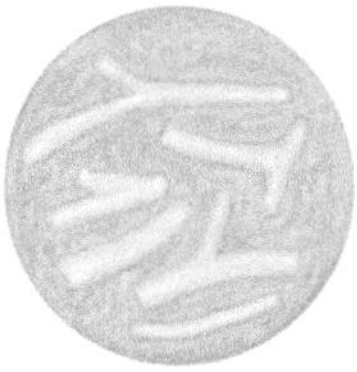	branch-like or gyrus-like pits	adenoma (59.7%) (almost tubulovillous adenoma) intramucosal adenocarcinoma (37.2%)
Type V	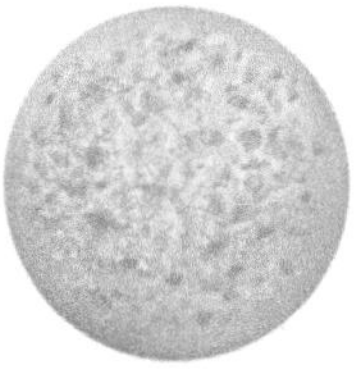	nonstructural pits	submucosal adenocarcinoma (62.5%)

Figure 5-1. Modified pit pattern classification. (Reprinted with permission from Kudo S. Endoscopic mucosal resection of flat and depressed types of early colorectal cancer. *Endoscopy*. 1993;25:455-461.)

detected by random or nontargeted biopsies) or raised (endoscopically visible and detected by targeted biopsies).[27] Dysplasia is defined as unequivocal neoplastic epithelial alteration without invasive growth.[34] In the general population, this lesion in called an *adenomatous polyp*, which is easily detectable on colonoscopy. In patients with IBD, the premalignant lesion is more broadly referred to as *dysplasia*. Dysplasia in IBD differs than in non-IBD as it is more often flat and difficult to detect on colonoscopy. Even so, it is important to remember that most dysplasia in IBD is visible.[35] Recent studies have demonstrated that approximately 75% of dysplasia in IBD is visible (raised) and only 25% is "invisible" (flat).[36,37]

Several guidelines for CRC prevention in IBD have been published over the past decade to assist gastroenterologists in approaching screening and surveillance colonoscopy in IBD (Table 5-2).[33,38-42] It is acknowledged that patients who have only had small intestinal CD without colonic involvement or patients with UC limited to the rectum are not considered to be at high risk for CRC and should be managed according to general population CRC screening guidelines.[1,5,27,33] Recommended guidelines are based on expert opinion, as there are no controlled trials.

Several definitions commonly used in surveillance guidelines should be noted and understood. A *screening* examination is defined as the initial colonoscopy performed solely to determine the presence or absence of histologic dysplasia and not to investigate symptoms.[33] A *surveillance* examination is defined as any and all subsequent colonoscopies with that indication. Although all guidelines agree that the initial screening examination should occur 8 to 10 years after the diagnosis of IBD to clarify the true extent of disease, they vary widely in the timing, frequency, and selection of patients for subsequent surveillance colonoscopies (see Table 5-2). Notable is the most recent British Society of Gastroenterology guidelines that risk stratify patients based on personal risk factors not previously used, including degree of inflammation, endoscopic findings, and family history.[38] This guideline extends the surveillance interval in the lowest risk patients out to 5 years, the longest of any guideline. Commonly, the surveillance interval is recommended to be between 1 and 2 years.

At present, no randomized studies have been performed documenting a reduction in the risk of developing or dying from CRC by surveillance colonoscopy. Such studies are unlikely to be performed because of feasibility.[43] Despite the lack of randomized controlled trials, surveillance colonoscopy is considered the primary methodology to detect dysplasia and prevent CRC in IBD, and it is endorsed by several gastroenterology societies (see Table 5-2).[27,33,38-42]

Evidence that surveillance colonoscopy reduces the risk of CRC and mortality consists of several observational case-control studies and case series.[15,44,45] Case-control studies have reported that a prior history of surveillance colonoscopy reduces the odds of CRC by 60% to 80%.[15,46] Case series have demonstrated that 5-year survival rates are higher for chronic UC patients with CRC detected within a surveillance program than for those who present with symptomatic cancers detected outside of a surveillance program.[44,45]

Table 5-2. Gastroenterology Society Guidelines for Screening and Surveillance Colonoscopy in Persons With Inflammatory Bowel Diseases

	FIRST COLONOSCOPY (SCREENING)	INTERVAL SUBSEQUENT COLONOSCOPY (SURVEILLANCE)
AGA and US Multisociety Task Force on Colorectal Cancer[42]	All patients 8 to 10 years after diagnosis	Surveillance with systemic biopsies should be *considered*
ACG (2004)[41] and ASGE (2006)[40]	All patients 8 to 10 years after diagnosis; immediately in PSC	Every 1 to 2 years (all patients)
Canadian Association of Gastroenterology (2004)-endorsement BSG 2002[39]	All patients 8 to 10 years after diagnosis	In pancolitis: every 3 years in second decade after diagnosis; every 2 years in third decade; every year after third decade In left sided: next colonoscopy at 15 years after diagnosis
Crohn's and Colitis Foundation[33]	All patients 8 to 10 years after diagnosis; immediately in PSC	Next 2 examinations in 1 to 2 years then every 1 to 3 years until 20 years duration, then return to every 1 to 2 years Yearly in PSC
BSG (2010)[38]	All patients 10 years after diagnosis to determine extent and endoscopic risk	Yearly: pancolitis with active/ moderate inflammation or stricture or PSC or history of dysplasia or FH CRC age <50 Every 3 years: pancolitis with mild inflammation or inflammatory polyps or FH CRC >50 years Every 5 years: quiescent pancolitis or left-sided colitis

ACG = American College of Gastroenterology; AGA = American Gastroenterological Association; ASGE = American Society of Gastrointestinal Endoscopy; BSG = British Society of Gastroenterology; CRC = colorectal cancer; FH = family history; PSC = primary sclerosing cholangitis.

Skeptics often highlight the failures of surveillance colonoscopy. A pooled analysis of prospective studies has shown that there is a high rate of coexisting cancer even when dysplasia is the worst histologic lesion detected at surveillance.[29] There are many instances of CRC developing even between closely spaced surveillance examinations.[29] In addition, physicians and patients do not adhere to recommended guidelines. For example, 88% of practicing gastroenterologists report to taking less than 15 biopsies per surveillance examination,[47] significantly fewer than the 33 biopsies required to exclude dysplasia with 90% confidence.[48] Data from 3 continents suggest gastroenterologists, when they find dysplasia, manage it in a manner inconsistent with current recommendations. A recent study showed that only 13% of British gastroenterologists offered colectomy for flat LGD. In the same study, 85% considered that LGD with DALM had a high risk of concurrent cancer; however, only 52% offered colectomy to this group.[49] Finally, adherence by patients to the rigorous (every 1 to 2 years) surveillance recommendations is poor, potentially negating the efficacy of any surveillance program.[50,51]

Results from a recently published 30-year surveillance program likely reflect the current clinical reality of surveillance colonoscopy,[8] both the good and the bad. The study showed a reduction in the incidence of CRC among patients enrolled in a surveillance program. The authors concluded that surveillance is effective in reducing the risk of CRC, thereby allowing the majority of patients to retain their colon. The same study, however, showed that 16 of 30 interval cancers occurred after a normal colonoscopy or were advanced (more than Duke C), showing that this procedure is not completely effective in protecting patients from CRC.[8] Moving forward, to improve the sensitivity and specificity of surveillance colonoscopy, it will be critical to test whether the use of vital stains and molecular markers, as well as standardizing surveillance technique and management of dysplasia, will allow further improvement in the efficacy of this procedure.

The recommended technique for performing surveillance colonoscopy is based on expert consensus and not rigorous trials.[33] Many experts recommend obtaining 4-quadrant biopsy specimens every 10 cm in flat mucosa using jumbo forceps (at least 32 biopsies). Biopsies every 5 cm should be considered in the lower sigmoid and rectum given the frequency of CRC is higher in this region.[52] Biopsies should be placed in separate containers and linked "geographically" to parts of the colon in case there is a need to examine an area in particular during a subsequent colonoscopy. Specimens from targeted biopsies of raised area or suspicious area and the surrounding mucosa should each be placed in separate containers.[33] Notable is the recent proposal that the current surveillance technique of white light colonoscopy with random biopsies be abandoned in favor of methods that use adjuncts to enhance the detection of flat or subtle dysplastic lesions.[37]

It should be noted that so-called flat, "invisible," or subtle dysplasia detection can be improved even without the use of adjuncts. Toruner et al reported on 635 patients with IBD who underwent surveillance colonoscopy and found that, while the number of random biopsies did not increase the detection of dysplasia, every additional minute of colonoscopy time increased the flat dysplasia diagnosis rate by 3.5%. No minimum or optimal withdrawal time has been suggested.[53]

With regard to adjuncts to enhance the detection of dysplasia, several approaches and strategies are under investigation, including chromoendoscopy, narrow-band imaging, autofluorescence, and confocal endomicroscopy. Of

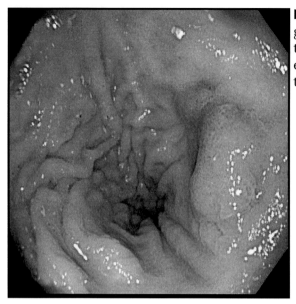

Figure 5-2. Endoscopic photograph of a DALM lesion in a patient with UC. Histopathologic examination showed adenomatous tissue with LGD.

these, chromoendoscopy appears to be the most likely to have widespread use in the near term. Chromoendoscopy involves the use of dye delivered through a fine mist spray catheter to coat the mucosa of the colon. The dye typically used in IBD surveillance is either an absorptive dye, such as methylene blue, or a contrast dye, such as indigo carmine. The spraying of dye on the mucosa has 2 purposes. The first is to improve detection of flat or subtle colonic lesions and therefore increase the sensitivity of surveillance colonoscopy. The second is to help in distinguishing between neoplastic and non-neoplastic lesions based on assessment of crypt architecture and modified pit pattern (Figure 5-2).[54]

Chromoendoscopy is inexpensive, does not require significant additional equipment and supplies, and appears safe.[55] There is a recent report of in vitro DNA damage with methylene blue at concentrations used in the colon; however, the clinical relevance of this report is unclear.[56]

Several prospective and randomized studies have now demonstrated chromoendoscopy results approximately 3-fold better detection rates of dysplasia compared to conventional white light colonoscopy with random 4-quadrant biopsies at 10-cm intervals.[37,57-60] Although not currently the standard of care, its use as an alternative to traditional white light endoscopy with random biopsies by persons trained in the technique is mentioned by several societies, including the Crohn's and Colitis Foundation of America,[33] European Crohn's and Colitis Organization,[61] British Society of Gastroenterology,[38] and American Gastroenterological Association.[27] With ongoing improvements in white light technology (high-definition and magnification colonoscopes), the next several years will determine whether chromoendoscopy will become the standard of care.[27]

Narrow-band imaging (virtual chromoendoscopy), which uses color filters or postprocessing techniques to create a pseudocolored image to enhance tissue vasculature and mucosal contours, is also a readily available and safe modality. Without additional data, it cannot be recommended at this time. A prospective randomized crossover trial showed that it is no better than standard white light colonoscopy for detecting dysplasia in IBD surveillance.[62]

MANAGEMENT/TREATMENT/OUTCOMES

Once dysplasia is detected, proper management going forward is critical. First, it is essential to confirm all abnormal findings with a second expert gastroenterology (GI) pathologist to correctly interpret and confirm the presence of dysplasia, as there is significant interobserver variation.[63,64] It is also essential to properly classify the type of dysplasia, as each type has its own natural history for harboring occult cancer or rapidly progressing to cancer.[29]

Dysplasia is typically categorized and managed by its histology (indefinite, low grade, high grade) and gross endoscopic appearance (flat and elevated). *Flat* dysplasia commonly refers to endoscopically undetected lesions found on nontargeted biopsies. *Raised* dysplasia commonly refers to endoscopically detected lesions found on targeted biopsies. Flat dysplasia is further characterized as unifocal or multifocal. Raised dysplasia, also called *polypoid dysplasia*, traditionally has been grouped into a large category of DALM. For at least the past 10 years, raised lesions appearing like sporadic adenomas have been separated into a distinct classification of DALM: "adenoma-like DALMs," reflecting smaller, discrete, and endoscopically resectable lesions in inflamed mucosa, without surrounding flat dysplasia.[65,66] This was the first acknowledgment that the DALM category was a heterogeneous group. At least 4 studies[65-68] have confirmed that the adenoma-like DALM does not have the malignant potential observed in the first series of DALMs published in 1981 among 12 patients with IBD.[69]

Indefinite Dysplasia in Flat Mucosa

Patients with indefinite dysplasia in flat mucosa should undergo a second surveillance colonoscopy. The time interval between examinations should be dictated by whether the pathologists reviewing the specimen believe it is likely positive or likely negative. Inflammation can sometimes obscure the determination; however, most pathologists can distinguish between reactive changes due to inflammation and true indefinite dysplasia (Figure 5-3A).[33]

Low-Grade Dysplasia in Flat Mucosa

Whether patients with flat LGD should undergo colectomy is widely debated.[34] A recent AGA medical position statement on the diagnosis and management of colorectal neoplasia in IBD concluded there was insufficient evidence to determine the balance of benefits and harms of colectomy for flat LGD (Figure 5-3B).[27]

Many centers refer patients with flat LGD for colectomy; some will repeat colonoscopy in 6 months. Proponents on both sides cite natural history studies to support their approach. Proponents of colectomy note that 3 studies

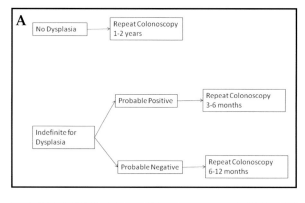

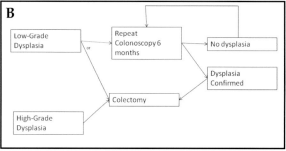

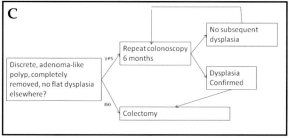

Figure 5-3. (A) CRC surveillance strategies in IBD. (B) Surveillance of flat dysplasia. (C) Dysplasia in a raised lesion (high or low grade).

show that the rate of progression from low-grade to advanced neoplasia (HGD or cancer) is approximately 55% at 5 years.[70-72] Furthermore, 19% of patients who undergo immediate colectomy may have an unrecognized CRC already present.[29] Proponents of watchful waiting cite different studies showing a lower rate of progression[73-75] and point out the inconsistencies in the diagnosis of LGD for predicting future cancer risk.[76] If a nonoperative strategy is pursued, a subsequent negative examination after LGD is not sufficiently reassuring to return to normal surveillance. A high level of vigilance is required, with frequent (<6 months) subsequent examinations.[52]

New data suggest that the key driver for recommending colectomy should not be the currently debated rate of long-term progression of dysplasia to CRC, but rather the increased rate of occult cancer and short-term progression to cancer.[77] Occult cancer (ie, cancer present but not detected at the time of surveillance colonoscopy) is present in 19% of IBD patients with flat LGD.[29] In a recently published decision analysis, immediate colectomy was the superior strategy in nearly every scenario where there was risk of occult cancer, primarily due to the lower mortality associated with early intervention. In fact, colectomy was superior even when the rate of progression to cancer over time was modeled to be 0%, further highlighting the importance of occult cancer in the management of dysplasia. Despite this, few patients undergo colectomy after a diagnosis of colorectal dysplasia. They report needing a much higher personal possibility of occult cancer than currently published estimates before agreeing to undergo colectomy.[51]

High-Grade Dysplasia in Flat Mucosa

There is consensus that patients with HGD in flat mucosa should undergo colectomy to treat undiagnosed synchronous cancer and prevent metachronous cancer.[27,33] Up to 42% of patients may already have an underlying CRC.[29] For those who do not, there is a high rate of progression to CRC (see Figure 5-3B).

Low-Grade or High-Grade Dysplasia in a Raised Lesion

This is the most likely scenario that is encountered during colonoscopy, as approximately 75% of dysplastic lesions are visible on routine surveillance colonoscopy.[36] The key consideration here is whether the endoscopist believes that the lesion represents an isolated polyp in a field of colitis that can be completely removed endoscopically (adenoma-like DALM) or whether the lesion is a raised polypoid lesion that either cannot be resected endoscopically or is within a greater field change of flat dysplasia (true DALM or nonadenoma DALM) (Figure 5-3C).[33]

A nonsurgical strategy can be pursued if polypectomy is complete, biopsies taken immediately surrounding the polyp are negative for dysplasia, and there is no additional dysplasia elsewhere in the colon. A surveillance colonoscopy should be repeated in 6 months with regular surveillance resumed if no dysplasia is found. Several studies have shown that polypectomy in such a group is associated with a low risk of developing CRC[65,66] up to a mean of 82 months.[68] The key concept is that the adenoma-like DALM must be completely removed. Vieth et al showed a high rate of progression to cancer among patients with raised lesions that were biopsied but not completely removed.[67]

In contrast, a surgical strategy (ie, colectomy) should be pursued under 2 circumstances: (1) the polypoid lesion cannot be completely resected or (2) even if it can be resected, dysplasia is present in biopsies of the surrounding flat mucosa or flat dysplasia is present as a distant site. Such raised dysplastic lesions would more appropriately be termed as DALM and not an adenoma-like DALM and would represent a high-risk, rather than a low-risk, dysplastic lesion. A nonadenoma DALM lesion is associated with a high risk of synchronous CRC (43%).[29]

The AGA recently concluded with grade A evidence (high certainty that the magnitude of net effects is substantial) that patients with IBD diagnosed with an adenoma-like DALM (adenoma DALM), and no evidence of flat dysplasia elsewhere in colon, could be managed safely with polypectomy and continued surveillance. In contrast, those diagnosed with a non–adenoma-like DALM (true DALM) should be treated with colectomy.[27]

SPECIAL TOPICS

Management of Adenomas Detected Outside Areas of Colitis

Adenomas detected outside of endoscopically and histologically abnormal areas of inflammation can be managed as a traditional adenoma, with complete excision and polypectomy considered definitive treatment. It should be remembered that many of these patients often are young, so that while the polyp excision was definitive therapy of the polyp, these patients independently may be at high risk for subsequent polyps and CRC based on the presence of polyps at a young age.

Surveillance in the Presence of Inflammatory Polyps and Strictures

Inflammatory polyps (pseudopolyps) are commonly encountered during surveillance. Although they do not specifically harbor any malignant potential, their presence is associated with a 2.5-fold increased risk of cancer, possibly as a marker of significant prior inflammation or because they may obscure true polyps.[15,78] Although classic-appearing pseudopolyps are evident based on appearance and do not have to be resected, if there is any concern whether a polypoid lesion represents a true polyp instead of an inflammatory polyp, one should consider biopsies or endoscopic resection of the lesion if feasible.

Occasionally multiple or massed pseudopolyps are encountered, raising concern about the ability to reliably distinguish between inflammatory and true dysplastic lesions or to sample all lesions. There is no best practice based on available literature.[33] Options include referral to an expert center with expertise in IBD, colectomy, segmental resection, complete polypectomy (if feasible), or routine surveillance of flat mucosa with removal of all suspicious polypoid lesions.[33]

Colonic strictures are occasionally encountered during surveillance. In patients with Crohn's colitis, strictures are often a consequence of the transmural nature of the disease itself and not a harbinger of CRC. In Crohn's colitis, if the endoscopist can bypass a stricture, extensive biopsies of the stricture and repeat endoscopic evaluation within 1 year if biopsies are negative for dysplasia is appropriate.[33] In contrast, a stricture in the setting of UC, which is a mucosal and not transmural process, is a strong indication for colectomy because of the high rate of underlying carcinoma. If colectomy is not performed and biopsies of the stricture are negative, a repeat examination should be performed within 3 to 4 months.[33] Anal strictures should be assessed by a surgeon with an examination under anesthesia to exclude malignancy with a repeat examination in 1 year.[33]

Chemoprevention

Chemoprevention refers to the use of a medication or other substance to reduce or prevent the development of cancer. The rationale for chemoprevention in IBD is based upon the premise that surveillance colonoscopy is not a perfect method of preventing CRC, and that it is possible and preferable to prevent neoplastic transformation of the colon from occurring in the first place.

It is important to note that much of the evidence for chemoprevention is based on small observational studies and biological plausibility. Therefore, it should be emphasized that this strategy, while promising, remains unproven. As a result, surveillance strategies should not be altered due to the consumption of putative chemopreventive agents.[33]

One IBD medication that has received significant attention for its possible role as a chemopreventive agent is 5-ASA. 5-ASA, a structural derivative of acetylsalicylic acid (aspirin), is a common anti-inflammatory therapy in IBD, particularly UC. Inflammation is a known risk factor for CRC, and 5-ASA shares several important anti-inflammatory and anticancer properties with aspirin and nonsteroidal anti-inflammatory medications (NSAIDs).[79] 5-ASA reduces oxidative stress, inhibits cell proliferation, and promotes apoptosis.

Many, but not all, observational studies have shown that use of 5-ASA reduces the risk of CRC.[11] In a pooled analysis, regular use of 5-ASA reduced the risk of CRC in chronic UC by approximately 50%, similar to what is observed with regular NSAID use in non-IBD patients.[11] At this time, it is premature to recommend the addition of 5-ASA for IBD patients on other IBD therapies solely for the chemopreventive benefit. However, 5-ASA prescribed for maintenance therapy in mild-moderate UC and Crohn's colitis is likely to yield a secondary benefit of CRC reduction.[27] Recent AGA guidelines rated the available evidence as grade B, suggesting there is moderate certainty that the magnitude of net benefits is moderate.[27]

Another medication that has been studied as a potential chemopreventive agent is ursodeoxycholic acid. Ursodeoxycholic acid is an exogenous bile acid used in PSC that reduces the concentration of toxic secondary bile acids in the colon. Secondary bile acids are carcinogenic and are increased in patients with cholestatic liver disease such as PSC. Two studies demonstrating its use were associated with a significant 80% reduced risk of CRC in IBD,[80,81] and a third demonstrated a nonsignificant 41% reduced risk.[82] It is currently recommended for the reduction of CRC risk in patients with IBD and PSC with a grade A endorsement (high certainty that the magnitude of net benefit is substantial).[27]

There are insufficient data on the efficacy of other anti-inflammatory agents (immunomodulators and steroids) for reducing the risk of CRC in IBD.[27] Folic acid supplements, calcium, vitamins, and statins have not been consistently associated with lower rates of CRC to recommend their routine use for this indication.[27]

☑ Key Points

☑ Chronic inflammation at surveillance colonoscopy is an important (and novel) etiologic risk factor for the development of CRC and suggests that reduction of background inflammation, perhaps via chronic use of medications used to keep IBD in remission, could also be a potentially important therapeutic strategy for reducing CRC risk.

☑ Despite the lack of randomized controlled trials, surveillance colonoscopy is considered the primary way to detect dysplasia and prevent CRC in IBD and is endorsed by several gastroenterology societies.

☑ The current surveillance technique consists of white light colonoscopy with random and targeted biopsies. With regard to adjuncts to enhance the detection of dysplasia, several approaches and strategies are under investigation.

☑ Once dysplasia is detected, it is critical to manage properly. First, it is essential to confirm all abnormal findings with a second expert gastrointestind pathologist to correctly interpret and confirm the presence of dysplasia, as there is significant interobserver variation. It is also essential to properly classify the type of dysplasia, as each type has its own natural history for harboring occult cancer or rapidly progressing to cancer.

☑ Patients with IBD diagnosed with an adenoma DALM, and no evidence of flat dysplasia elsewhere in the colon, can be managed safely with polypectomy and continued surveillance. In contrast, those diagnosed with a true DALM should be treated with colectomy.

References

1. Ekbom A, Helmick C, Zack M, Adami HO. Ulcerative colitis and colorectal cancer. A population-based study. *N Engl J Med.* 1990;323:1228-1233.
2. Ekbom A, Helmick C, Zack M, Adami HO. Increased risk of large-bowel cancer in Crohn's disease with colonic involvement. *Lancet.* 1990;336:357-359.
3. Clevers H. Colon cancer—understanding how NSAIDs work. *N Engl J Med.* 2006;354:761-763.
4. Eaden JA, Abrams KR, Mayberry JF. The risk of colorectal cancer in ulcerative colitis: a meta-analysis. *Gut.* 2001;48:526-535.
5. Canavan C, Abrams KR, Mayberry J. Meta-analysis: colorectal and small bowel cancer risk in patients with Crohn's disease. *Aliment Pharmacol Ther.* 2006;23:1097-1104.
6. Winther KV, Jess T, Langholz E, Munkholm P, Binder V. Long-term risk of cancer in ulcerative colitis: a population-based cohort study from Copenhagen County. *Clin Gastroenterol Hepatol.* 2004;2:1088-1095.

7. Jess T, Loftus EV Jr, Velayos FS, et al. Risk of intestinal cancer in inflammatory bowel disease: a population-based study from Olmsted County, Minnesota. *Gastroenterology.* 2006;130:1039-1046.

8. Rutter MD, Saunders BP, Wilkinson KH, et al. Thirty-year analysis of a colonoscopic surveillance program for neoplasia in ulcerative colitis. *Gastroenterology.* 2006;130:1030-1038.

9. Soderlund S, Brandt L, Lapidus A, et al. Decreasing time-trends of colorectal cancer in a large cohort of patients with inflammatory bowel disease. *Gastroenterology.* 2009;136:1561-1567.

10. Munkholm P. Review article: the incidence and prevalence of colorectal cancer in inflammatory bowel disease. *Aliment Pharmacol Ther.* 2003;18(suppl 2):1-5.

11. Velayos FS, Terdiman JP, Walsh JM. Effect of 5-aminosalicylate use on colorectal cancer and dysplasia risk: a systematic review and metaanalysis of observational studies. *Am J Gastroenterol.* 2005;100:1345-1353.

12. Soetikno RM, Lin OS, Heidenreich PA, Young HS, Blackstone MO. Increased risk of colorectal neoplasia in patients with primary sclerosing cholangitis and ulcerative colitis: a meta-analysis. *Gastrointest Endosc.* 2002;56:48-54.

13. Askling J, Dickman PW, Karlen P, et al. Family history as a risk factor for colorectal cancer in inflammatory bowel disease. *Gastroenterology.* 2001;120:1356-1362.

14. Pinczowski D, Ekbom A, Baron J, Yuen J, Adami HO. Risk factors for colorectal cancer in patients with ulcerative colitis: a case-control study. *Gastroenterology.* 1994;107:117-120.

15. Velayos FS, Loftus EV Jr, Jess T, et al. Predictive and protective factors associated with colorectal cancer in ulcerative colitis: a case-control study. *Gastroenterology.* 2006;130:1941-1949.

16. Siegel CA, Sands BE. Risk factors for colorectal cancer in Crohn's colitis: a case-control study. *Inflamm Bowel Dis.* 2006;12:491-496.

17. Rutter M, Saunders B, Wilkinson K, et al. Severity of inflammation is a risk factor for colorectal neoplasia in ulcerative colitis. *Gastroenterology.* 2004;126:451-459.

18. Heuschen UA, Hinz U, Allemeyer EH, et al. Backwash ileitis is strongly associated with colorectal carcinoma in ulcerative colitis. *Gastroenterology.* 2001;120:841-847.

19. Itzkowitz S. Colon carcinogenesis in inflammatory bowel disease: applying molecular genetics to clinical practice. *J Clin Gastroenterol.* 2003;36:S70-S74.

20. Itzkowitz SH, Harpaz N. Diagnosis and management of dysplasia in patients with inflammatory bowel diseases. *Gastroenterology.* 2004;126:1634-1648.

21. Itzkowitz SH, Yio X. Inflammation and cancer IV. Colorectal cancer in inflammatory bowel disease: the role of inflammation. *Am J Physiol Gastrointest Liver Physiol.* 2004;287: G7-G17.

22. Brentnall TA, Crispin DA, Rabinovitch PS, et al. Mutations in the p53 gene: an early marker of neoplastic progression in ulcerative colitis. *Gastroenterology.* 1994;107:369-378.

23. Eaden J, Abrams K, Ekbom A, Jackson E, Mayberry J. Colorectal cancer prevention in ulcerative colitis: a case-control study. *Aliment Pharmacol Ther.* 2000;14:145-153.

24. Rubin DT, Huo D, Rothe JA, et al. Increased inflammatory activity is an independent risk factor for dysplasia and colorectal cancer in ulcerative colitis: a case-control analysis with blinded prospective pathology review (Abstract 14). *Gastroenterology.* 2006;130:A2.

25. Bansal R, Itzkowitz S, Harpaz N, et al. Severity of inflammation predicts progression to colorectal neoplasia in ulcerative colitis. *Am J Gastroenterol.* 2005;100:S289.

26. Gupta RB, Harpaz N, Itzkowitz S, et al. Histologic inflammation is a risk factor for progression to colorectal neoplasia in ulcerative colitis: a cohort study. *Gastroenterology.* 2007;133:1099-1105.

27. Farraye FA, Odze RD, Eaden J, et al. AGA medical position statement on the diagnosis and management of colorectal neoplasia in inflammatory bowel disease. *Gastroenterology.* 2010;138:738-745.

28. Ullman T, Odze R, Farraye FA. Diagnosis and management of dysplasia in patients with ulcerative colitis and Crohn's disease of the colon. *Inflamm Bowel Dis.* 2009;15:630-638.

29. Bernstein CN, Shanahan F, Weinstein WM. Are we telling patients the truth about surveillance colonoscopy in ulcerative colitis? *Lancet.* 1994;343:71-74.

30. Delaunoit T, Limburg PJ, Goldberg RM, Lymp JF, Loftus EV Jr. Colorectal cancer prognosis among patients with inflammatory bowel disease. *Clin Gastroenterol Hepatol*. 2006;4: 335-342.

31. Jensen AB, Larsen M, Gislum M, et al. Survival after colorectal cancer in patients with ulcerative colitis: a nationwide population-based Danish study. *Am J Gastroenterol*. 2006;101: 1283-1287.

32. Watanabe T, Konishi T, Kishimoto J, Kotake K, Muto T, Sugihara K; Japanese Society for Cancer of the Colon and Rectum. Ulcerative colitis-associated colorectal cancer shows a poorer survival than sporadic colorectal cancer: a nationwide Japanese study. *Inflamm Bowel Dis*. 2011;17(3):802-808.

33. Itzkowitz SH, Present DH. Consensus conference: colorectal cancer screening and surveillance in inflammatory bowel disease. *Inflamm Bowel Dis*. 2005;11:314-321.

34. Bernstein CN. A Balancing view: dysplasia surveillance in ulcerative colitis—sorting the pro from the con. *Am J Gastroenterol*. 2004;99:1636-1637.

35. Rubin DT, Rothe JA, Hetzel JT, Cohen RD, Hanauer SB. Are dysplasia and colorectal cancer endoscopically visible in patients with ulcerative colitis? *Gastrointest Endosc*. 2007;65:998-1004.

36. Rutter MD, Saunders BP, Wilkinson KH, Kamm MA, Williams CB, Forbes A. Most dysplasia in ulcerative colitis is visible at colonoscopy. *Gastrointest Endosc*. 2004;60:334-339.

37. Marion JF, Waye JD, Present DH, et al. Chromoendoscopy-targeted biopsies are superior to standard colonoscopic surveillance for detecting dysplasia in inflammatory bowel disease patients: a prospective endoscopic trial. *Am J Gastroenterol*. 2008;103:2342-2349.

38. Cairns SR, Scholefield JH, Steele RJ, et al. Guidelines for colorectal cancer screening and surveillance in moderate and high risk groups (update from 2002). *Gut*. 2010;59: 666-689.

39. Eaden JA, Mayberry JF. Guidelines for screening and surveillance of asymptomatic colorectal cancer in patients with inflammatory bowel disease. *Gut*. 2002;51(suppl 5): V10-V12.

40. Davila RE, Rajan E, Baron TH, et al. ASGE guideline: colorectal cancer screening and surveillance. *Gastrointest Endosc*. 2006;63:546-557.

41. Kornbluth A, Sachar DB. Ulcerative colitis practice guidelines in adults (update): American College of Gastroenterology, Practice Parameters Committee. *Am J Gastroenterol*. 2004;99:1371-1385.

42. Winawer S, Fletcher R, Rex D, et al. Colorectal cancer screening and surveillance: clinical guidelines and rationale—update based on new evidence. *Gastroenterology*. 2003;124:544-560.

43. Bernstein CN. Challenges in designing a randomized trial of surveillance colonoscopy in IBD. *Inflamm Bowel Dis*. 1998;4:132-141.

44. Choi PM, Nugent FW, Schoetz DJ Jr, Silverman ML, Haggitt RC. Colonoscopic surveillance reduces mortality from colorectal cancer in ulcerative colitis. *Gastroenterology*. 1993;105:418-424.

45. Connell WR, Lennard-Jones JE, Williams CB, Talbot IC, Price AB, Wilkinson KH. Factors affecting the outcome of endoscopic surveillance for cancer in ulcerative colitis. *Gastroenterology*. 1994;107:934-944.

46. Karlen P, Kornfeld D, Brostrom O, Lofberg R, Persson PG, Ekbom A. Is colonoscopic surveillance reducing colorectal cancer mortality in ulcerative colitis? A population based case control study. *Gut*. 1998;42:711-714.

47. Eaden JA, Ward BA, Mayberry JF. How gastroenterologists screen for colonic cancer in ulcerative colitis: an analysis of performance. *Gastrointest Endosc*. 2000;51:123-128.

48. Rubin CE, Haggitt RC, Burmer GC, et al. DNA aneuploidy in colonic biopsies predicts future development of dysplasia in ulcerative colitis. *Gastroenterology*. 1992;103:1611-1620.

49. Thomas T, Nair P, Dronfield MW, Mayberry JF. Management of low and high-grade dysplasia in inflammatory bowel disease: the gastroenterologists' perspective and current practice in the United Kingdom. *Eur J Gastroenterol Hepatol*. 2005;17:1317-1324.

50. Velayos FS, Liu L, Lewis JD, et al. Prevalence of colorectal cancer surveillance for ulcerative colitis in an integrated health care delivery system. *Gastroenterology*. 2010;139:1511-1518.

51. Awais D, Velayos F, Ullman T, Higgins PD. Colon cancer risk perception in ulcerative colitis: patients overestimate the risk, but disagree with the therapy. *Gastroenterology.* 2009;136:A198-A199.

52. Woolrich AJ, DaSilva MD, Korelitz BI. Surveillance in the routine management of ulcerative colitis: the predictive value of low-grade dysplasia. *Gastroenterology.* 1992;103:431-438.

53. Toruner M, Harewood GC, Loftus EV Jr, et al. Endoscopic factors in the diagnosis of colorectal dysplasia in chronic inflammatory bowel disease. *Inflamm Bowel Dis.* 2005; 11:428-434.

54. Kudo S. Endoscopic mucosal resection of flat and depressed types of early colorectal cancer. *Endoscopy.* 1993;25:455-461.

55. Wong Kee Song LM, Adler DG, Chand B, et al. Chromoendoscopy. *Gastrointest Endosc.* 2007;66:639-649.

56. Davies J, Burke D, Olliver JR, Hardie LJ, Wild CP, Routledge MN. Methylene blue but not indigo carmine causes DNA damage to colonocytes in vitro and in vivo at concentrations used in clinical chromoendoscopy. *Gut.* 2007;56:155-156.

57. Hurlstone DP, McAlindon ME, Sanders DS, Koegh R, Lobo AJ, Cross SS. Further validation of high-magnification chromoscopic-colonoscopy for the detection of intraepithelial neoplasia and colon cancer in ulcerative colitis. *Gastroenterology.* 2004;126:376-378.

58. Kiesslich R, Fritsch J, Holtmann M, et al. Methylene blue-aided chromoendoscopy for the detection of intraepithelial neoplasia and colon cancer in ulcerative colitis. *Gastroenterology.* 2003;124:880-888.

59. Hurlstone DP, Sanders DS, Lobo AJ, McAlindon ME, Cross SS. Indigo carmine-assisted high-magnification chromoscopic colonoscopy for the detection and characterisation of intraepithelial neoplasia in ulcerative colitis: a prospective evaluation. *Endoscopy.* 2005; 37:1186-1192.

60. Rutter MD, Saunders BP, Schofield G, Forbes A, Price AB, Talbot IC. Pancolonic indigo carmine dye spraying for the detection of dysplasia in ulcerative colitis. *Gut.* 2004;53:256-260.

61. Livia B, Pierre M, Simon T, et al. European evidence-based consensus on the management of ulcerative colitis: special situations. *J Crohns Colitis.* 2008;2:63-92.

62. Dekker E, van den Broek FJ, Reitsma JB, et al. Narrow-band imaging compared with conventional colonoscopy for the detection of dysplasia in patients with longstanding ulcerative colitis. *Endoscopy.* 2007;39:216-221.

63. Eaden J, Abrams K, McKay H, Denley H, Mayberry J. Inter-observer variation between general and specialist gastrointestinal pathologists when grading dysplasia in ulcerative colitis. *J Pathol.* 2001;194:152-157.

64. Farraye FA, Odze RD, Eaden J, Itzkowitz SH. AGA technical review on the diagnosis and management of colorectal neoplasia in inflammatory bowel disease. *Gastroenterology.* 2010;138:746-774.

65. Engelsgjerd M, Farraye FA, Odze RD. Polypectomy may be adequate treatment for adenoma-like dysplastic lesions in chronic ulcerative colitis. *Gastroenterology.* 1999;117:1288-1294.

66. Rubin PH, Friedman S, Harpaz N, et al. Colonoscopic polypectomy in chronic colitis: conservative management after endoscopic resection of dysplastic polyps. *Gastroenterology.* 1999;117:1295-1300.

67. Vieth M, Behrens H, Stolte M. Sporadic adenoma in ulcerative colitis: endoscopic resection is an adequate treatment. *Gut.* 2006;55:1151-1155.

68. Odze RD, Farraye FA, Hecht JL, Hornick JL. Long-term follow-up after polypectomy treatment for adenoma-like dysplastic lesions in ulcerative colitis. *Clin Gastroenterol Hepatol.* 2004;2:534-541.

69. Blackstone MO, Riddell RH, Rogers BH, Levin B. Dysplasia-associated lesion or mass (DALM) detected by colonoscopy in long-standing ulcerative colitis: an indication for colectomy. *Gastroenterology.* 1981;80:366-374.

70. Connell WR, Talbot IC, Harpaz N, et al. Clinicopathological characteristics of colorectal carcinoma complicating ulcerative colitis. *Gut.* 1994;35:1419-1423.

71. Ullman T, Croog V, Harpaz N, Sachar D, Itzkowitz S. Progression of flat low-grade dysplasia to advanced neoplasia in patients with ulcerative colitis. *Gastroenterology.* 2003;125: 1311-1319.

72. Ullman TA, Loftus EV Jr, Kakar S, Burgart LJ, Sandborn WJ, Tremaine WJ. The fate of low grade dysplasia in ulcerative colitis. *Am J Gastroenterol.* 2002;97:922-927.

73. Lindberg B, Persson B, Veress B, Ingelman-Sundberg H, Granqvist S. Twenty years' colonoscopic surveillance of patients with ulcerative colitis. Detection of dysplastic and malignant transformation. *Scand J Gastroenterol.* 1996;31:1195-1204.

74. Befrits R, Ljung T, Jaramillo E, Rubio C. Low-grade dysplasia in extensive, long-standing inflammatory bowel disease: a follow-up study. *Dis Colon Rectum.* 2002;45:615-620.

75. Lim CH, Dixon MF, Vail A, Forman D, Lynch DA, Axon AT. Ten year follow up of ulcerative colitis patients with and without low grade dysplasia. *Gut.* 2003;52:1127-1132.

76. van Schaik FD, ten Kate FJ, Offerhaus GJ, et al. Dutch initiative on Crohn and colitis. *Inflamm Bowel Dis.* 2011;17(5):1108-1116.

77. Nguyen GC, Frick KD, Dassopoulos T. Medical decision analysis for the management of unifocal, flat, low-grade dysplasia in ulcerative colitis. *Gastrointest Endosc.* 2009;69:1299-1310.

78. Rutter MD, Saunders BP, Wilkinson KH, et al. Cancer surveillance in longstanding ulcerative colitis: endoscopic appearances help predict cancer risk. *Gut.* 2004;53:1813-1816.

79. Allgayer H. Review article: mechanisms of action of mesalazine in preventing colorectal carcinoma in inflammatory bowel disease. *Aliment Pharmacol Ther.* 2003;18(suppl 2):10-14.

80. Tung BY, Emond MJ, Haggitt RC, et al. Ursodiol use is associated with lower prevalence of colonic neoplasia in patients with ulcerative colitis and primary sclerosing cholangitis. *Ann Intern Med.* 2001;134:89-95.

81. Pardi DS, Loftus EV Jr, Kremers WK, Keach J, Lindor KD. Ursodeoxycholic acid as a chemopreventive agent in patients with ulcerative colitis and primary sclerosing cholangitis. *Gastroenterology.* 2003;124:889-893.

82. Wolf JM, Rybicki LA, Lashner BA. The impact of ursodeoxycholic acid on cancer, dysplasia and mortality in ulcerative colitis patients with primary sclerosing cholangitis. *Aliment Pharmacol Ther.* 2005;22:783-788.

SUGGESTED READINGS

Bernstein CN, Shanahan F, Weinstein WM. Are we telling patients the truth about surveillance colonoscopy in ulcerative colitis? *Lancet.* 1994;343(8889):71-74.

Canavan C, Abrams KR, Mayberry J. Meta-analysis: colorectal and small bowel cancer risk in patients with Crohn's disease. *Aliment Pharmacol Ther.* 2006;23(8):1097-1104.

Ekbom A, Helmick C, Zack M. Increased risk of large-bowel cancer in Crohn's disease with colonic involvement. *Lancet.* 1990;336(8711):357-359.

Ekbom A, Helmick C, Zack M, Adami HO. Ulcerative colitis and colorectal cancer. A population-based study. *N Engl J Med.* 1990;323(18):1228-1233.

Engelsgjerd M, Farraye FA, Odze RD. Polypectomy may be adequate treatment for adenoma-like dysplastic lesions in chronic ulcerative colitis. *Gastroenterology.* 1999;117(6):1288-1294.

Farraye FA, Odze RD, Eaden J, et al. AGA medical position statement on the diagnosis and management of colorectal neoplasia in inflammatory bowel disease. *Gastroenterology.* 2010; 138(2):738-745.

Itzkowitz SH, Present DH. Consensus conference: colorectal cancer screening and surveillance in inflammatory bowel disease. *Inflamm Bowel Dis.* 2005;11(3):314-321.

Marion JF, Waye JD, Present DH, et al. Chromoendoscopy-targeted biopsies are superior to standard colonoscopic surveillance for detecting dysplasia in inflammatory bowel disease patients: a prospective endoscopic trial. *Am J Gastroenterol.* 2008;103(9):2342-2349.

Rubin PH, Friedman S, Harpaz N, et al. Colonoscopic polypectomy in chronic colitis: conservative management after endoscopic resection of dysplastic polyps. *Gastroenterology.* 1999;117(6):1295-1300.

Rutter M, Saunders B, Wilkinson K, et al. Severity of inflammation is a risk factor for colorectal neoplasia in ulcerative colitis. *Gastroenterology.* 2004;126(2):451-459.

Rutter MD, Saunders BP, Wilkinson KH, et al. Thirty-year analysis of a colonoscopic surveillance program for neoplasia in ulcerative colitis. *Gastroenterology.* 2006;130(4):1030-1038.

Velayos FS, Loftus EV Jr, Jess T. Predictive and protective factors associated with colorectal cancer in ulcerative colitis: a case-control study. *Gastroenterology.* 2006;130(7):1941-1949.

Infections in IBD
Clostridium difficile *and* Cytomegalovirus

Ashwin N. Ananthakrishnan, MD, MPH

Inflammatory bowel diseases (IBDs), comprising Crohn's disease (CD) and ulcerative colitis (UC), are lifelong immunologically mediated disorders affecting the gastrointestinal tract. With an onset often during young adulthood, IBD has a relapsing-remitting course. The majority of relapses relate to the underlying disease, but in a significant proportion of patients, disease flares are triggered by, or are due to, superimposed gastrointestinal infections. The 2 most well recognized among such infections are those due to *Clostridium difficile* and cytomegalovirus (CMV).

CLOSTRIDIUM DIFFICILE INFECTION

The past 2 decades have seen an alarming rise in the incidence of *C difficile* among hospitalized patients.[1-3] Initially recognized as the etiologic agent for antibiotic-associated pseudomembranous colitis,[4] *C difficile* is the most common cause of health care–associated diarrhea. Also concerning is the rising incidence of *C difficile* as a community-acquired infection in populations not previously considered high risk.[5] One such at-risk cohort that is being increasingly recognized to be susceptible to the adverse impact of *C difficile* infection (CDI) consists of patients with underlying IBD.[6] It is essential for the clinician to have a high index of suspicion for CDI in IBD patients for the following reasons: (1) the clinical presentation of CDI and IBD flares are similar, but treatment pathways are markedly divergent, (2) there is significant morbidity and mortality associated with CDI in patients with IBD, and (3) early and effective antibiotic therapy often avoids adverse outcomes including the need for hospitalization or colectomy.

Regueiro MD, Swoger JM, eds.
Clinical Challenges and Complications of IBD (pp 101-124).
© 2013 Taylor & Francis Group.

Pathogenesis

C difficile is a gram-positive, spore-forming anaerobe identified in 1978 by Bartlett et al to be the causative organism for antibiotic-associated pseudo-membranous colitis.[4] It is a toxigenic bacterium that exerts its effect primarily through the production of 2 cytotoxins: toxins A and B, encoded by the genes tcd A and tcd B, respectively, and located within the 19.6-kb pathogenicity locus (PaLoc).[7,8] After receptor-mediated endocytosis, the toxins lead to pore formation, glycosylation of the structural rho and ras proteins, disruption of the epithelial cytoskeleton and intercellular tight junctions, which leads to the voluminous watery diarrhea often associated with CDI.[7,8] Although toxin A was previously considered the primary toxin of interest, recent research suggests that significant infection can occur with strains that produce toxin B alone,[7] accounting for up to 7% of all CDIs.[9,10] Several other toxins have also been described but their roles are less clearly defined. The newly described binary toxin (CDT) encoded within a distinct locus (CdtLoc) appears to interfere with the regulation of tcd A and tcd B, leading to highly toxigenic strains producing a greater quantity of toxins A and B and to more severe disease.[7,11]

Recent studies have also highlighted the development of novel epidemic strains of *C difficile*, the most prominent being BI/NAP1/027 (restriction-endonuclease analysis group BI, North American pulsed-field gel electrophoresis type 1, polymerase chain reaction ribotype 027).[12,13] This newly described ribotype of *C difficile* was responsible for severe outbreaks, initially in the Quebec province of Canada, but subsequently noted from other parts of the world. The impact of this strain on IBD patients is yet to be defined; however, initial reports do not suggest an increased frequency of occurrence.[14] A second epidemic strain described from the Netherlands, ribotype 078, may cause severe community-acquired disease among younger patients.[15]

Prevalence

Early studies reported *C difficile* infrequently among IBD patients presenting with a disease flare.[16-19] However, paralleling the rising tide of CDI in the general population, the past decade has seen a string of reports highlighting the increase in incidence of *C difficile* among patients with IBD.[14,20-24] A single-center study by Rodemann et al demonstrated a doubling of incidence of CDI among patients with CD (from 9.5 to 22.3 per 1000 admissions) and a tripling among those with UC (from 18.4 to 57.6 per 1000 admissions) from 1998 to 2004.[24] Other single-center studies reported similar rising trends,[21] a finding subsequently corroborated from a national hospitalization discharge database by Ananthakrishnan et al using the Nationwide Inpatient Sample.[20] Ongoing analysis since the publication of that study has shown a continued upward trend till at least 2007 (the most recent data available). Although these prevalence estimates utilize the entire IBD population as the denominator, restricting analysis only to patients presenting with symptoms of a disease flare led to a prevalence of 47% among 99 UC patients admitted to Mount

Table 6-1. Risk Factors for Clostridium difficile Infection	
HOST FACTORS	ENVIRONMENTAL FACTORS
Age Comorbidities Host immune response Colonic disease UC>CD Disease severity	Antibiotic use Immunosuppressive therapy C difficile strain—BI/NAP 1/027 Contact with health care workers
CD = Crohn's disease; UC = ulcerative colitis	

Sinai hospital.[22] The pediatric IBD population is not excluded from the rising incidence of CDI with a rate of 25% being reported from a single pediatric IBD center in Italy.[25] The reason behind this continuing rise is yet to be clearly defined. There are several likely factors including host susceptibility (increasing age of IBD population, use of immunosuppression), widespread use of broad-spectrum antibiotics, frequent health care contact, as well as variation in C difficile itself, leading to strains with greater pathogenicity and propensity to cause community-acquired infections even in the absence of the traditional risk factors.

RISK FACTORS

The risk factors for acquisition of C difficile can be divided into host factors and those related to the environment (Table 6-1).

Intrinsic (Host) Factors

Older age and greater comorbidity are well-recognized risk factors for CDI and may be associated with a higher likelihood of an adverse outcome.[2,23,26,27] Host immunity also plays a role in CDI pathogenesis with individuals producing lower level of antibodies to C difficile toxins being more likely to develop symptomatic disease.[28,29]

There are several disease-specific risk factors for CDI in patients with IBD. Presence of colonic disease confers a 3-fold greater risk (odds ratio [OR] 3.12, 95% confidence interval [CI] 1.22 to 8.02).[21] More extensive colonic disease is associated with a greater risk for CDI.[30] However, this does not seem to be an essential factor, as cases of CDI have been reported from ileal pouches and small bowel stomas in patients who have undergone colectomy. CDI is also more common in patients with UC compared to those with CD.[20] The role of disease activity in conferring CDI risk is less clear as there are no prospective studies available to answer this question. Patients with CDI tend to have more severe disease[25]; however, whether this is a consequence of or a risk factor for CDI is yet to be defined.

Extrinsic Factors

The classically described risk factor for CDI is use of broad-spectrum antibiotics.[2,26,27] By suppressing normal intestinal flora, this allows for the proliferation of *C difficile*, a more resistant organism, within the intestine. First described with the use of clindamycin,[4] CDI can be associated with the use of any broad-spectrum antibiotic. Recent attention has been focused on the widespread use of fluoroquinolones as a risk factor[31,32]; hospital-wide increases in prescription of these broad-spectrum antibiotics have resulted in a significant increase in the rate of CDI. Conversely, policies that aim to limit the use of broad-spectrum agents and use more selective antibiotics, thus decreasing the selective pressure exerted by the broad-spectrum agents, may be helpful in curtailing local epidemics of CDI. Therapeutic immunosuppression associated with organ transplant and systemic chemotherapy is another well-recognized factor that increases the risk of CDI.[26,27] This is an especially important risk factor in IBD patients, as a significant proportion of them are immunosuppressed, either due to medications or due to the disease itself. In the study by Issa et al, use of maintenance immunosuppressive therapy was associated with a nearly 3-fold increase in CDI (OR 2.58, 95% CI 1.28 to 5.12),[21] a finding confirmed by other subsequent studies.[14] Other medications that have been proposed to increase the risk for CDI, such as proton pump inhibitor[33] therapy, have not consistently been shown to be risk factors in the IBD population.[34]

CLINICAL FEATURES

The signs and symptoms of CDI are often indistinguishable from that of an IBD flare. Watery diarrhea with or without overt bleeding, abdominal pain and tenderness, and systemic symptoms of fever or malaise may be seen with both conditions. Laboratory evaluation may reveal leukocytosis, anemia, or hypoalbuminemia, representing prolonged poorly controlled disease. Unexplained leukocytosis or systemic symptoms in a hospitalized IBD patient should prompt investigation for CDI. Radiologic evaluation may yield supportive information with computed tomography scans being preferred to demonstrate extent and severity of colitis demonstrated in the form of colonic wall thickening and enhancement. Plain films are usually sufficient to make the diagnosis of toxic megacolon or free perforation in the patients with fulminant disease. Radiologic imaging is also useful to rule out other potential causes for symptoms, such as bowel obstruction or fistulizing disease.

Endoscopic evaluation is useful in identifying severity of disease, but plays a limited role in diagnosing CDI as the findings of erythema, exudates, and ulcerations are nonspecific and fail to differentiate IBD disease activity from CDI. The classically described sign of CDI is the pseudomembrane, which consists of necrotic debris and sloughed mucosa[26] (Figure 6-1). This correlates histologically with the "volcano" lesion, an eruption of inflammatory cell infiltrate in the setting of mucosal ulceration. However, pseudomembranes appear

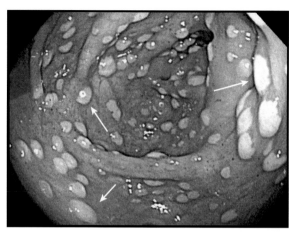

Figure 6-1. Endoscopic image showing *C difficile* colitis in a patient with UC. Note the multiple pseudomembranes (arrows) typically seen in this condition. (Reprinted with permission of Jason M. Swoger, MD, MPH.)

to be rarely seen in IBD patients with CDI. In 2 recent studies providing endoscopic information, pseudomembranes were not seen in any of the IBD patients with CDI.[14,21]

IMPACT OF *CLOSTRIDIUM DIFFICILE* INFECTION ON IBD OUTCOMES

There is a growing body of evidence on the impact of CDI on patients with IBD. In an analysis using the Nationwide Inpatient Sample, Ananthakrishnan et al demonstrated that IBD patients with CDI have a 4-fold greater inhospital mortality (OR 4.7, 95% CI 2.9 to 7.9) compared to IBD patients without CDI.[20] In addition, IBD patients with CDI may also have a substantial risk of requiring colectomy. In another series from the same institution, up to 45% of patients required emergent colectomy[21]; the rate in a second study of UC patients was 23%.[22] IBD patients with CDI may have a 6-fold increase in colectomy risk (OR 6.6, 95% CI 4.7 to 9.3) compared to non-IBD patients, and have a 40% to 60% increase in the length of hospital stay and hospitalization charges.[20,23] Beyond the short-term impact, IBD patients may also have a more long-term modification of their disease course after a single episode of CDI, although further research is needed to answer this question. Up to half the IBD patients with CDI may require an escalation of their medical maintenance therapy in the year following the episode of CDI compared to the year prior.[35] Other studies have shown an increased need for emergency room visits related to patients' disease activity in the year following CDI.[22]

DIAGNOSIS

The diagnosis of CDI depends on the demonstration of toxin, or the toxin-producing bacterial strain in the stool.[36,37] The gold standard is culture of the organism from the stool; however, this lacks the ability to distinguish toxigenic from non–toxin-producing strains and needs to be combined with cell culture cytotoxicity assay for detection of toxin.[26,27,38] These tests are also time consuming and require significant technical expertise, precluding widespread use. More recent testing has relied on using enzyme immunosorbent assay (EIA) tests for direct detection of the *C difficile* toxins. Earlier generation EIAs detected only toxin A, thus missing a significant proportion of infections that were due to strains producing toxin B alone. The widely used newer generation EIAs have substantially greater sensitivity and specificity. The positive and negative predictive values depend on the prevalence of CDI in the population being tested and vary from 52% to 95% and 70% to 100%, respectively.[26,27,36,37] A more recent tool for the diagnosis of *C difficile* uses real-time PCR to demonstrate the toxin-producing genes (tcd B, tcd C) and has a greater sensitivity (85% to 100%), specificity, and positive and negative predictive values compared to the EIA tests.[37] The diagnostic yield of any of the above tests may be improved by multiple-sample testing depending on the clinical scenario.[21] In a patient with low pretest probability, a single negative EIA may be sufficient to rule out CDI. However, in individuals with a high pretest probability, testing of multiple samples may be necessary to confidently rule out CDI. Issa et al demonstrated that the yield of EIA increases from 54% to 92% when the number of samples tested increased from 1 to 4.[21]

TREATMENT

Initial Episode

The 2 options available for the treatment of the initial episode of CDI are metronidazole and vancomycin, of which only the latter has received approval from the Food and Drug Administration for this use (Table 6-2).[2,27,39,40] Cessation of the offending antibiotic should be recommended in all cases, as in a small fraction of patients this may be the only necessary step to treat CDI.[14] The vast majority of patients will require therapy with either metronidazole or vancomycin. Metronidazole may be used in a dose of 500 mg every 8 hours administered orally or intravenously. Metronidazole is much less expensive than vancomycin ($20 for a 10-day course compared to $300 to $600 for oral vancomycin) but may be associated with gastrointestinal adverse effects, neuropathy with long-term use, and potentially greater rates of treatment failure.[41] Vancomycin is administered orally in a dose of 125 to 500 mg every 6 hours.[36] Both these agents act locally by achieving adequate concentration within the colonic lumen; vancomycin achieves a greater fecal concentration-to-maximum minimal inhibitory concentration ratio than metronidazole.[41] Intravenous vancomycin is not secreted into the colonic lumen and has no role in the treatment of CDI.

The choice of the initial antibiotic depends on the severity of the underlying CDI.[41-43] Two studies have yielded data on their comparative efficacy in severe disease. Zar et al used a scoring system composed of fever, leukocytosis, age, albumin, and presence of pseudomembranes to stratify severity of CDI.[44] In patients with mild disease, both vancomycin and metronidazole had

Table 6-2. Recommendations for the Treatment of Clostridium difficile Infection

Type of Infection	Treatment Course

Initial diagnosis	Stop offending antibiotic
	Metronidazole (IV or PO)—500 mg every 8 hours
	Vancomycin (PO)—125 to 500 mg every 6 hours*
	
	Possible benefit
	Probiotics—*S boulardii*
	Bile-salt binding resins (cholestyramine)
	Antibiotics
	   Teicoplanin
	   Nitazoxanide

Refractory disease	Vancomycin (PO)—500 mg every 6 hours Metronidazole (IV)—500 mg every 8 hours Vancomycin (per rectum)—0.5 to 1 g in 100 to 1000 mL NS IVIG—150 to 400 mg/kg Fecal biotherapy Colectomy
Recurrent infection	Vancomycin (PO) taper—4 to 8 week course Rifaximin—2 to 4 weeks following vancomycin Probiotics—*S boulardii* IVIG Rifampin Monoclonal antibody against toxins A and B

g = gram; IV = intravenous; IVIG = intravenous immunoglobulin; mg = milligram; NS = normal saline; PO = oral; PR = per rectum
*Vancomycin may be more effective initial therapy in patients with severe disease.

comparable efficacy (98% versus 90%, $P = 0.36$), but vancomycin was significantly superior in those with severe disease (97% versus 76%, $P = 0.02$).[44] A second study comparing the 2 agents with tolevamer also showed a significantly superior efficacy with vancomycin in those with severe, but not mild or moderate, disease.[45] There are limited data on the efficacy of these agents specifically in the IBD population, particularly with regard to what constitutes severe disease. Arguably patients requiring hospitalization represent a more severe cohort who may warrant initial therapy with vancomycin, while ambulatory patients with mild disease may be treated with oral metronidazole.

Other agents that have been used for treatment of CDI but not used widely include probiotics (particularly *Saccharomyces boulardii*), anion binding resins (cholestyramine, colestipol), and antibiotics such as teicoplanin and nitazoxanide.[40,43] There are limited data on utilizing these agents as monotherapy in patients with IBD.

As CDI often mimics or is accompanied by an IBD flare, and immunosuppression is a risk factor for worse outcomes from CDI, the difficult question on what to do with immunosuppressive therapy in IBD patients with CDI often arises. There are limited high-quality data to answer this question. In a retrospective study by Ben-Horin et al, patients with combined antibiotic and immunosuppressive treatment had worse outcomes compared to those treated with antibiotics alone.[46] However, the retrospective study design made it difficult to exclude confounding by indication, where combined therapy may have been administered to sicker patients who are independently at a higher risk of adverse outcomes. Overall, it is our practice to avoid escalating immunosuppressive therapy in IBD patients with active untreated CDI while minimizing the dose of systemic steroids. However, in patients with fulminant disease, it may often be essential to concurrently use both medications or even initiate anti-tumor necrosis factor (TNF) therapy.

Refractory Disease

Patients with disease refractory to metronidazole may be switched to oral vancomycin therapy. For those not responding to low-dose vancomycin, a higher dose (500 mg orally every 6 hours) may be effective. Patients with slow intestinal transit or ileus may not achieve adequate colonic luminal concentration with oral vancomycin; in such patients intravenous metronidazole may be added as adjunct therapy.[36] Another option in such patients is intracolonic administration of vancomycin, using a rectal tube or Foley catheter, at a dose of 0.5 to 1 g of drug mixed in 100 to 1000 mL of normal saline.[27,39,43] This may be administered 2 to 4 times daily and has achieved good response in small case series. Yet another therapeutic option in those with severe, refractory disease is intravenous immunoglobulin (IVIG).[47] In a case series, 14 patients who had failed a median of 3 courses of metronidazole or vancomycin were given IVIG 150 or 400 mg/kg as a single infusion. After a median of 10 days (range 2 to 26 days), 9 patients (64%) responded while 4 patients died of other causes.[48] A second, larger case series yielded a success rate of only 43%, demonstrating the severity of both concurrent illness and CDI in this refractory cohort.[49] Fecal biotherapy (nasoduodenal or colonic administration) with healthy donor feces has shown promising results (80% to 90% success rate) and works on the principle of reconstituting normal intestinal flora.[2] There is limited experience with this therapy in IBD.

Early surgical consultation is essential in patients with refractory disease, as delayed surgery may be associated with substantial morbidity and morbidity. The procedure of choice is total or subtotal colectomy with an end ileostomy, as segmental resection is often associated with worse outcomes.

Recurrent Infection

The rate of recurrence of CDI after the initial episode is 15% to 35% with a higher rate after the first recurrence (35% to 60%).[27] The risk factors for recurrent disease include continued use of antibiotics (OR 4.23, 95% CI 2.10 to 8.55), antacid use (OR 2.15, 95% CI 1.13 to 4.08), and older age (OR 1.62, 95% CI 1.11 to 2.36).[50] The rate of recurrence in IBD patients seems to be similar to the non-IBD cohort.[21] In patients with mild disease, retreatment with the initial antibiotic has been recommended, although switching to vancomycin in patients previously treated with metronidazole is a reasonable alternative.[36] A prolonged course of vanco-mycin with a gradual taper over several weeks has achieved success in a cohort of patients.[51] Another antibiotic that has been used for recurrent disease is rifaxi-min, a nonabsorbed oral antibiotic that may be administered as a "chaser" for 2 to 4 weeks following a course of vancomycin.[52,53] Probiotics, in particular *S boulardii*, have also been shown to reduce the rate of recurrence from 50% to 17%.[54] IVIG and rifampin are other alternatives that have been tried in small series.[51] A recent phase II trial randomized 200 patients to a single infusion of a monoclonal anti-body against toxins A and B compared to placebo. The rate of recurrence was significantly lower in the antibody group (7%) compared to placebo (25%).[55]

Addressing modifiable risk factors (antibiotic use) and potential environ-mental sources of reinfection are essential to decrease risk of recurrent disease. Strict hand hygiene and hand-washing techniques should be emphasized to both the patient and family members. Appropriate isolation and decontamina-tion procedures should be followed in health care settings.

CLOSTRIDIUM DIFFICILE POUCHITIS AND ENTERITIS

CDI has been reported in the pouches of patients who have undergone total proctocolectomy with ileal pouch-anal anastomosis for refractory UC.[56-58] In the study by Shen and colleagues, nearly one-fifth (18.3%) of 115 patients with an ileo-anal pouch were positive for *C difficile* using enzyme-linked immunosor-bent assay.[58] CDI has also been reported from diverted bowel and causes severe enteritis in patients with an end ileostomy.[59-61] The treatment for patients with either of these conditions is similar to the treatment of *C difficile* colitis.

Infection Control

Appropriate infection control measures are an essential part of the manage-ment of CDI in the health care setting.[62,63] Quaternary ammonium–based solutions are not as effective as hypochlorite, which should be the preferred antispectic for decontamination.[36,62] Vigorous soap-and-water hand washing is essential before and after contact with each patient with suspected CDI, as alcohol-based hand rubs may not be effective against *C difficile* spores.[64] In gastrointestinal units, standard endoscope decontamination procedures may be followed.[62]

CYTOMEGALOVIRUS INFECTIONS

CMV is a 230-kb double-stranded DNA virus belonging to the *Herpesviridae* family.[65] The first report of CMV infection in a patient with UC was by Powell et al in 1961.[66] Despite several subsequent reports of such infections in

IBD patients,[67] several questions about the exact relationship between CMV and IBD remain unanswered. Some authors have questioned whether CMV is a true pathogen or represents a secondary opportunistic infection in the setting of severe disease in patients with steroid-refractory colitis.[68] However, several lines of evidence support the true pathogenic role of CMV in severe colitis. The high incidence of adverse outcomes in patients with severe IBD who develop CMV infection, and the good response to specific antiviral therapy without need for escalation of immunosuppression, support the hypothesis that CMV represents a true pathogenic infection in patients with severe colitis. The role of CMV is less clear in those with milder colitis responsive to steroids or conventional immunosuppressive therapy.

PATHOGENESIS

Serological evidence of prior CMV infection may be seen in 40% to 100% of the population,[69] with a similar seroprevalence in IBD patients compared to controls.[70] Like other members of the *Herpesviridae* family, CMV has a predilection for remaining latent following an initial primary infection, with the potential for subsequent reactivation.[67,68,71] Several mechanisms have been proposed to explain this. These include suppression of the antigen presentation by the major histocompatibility complex antigens, neutralization of host antibodies, interference with the cytotoxic function of the natural killer lymphocyte (a key member of antiviral defense), and inhibition of host expression of inflammatory cytokines.[68] In HIV patients, CD4+ T-cell count is important in disease pathogenesis, with CMV disease being seen with CD4+ T-cell counts below 100/μL.[65] Transmission of CMV is primarily through nonsexual contact with bodily fluids.

CMV has a tropism toward inflamed tissue.[72-74] In animal models, CMV tends to infect rapidly proliferating cells in granulation tissue.[74] In endoscopic biopsies, CMV immunostaining is often positive within the vascular endothelial cell or within the lamina propria/submucosa of inflamed areas[72] and is rarely found in areas without inflammation. The affinity of CMV to endothelial cells enables it to play a direct role in production of inflammatory cytokines when reactivated, setting up a cycle of leukocyte adhesion, migration, and local inflammation.[67,75] Proinflammatory cytokines including TNF-α induce reactivation of CMV,[67] which induces migration of monocytes to colonic tissue and differentiation into macrophages, which also function as reservoirs for CMV.[67,73] The tropism of CMV to the inflamed colon is further supported by the fact that patients who undergo proctocolectomy for refractory disease do not require further antiviral therapy.[76]

PREVALENCE

The prevalence of CMV disease in IBD is difficult to estimate for several reasons. Tertiary referral center cohorts may suffer from referral biases. Papadakis et al calculated a prevalence of 0.53% among their cohort of 1895 patients.[77]

However, this was not an accurate prevalence estimate as only a small fraction of patients were tested for CMV. Comparing prevalence across studies is also subject to potential errors as studies differ based on their definition of CMV infection. Several studies required demonstration of CMV in colonic tissue,[70,72,78,79] whereas in other studies, demonstrating the presence of viremia was considered sufficient evidence for CMV disease.[80] However, there are a few prospective studies that provide reliable prevalence estimates. Domenech et al assembled a cohort of UC patients categorized as having severe colitis responsive to intravenous steroids ($n = 25$), steroid-refractory colitis ($n = 19$), inactive disease treated with azathioprine ($n = 25$) or mesalamine ($n = 25$), and healthy controls ($n = 25$).[70] Despite a similar seroprevalence (CMV-IgG +) in all 5 groups, ranging from 61% to 76%, CMV disease was found in 6 patients, all of whom belonged to the steroid-refractory group (32%). In an earlier Italian series by Cottone et al, 7 of 19 (30%) patients with steroid-refractory severe colitis were positive for CMV on rectal biopsy.[78] A second Italian prospective by Criscuoli et al identified CMV infection in 21% of patients admitted with acute severe colitis and 33% of those with steroid-refractory disease.[79] Several retrospective reports also arrived at similar prevalence estimates of CMV disease between 20% and 40% among patients hospitalized with steroid-refractory UC.[72,76,81] Studies examining colectomy specimens have reported similar prevalence among those with disease severe enough to require surgery.[76]

CLINICAL FEATURES

The vast majority of CMV infections in immunocompetent adults are asymptomatic. Some patients present with a mononucleosis-like syndrome, with fever, lymphadenopathy, and myalgias. This illness usually has a self-limiting course and rarely requires antiviral therapy. In contrast, immunosuppressed individuals are more likely to develop symptomatic disease related to primary or reactivated CMV infection and can suffer a variety of end-organ manifestations, including retinitis, encephalitis, hepatitis, and colitis. The majority of reports of CMV colitis complicating IBD patients are in patients with long-established disease, although in one series 4 of 16 patients with CMV infection were newly diagnosed with UC.[82]

Symptoms of CMV colitis are often indistinguishable from that of underlying IBD activity and include diarrhea with or without overt gastrointestinal bleeding, abdominal pain, and fatigue. A high fever is seen more commonly with CMV infection than with active IBD alone and may also represent primary CMV infection.[74,77] The spectrum of disease can range from asymptomatic infection to fulminant colitis and toxic megacolon,[83] and a mortality rate up to 33% in the era prior to antiviral therapy.[84] Untreated CMV infection has been shown to be associated with a high rate of colectomy,[70,82,84] although it is unclear if this rate is in excess of those with CMV-negative steroid-refractory disease.[68] Upper gastrointestinal involvement may also be seen with CMV infection, although it appears to be less common in the IBD population compared to colonic disease.

Figure 6-2. Endoscopic image of CMV colitis in a patient with underlying UC. The CMV-associated ulcers are often deep and cratered, with a characteristic "punched out" appearance. (Reprinted with permission of Jason M. Swoger, MD, MPH.)

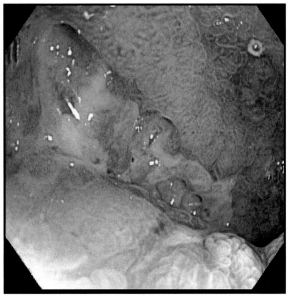

Endoscopic evaluation may reveal erythema, exudates, and erosions with scattered ulcerations, sometimes deep, that may be difficult to differentiate from active IBD[85] (Figure 6-2). The more significant role for endoscopy is to obtain biopsies to demonstrate CMV in the colon. Biopsies from inflamed tissue or from the center of ulcer beds have a higher diagnostic yield, as CMV DNA is often not detected in the uninflammed mucosa.[73] Up to one-third of CMV infections may involve the right colon alone in non-IBD patients.[86] However, the risks of performing a full colonoscopy compared to a flexible sigmoidoscopy should be carefully weighed in patients with severe active colitis who may be at a high risk for procedure-related perforation. In the vast majority of cases, a flexible sigmoidoscopy will be sufficient both to assess severity of colitis and obtain biopsies to diagnose CMV. CMV infection has also been reported in the pediatric age group[87] and in IBD patients with refractory pouchitis[88] and should be considered as a potential etiologic agent in refractory disease in such cohorts.

RISK FACTORS

Some reports suggested an increased risk for infection and adverse outcomes in older patients[80,82] and women,[81,82] although others have failed to find such associations.[73,89] The extent of underlying colitis also does not appear to influence risk of CMV.[73,80,89] CMV is more common in patients with UC compared to CD, suggesting an association with active colonic disease.[89] Therapeutic immunosuppression, malnutrition associated with disease activity, and impaired natural killer cell function have all been proposed as risk factors for CMV in patients with IBD. The risk associated with azathioprine use appears to be low.[70,76,78,90] One consistent association that has been demonstrated is with steroid-refractory disease. This appears to be independent of the potential confounding effect of disease activity because patients with acute severe colitis requiring hospitalization who respond to intravenous steroid therapy appear to be at a lower risk for developing CMV colitis than those with steroid-refractory disease.[70] Whether the CMV infection contributes to the steroid refractoriness, or if use of high-dose steroids predisposes to acquiring "secondary" CMV infection, is not yet clear. The impact of the newer antibodies to anti-TNF-α or other biological therapies on the risk of CMV infection is unclear, but they appear to be safe in preliminary studies.[91]

DIAGNOSIS

Two important disease states that merit distinguishing are *CMV infection* and *CMV disease*.[65,71] CMV infection may be either *latent* (positive serology but no evidence of active viral replication) or *active* (there is evidence of active viral replication in the peripheral blood or tissues). Active CMV disease refers to a state with clinical signs and symptoms of disease and requires the demonstration of virus within the end-organ tissues. There are several tools available to diagnose CMV infection, each with their pros and cons (Table 6-3).

◊ Serology: Demonstration of CMV IgG antibodies has a limited role in diagnosing active CMV infection owing to the high seroprevalence in the population and the inability to distinguish past from current infection. A majority of the patients who develop CMV colitis are IgG positive,[70] suggesting a potential role of IgG as a "screening" test to identify the population at risk.[92] Demonstrating a 4-fold rise in the CMV IgG titer may be useful in diagnosing active infection but is limited by the lack of availability of such paired samples.[71] On the other hand, CMV IgM antibodies may represent active infection but titers may remain elevated for a few months after active infection (false positive) or may remain negative in the immunosuppressed IBD patients (false negative).

◊ CMV antigenemia: Demonstration of the CMV late structural protein pp65 antigen using immunofluoresecent monoclonal antibodies has greater utility than conventional serology, with a sensitivity of 60% to 100% and a higher specificity of 83% to 100%.[65,68,71] However, it may not always correlate well with active CMV colitis. In the series by Domenech et al, 4 of 6 patients with CMV demonstrated on colonic tissue had negative CMV pp65 antigenemia.[70] Only a minority of patients with demonstrable CMV DNA in colonic tissue are positive for CMV antigenemia.[73]

◊ CMV culture: This may be performed in blood or tissue specimens and was previously considered the gold standard. However, there are several limitations to this test, including prolonged turnaround time (1-to 3-week incubation period) and lower sensitivity.[65,71] Conventional cultures require demonstration of CMV cytopathic effect on fibroblast tissue culture. Modifications of this technique include the shell vial

Table 6-3. Diagnostic Modalities for Cytomegalovirus Infection in Inflammatory Bowel Disease Patients

DIAGNOSTIC TOOLS	CHARACTERISTICS
Serology IgG	Limited role Need paired titers to distinguish current from prior infection
IgM	Marker of active infection May remain elevated for months (false positive) May not rise in immunosuppressed patients (false negative)
CMV antigenemia (pp65)	Sensitivity 60% to 100%, specificity 83% to 100% Poor correlation with active CMV colitis
Culture	Low sensitivity, long turnaround time (1 to 3 weeks) More rapid results with shell vial culture (24 to 48 hours)
Histology	Gold standard IHC increases sensitivity
PCR DNA tests Serum	Sensitivity 65% to 100%, specificity 40% to 92% Difficult to interpret—no established threshold for diagnosis
Colonic tissue	High sensitivity False positive if no histologic evidence of disease
Stool	Sensitivity 83% and specificity 93% (versus colonic DNA) Noninvasive

CMV = cytomegalovirus; IBD = inflammatory bowel disease; Ig = immunoglobulin; IHC = immunohistochemistry; PCR = polymerase chain reaction

culture, where the presence of CMV is demonstrated using immuno-fluoresecent monoclonal antibodies to early antigens. This technique provides rapid results within 24 to 48 hours.[65,71]

◊ Histology: Histologic demonstration of CMV in the colon is considered the gold standard for diagnosis of CMV colitis (Figure 6-3). The classic histopathologic changes are enlarged cells (2 to 4 times normal), with eosinophilic intranuclear inclusions and a surrounding halo ("owl's eye" appearance).[68,71,72] Intracytoplasmic inclusions may also frequently be seen. Immunohistochemistry (IHC) is a modification that utilizes

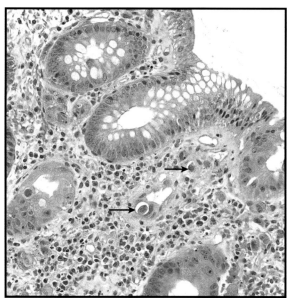

Figure 6-3. Intact colonic epithelium with increased inflammatory cells within lamina propria showing characteristic cellular changes in the colonic epithelium and stromal cells consistent with CMV infection. The arrows point to the characteristic "owl's eye" appearance and smudgy nuclear features often seen with CMV infections. (Hematoxylin and eosin stain, 400) (Reprinted with permission of Jason M. Swoger, MD, MPH.)

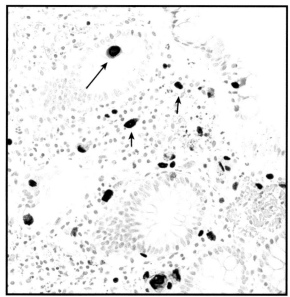

Figure 6-4. Immunohistochemical staining of a colonic mucosal biopsy in a patient with CMV colitis, showing multiple CMV infected cells (arrows). (Reprinted with permission of Jason M. Swoger, MD, MPH.)

monoclonal antibodies against CMV early antigens and is more sensitive than conventional hematoxylin and eosin histology (Figure 6-4). In one series, IHC was positive for CMV in 10 of 40 patients with steroid-refractory colitis while conventional histology identified CMV in only 2 of these patients.[72]

◊ CMV PCR DNA tests: PCR techniques can be used to demonstrate CMV in blood, body fluids, and tissue. It has a high sensitivity (65% to 100%) and specificity (40% to 92%) and is currently the most sensitive test for detecting CMV in blood or plasma.[71,73] CMV viral loads in plasma are lower than in whole blood. Despite the good performance of peripheral blood CMV PCR as a diagnostic tool, one limitation is that without appropriate threshold cutoffs to diagnose active infection, low viral loads are sometimes difficult to interpret, while high viral loads are more likely to represent active disease. Matsuoka et al prospectively studied 69 UC patients with moderate to severe disease. CMV PCR was positive at least once in 52% of the seropositive patients during the 8-week study. However, viral loads remained low, and none of the patients had demonstrable CMV infection on colonic biopsy specimens. Furthermore, three-quarters of the patients (72%) achieved clinical remission with conventional immunosuppressive therapy and without antiviral agents.[80] Kandiel et al proposed a plasma CMV DNA level of 5000 copies/mL (or whole blood copies of 25,000 copies/mL) or greater to represent active CMV infection meriting antiviral treatment in patients with IBD.[71]

◊ CMV DNA PCR in colonic biopsies is likely the most sensitive test for diagnosing CMV colitis but may be associated with false positives[68] in the absence of histologic evidence of disease. Stool CMV DNA testing is another promising tool for the diagnosis of CMV infection in the colon and is more organ specific than peripheral blood. Stool CMV DNA has a sensitivity and specificity of 83% and 93% compared to CMV DNA detection in colonic biopsy tissue[93] and has the added advantages of being noninvasive and less subject to sampling errors[76] than endoscopic biopsies.

CLINICAL COURSE AND TREATMENT

Not all IBD patients with CMV infection require treatment. Those with disease responsive to steroids or conventional immunosuppressive therapy appear to have a favorable clinical course even without antiviral treatment.[72,79,94] On the other hand, steroid-refractory patients who develop CMV colitis have a high risk of colectomy, which is reduced significantly by antiviral therapy. The treatment of choice is ganciclovir in a dose of 5 mg/kg intravenously every 12 hours for a 2- to 3-week period. If the patient is responding after 3 to 5 days, it may be switched to oral valganciclovir to complete the course. In patients who are intolerant or not responding to ganciclovir, foscarnet (90 mg/kg every 12 hours or 60 mg/kg every 8 hours) may be used for a similar treatment duration. Both therapies can have significant side effects including myelosuppression (up to 40% with ganciclovir use), nephrotoxicity (foscarnet), and central nervous system effects (foscarnet). Over two-thirds of patients (67% to 100%) respond with antiviral therapy, with or without reduction in immunosuppression,[68,70,72,73,77-79,95] although up to one-quarter of the patients do not respond to medical therapy and require colectomy.[70,78,95] It is important to remember that a significant proportion of the IBD patients with CMV colitis who require

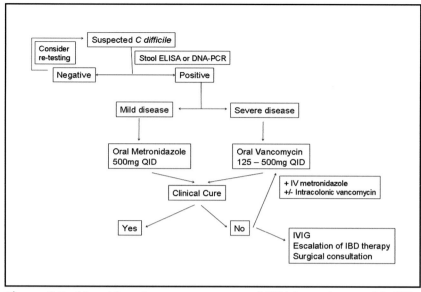

Figure 6-5. Algorithm for management of CDI in patients with IBD. (Reprinted with permission of Jason M. Swoger, MD, MPH.) ELISA = enzyme-linked immunosorbent assay; DNA-PCR = deoxyribonucleic acid-polymerase chain reaction; QID = four times a day; IV = intravenous; IVIG = intravenous immunoglobin

colectomy do so prior to antiviral therapy being initiated[70,82] emphasizing the importance of having a high index of suspicion for early diagnosis and treatment of CMV in steroid-refractory IBD patients.

CONCLUSION

Both *C difficile* and CMV infections lead to refractory disease and significant morbidity in IBD patients and often mimic IBD activity. A high index of suspicion for these infectious complications is essential as substantial benefit can be achieved with early institution of appropriate targeted therapy in either scenario. All IBD patients hospitalized with a disease flare should undergo stool testing for *C difficile* toxin (Figure 6-5). IBD patients with *C difficile* should be started on metronidazole or vancomycin (preferred in those with severe disease). Those with severe colitis refractory to 3 to 7 days of intravenous steroids or anti-TNF therapy should undergo a flexible sigmoidoscopy for obtaining biopsies to look for CMV in colonic tissue (Figure 6-6). Preferred modalities for diagnosis include either CMV DNA PCR in colonic biopsy specimens or IHC. Patients with steroid-refractory colitis and demonstrable CMV disease should receive treatment initially with intravenous ganciclovir and may be switched to oral therapy once they exhibit a response. Early comanagement with surgeons is essential in those with severe disease. Further research is needed focusing on the efficacy of individual agents and treatment algorithms for both CMV and CDI in the IBD population.

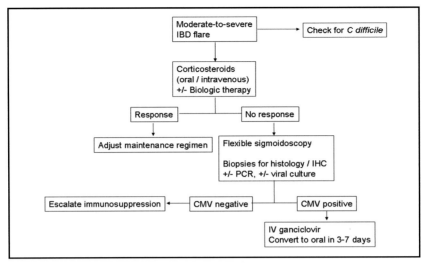

Figure 6-6. Algorithm for management of CMV infection in patients with IBD. (Reprinted with permission of Jason M. Swoger, MD, MPH.) IHC = immunohistochemistry; PCR = polymerase chain reaction; CMV = cytomegalovirus; IV = intravenous

☑Key Points

☑ The incidence of CDI is rising in the hospital setting. Additionally, the incidence of CDI among IBD patients in the community setting, even in the absence of antibiotic exposure, has shown a significant increase.

☑ The clinical symptoms due to CDI and CMV infection are largely indistinguishable from those of an IBD flare. These infectious entities need to be considered and evaluated for early in the hospital course.

☑ The initial treatment of CDI should be oral metronidazole or vancomycin, with the latter having been shown to be more effective in patients with risk factors for severe disease.

☑ CMV infection in IBD patients is associated with steroid-refractory disease and should be considered as a complicating factor in the appropriate clinical scenario.

☑ The diagnosis of CMV is challenging, with multiple different diagnostic tools available. The gold standard for diagnosis is the demonstration of CMV in colonic tissue, with IHC increasing diagnostic sensitivity.

☑ Not all patients with CMV infection require treatment. However, treating CMV colitis in steroid-refractory patients is associated with a decreased colectomy rate.

References

1. McDonald LC, Owings M, Jernigan DB. *Clostridium difficile* infection in patients discharged from US short-stay hospitals, 1996-2003. *Emerg Infect Dis.* 2006;12:409-415.

2. McFarland LV. Renewed interest in a difficult disease: *Clostridium difficile* infections—epidemiology and current treatment strategies. *Curr Opin Gastroenterol.* 2009;25:24-35.

3. Pepin J, Valiquette L, Alary ME, et al. *Clostridium difficile*-associated diarrhea in a region of Quebec from 1991 to 2003: a changing pattern of disease severity. *CMAJ.* 2004;171:466-472.

4. Bartlett JG, Chang TW, Gurwith M, Gorbach SL, Onderdonk AB. Antibiotic-associated pseudomembranous colitis due to toxin-producing clostridia. *N Engl J Med.* 1978;298: 531-514.

5. Pituch H. *Clostridium difficile* is no longer just a nosocomial infection or an infection of adults. *Int J Antimicrob Agents.* 2009;33(suppl 1):S42-S45.

6. Ananthakrishnan AN, Issa M, Binion DG. *Clostridium difficile* and inflammatory bowel disease. *Gastroenterol Clin North Am.* 2009;38:711-728.

7. Rupnik M, Wilcox MH, Gerding DN. *Clostridium difficile* infection: new developments in epidemiology and pathogenesis. *Nat Rev Microbiol.* 2009;7:526-536.

8. Voth DE, Ballard JD. *Clostridium difficile* toxins: mechanism of action and role in disease. *Clin Microbiol Rev.* 2005;18:247-263.

9. Drudy D, Harnedy N, Fanning S, O'Mahony R, Kyne L. Isolation and characterisation of toxin A-negative, toxin B-positive *Clostridium difficile* in Dublin, Ireland. *Clin Microbiol Infect.* 2007;13:298-304.

10. Johnson S, Kent SA, O'Leary KJ, et al. Fatal pseudomembranous colitis associated with a variant *Clostridium difficile* strain not detected by toxin A immunoassay. *Ann Intern Med.* 2001;135:434-438.

11. Rupnik M, Grabnar M, Geric B. Binary toxin producing *Clostridium difficile* strains. *Anaerobe.* 2003;9:289-294.

12. McDonald LC, Killgore GE, Thompson A, et al. An epidemic, toxin gene-variant strain of *Clostridium difficile. N Engl J Med.* 2005;353:2433-2441.

13. Warny M, Pepin J, Fang A, et al. Toxin production by an emerging strain of *Clostridium difficile* associated with outbreaks of severe disease in North America and Europe. *Lancet.* 2005;366:1079-1084.

14. Bossuyt P, Verhaegen J, Van Assche G, Rutgeerts P, Vermeire S. Increasing incidence of *Clostridium difficile*-assiociated diarrhea in inflammatory bowel disease. *J Crohns Colitis.* 2009;3:4-7.

15. Goorhuis A, Bakker D, Corver J, et al. Emergence of *Clostridium difficile* infection due to a new hypervirulent strain, polymerase chain reaction ribotype 078. *Clin Infect Dis.* 2008;47:1162-1170.

16. Gryboski JD. *Clostridium difficile* in inflammatory bowel disease relapse. *J Pediatr Gastroenterol Nutr.* 1991;13:39-41.

17. Mylonaki M, Langmead L, Pantes A, Johnson F, Rampton DS. Enteric infection in relapse of inflammatory bowel disease: importance of microbiological examination of stool. *Eur J Gastroenterol Hepatol.* 2004;16:775-778.

18. Rolny P, Jarnerot G, Mollby R. Occurrence of *Clostridium difficile* toxin in inflammatory bowel disease. *Scand J Gastroenterol.* 1983;18:61-64.

19. Weber P, Koch M, Heizmann WR, Scheurlen M, Jenss H, Hartmann F. Microbic superinfection in relapse of inflammatory bowel disease. *J Clin Gastroenterol.* 1992;14:302-308.

20. Ananthakrishnan AN, McGinley EL, Binion DG. Excess hospitalisation burden associated with *Clostridium difficile* in patients with inflammatory bowel disease. *Gut.* 2008;57: 205-210.

21. Issa M, Vijayapal A, Graham MB, et al. Impact of *Clostridium difficile* on inflammatory bowel disease. *Clin Gastroenterol Hepatol.* 2007;5:345-351.

22. Jodorkovsky D, Young Y, Abreu MT. Clinical outcomes of patients with ulcerative colitis and co-existing *Clostridium difficile* infection. *Dig Dis Sci.* 2010;55(2):415-420.

23. Nguyen GC, Kaplan GG, Harris ML, Brant SR. A national survey of the prevalence and impact of *Clostridium difficile* infection among hospitalized inflammatory bowel disease patients. *Am J Gastroenterol.* 2008;103:1443-1450.

24. Rodemann JF, Dubberke ER, Reske KA, Seo da H, Stone CD. Incidence of *Clostridium difficile* infection in inflammatory bowel disease. *Clin Gastroenterol Hepatol.* 2007;5:339-344.

25. Pascarella F, Martinelli M, Miele E, Del Pezzo M, Roscetto E, Staiano A. Impact of *Clostridium difficile* infection on pediatric inflammatory bowel disease. *J Pediatr.* 2009;154:854-858.

26. Bartlett JG, Gerding DN. Clinical recognition and diagnosis of *Clostridium difficile* infection. *Clin Infect Dis.* 2008;46(suppl 1):S12-S18.

27. Kelly CP. A 76-year-old man with recurrent *Clostridium difficile*-associated diarrhea: review of *C difficile* infection. *JAMA.* 2009;301:954-962.

28. Kyne L, Warny M, Qamar A, Kelly CP. Asymptomatic carriage of *Clostridium difficile* and serum levels of IgG antibody against toxin A. *N Engl J Med.* 2000;342:390-397.

29. Kyne L, Warny M, Qamar A, Kelly CP. Association between antibody response to toxin A and protection against recurrent *Clostridium difficile* diarrhoea. *Lancet.* 2001;357:189-193.

30. Powell N, Jung SE, Krishnan B. *Clostridium difficile* infection and inflammatory bowel disease: a marker for disease extent? *Gut.* 2008;57:1183-1184.

31. Gaynes R, Rimland D, Killum E, et al. Outbreak of *Clostridium difficile* infection in a long-term care facility: association with gatifloxacin use. *Clin Infect Dis.* 2004;38:640-645.

32. Pepin J, Saheb N, Coulombe MA, et al. Emergence of fluoroquinolones as the predominant risk factor for *Clostridium difficile*-associated diarrhea: a cohort study during an epidemic in Quebec. *Clin Infect Dis.* 2005;41:1254-1260.

33. Dial S, Alrasadi K, Manoukian C, Huang A, Menzies D. Risk of *Clostridium difficile* diarrhea among hospital inpatients prescribed proton pump inhibitors: cohort and case-control studies. *CMAJ.* 2004;171:33-38.

34. Arif M, Weber LR, Knox JF, et al. Patterns of proton pump inhibitor use in inflammatory bowel disease and concomitant risk of *Clostridium difficile* infection. *Gastroenterology.* 2007;132:A513.

35. Chiplunker A, Ananthakrishnan AN, Beaulieu DB, et al. Long-term impact of *Clostridium difficile* on inflammatory bowel disease. *Gastroenterology.* 2009;136(suppl 1):S1145.

36. Cohen SH, Gerding DN, Johnson S, et al. Clinical practice guidelines for *Clostridium difficile* infection in adults: 2010 update by the society for healthcare epidemiology of America (SHEA) and the infectious diseases society of America (IDSA). *Infect Control Hosp Epidemiol.* 2010;31:431-455.

37. Crobach MJ, Dekkers OM, Wilcox MH, Kuijper EJ. European Society of Clinical Microbiology and Infectious Diseases (ESCMID): data review and recommendations for diagnosing *Clostridium difficile*-infection (CDI). *Clin Microbiol Infect.* 2009;15:1053-1066.

38. Kelly CP, LaMont JT. *Clostridium difficile* infection. *Annu Rev Med.* 1998;49:375-390.

39. Gerding DN, Muto CA, Owens RC Jr. Treatment of *Clostridium difficile* infection. *Clin Infect Dis.* 2008;46(suppl 1):S32-S42.

40. Leffler DA, Lamont JT. Treatment of *Clostridium difficile*-associated disease. *Gastroenterology.* 2009;136:1899-1912.

41. Pepin J. Vancomycin for the treatment of *Clostridium difficile* infection: for whom is this expensive bullet really magic? *Clin Infect Dis.* 2008;46:1493-1498.

42. Bartlett JG. The case for vancomycin as the preferred drug for treatment of *Clostridium difficile* infection. *Clin Infect Dis.* 2008;46:1489-1492.

43. Bauer MP, van Dissel JT, Kuijper EJ. *Clostridium difficile*: controversies and approaches to management. *Curr Opin Infect Dis.* 2009;22:517-524.

44. Zar FA, Bakkanagari SR, Moorthi KM, Davis MB. A comparison of vancomycin and metronidazole for the treatment of *Clostridium difficile*-associated diarrhea, stratified by disease severity. *Clin Infect Dis.* 2007;45:302-307.

45. Louie T. *Results of a phase III trial comparing tolevamer, vancomycin and metronidazole in Clostridium difficile-associated diarrhea (CDAD) [abstract k-4259].* Program and abstracts of the 47th Interscience Conference on Antimicrobial Agents and Chemotherapy (Washington DC). Herndon, VA: ASM Press; 2007.

46. Ben-Horin S, Margalit M, Bossuyt P, et al. Combination immunomodulator and antibiotic treatment in patients with inflammatory bowel disease and *Clostridium difficile* infection. *Clin Gastroenterol Hepatol*. 2009;7:981-987.

47. Salcedo J, Keates S, Pothoulakis C, et al. Intravenous immunoglobulin therapy for severe *Clostridium difficile* colitis. *Gut*. 1997;41:366-370.

48. McPherson S, Rees CJ, Ellis R, Soo S, Panter SJ. Intravenous immunoglobulin for the treatment of severe, refractory, and recurrent *Clostridium difficile* diarrhea. *Dis Colon Rectum*. 2006;49:640-645.

49. Abougergi MS, Broor A, Cui W, Jaar BG. Intravenous immunoglobulin for the treatment of severe *Clostridium difficile* colitis: an observational study and review of the literature. *J Hosp Med*. 2010;5:E1-E9.

50. Garey KW, Sethi S, Yadav Y, DuPont HL. Meta-analysis to assess risk factors for recurrent *Clostridium difficile* infection. *J Hosp Infect*. 2008;70:298-304.

51. Johnson S. Recurrent *Clostridium difficile* infection: a review of risk factors, treatments, and outcomes. *J Infect*. 2009;58:403-410.

52. Johnson S, Schriever C, Galang M, Kelly CP, Gerding DN. Interruption of recurrent *Clostridium difficile*-associated diarrhea episodes by serial therapy with vancomycin and rifaximin. *Clin Infect Dis*. 2007;44:846-848.

53. Johnson S, Schriever C, Patel U, Patel T, Hecht DW, Gerding DN. Rifaximin redux: treatment of recurrent *Clostridium difficile* infections with rifaximin immediately post-vancomycin treatment. *Anaerobe*. 2009;15:290-291.

54. McFarland LV. Meta-analysis of probiotics for the prevention of antibiotic associated diarrhea and the treatment of *Clostridium difficile* disease. *Am J Gastroenterol*. 2006;101:812-822.

55. Lowy I, Molrine DC, Leav BA, et al. Treatment with monoclonal antibodies against *Clostridium difficile* toxins. *N Engl J Med*. 2010;362:197-205.

56. Mann SD, Pitt J, Springall RG, Thillainayagam AV. *Clostridium difficile* infection—an unusual cause of refractory pouchitis: report of a case. *Dis Colon Rectum*. 2003;46:267-270.

57. Shen B, Goldblum JR, Hull TL, Remzi FH, Bennett AE, Fazio VW. *Clostridium difficile*-associated pouchitis. *Dig Dis Sci*. 2006;51:2361-2364.

58. Shen BO, Jiang ZD, Fazio VW, et al. *Clostridium difficile* infection in patients with ileal pouch-anal anastomosis. *Clin Gastroenterol Hepatol*. 2008;6:782-788.

59. Lundeen SJ, Otterson MF, Binion DG, Carman ET, Peppard WJ. *Clostridium difficile* enteritis: an early postoperative complication in inflammatory bowel disease patients after colectomy. *J Gastrointest Surg*. 2007;11:138-142.

60. Vesoulis Z, Williams G, Matthews B. Pseudomembranous enteritis after proctocolectomy: report of a case. *Dis Colon Rectum*. 2000;43:551-554.

61. Yee HF Jr, Brown RS Jr, Ostroff JW. Fatal *Clostridium difficile* enteritis after total abdominal colectomy. *J Clin Gastroenterol*. 1996;22:45-47.

62. Gerding DN, Muto CA, Owens RC Jr. Measures to control and prevent *Clostridium difficile* infection. *Clin Infect Dis*. 2008;46(suppl 1):S43-S49.

63. Vonberg RP, Kuijper EJ, Wilcox MH, et al. Infection control measures to limit the spread of *Clostridium difficile*. *Clin Microbiol Infect*. 2008;14(suppl 5):2-20.

64. Oughton MT, Loo VG, Dendukuri N, Fenn S, Libman MD. Hand hygiene with soap and water is superior to alcohol rub and antiseptic wipes for removal of *Clostridium difficile*. *Infect Control Hosp Epidemiol*. 2009;30:939-944.

65. de la Hoz RE, Stephens G, Sherlock C. Diagnosis and treatment approaches of CMV infections in adult patients. *J Clin Virol*. 2002;25(suppl 2):S1-S12.

66. Powell RD, Warner NE, Levine RS, Kirsner JB. Cytomegalic inclusion disease and ulcerative colitis; report of a case in a young adult. *Am J Med*. 1961;30:334-340.

67. Hommes DW, Sterringa G, van Deventer SJ, Tytgat GN, Weel J. The pathogenicity of cytomegalovirus in inflammatory bowel disease: a systematic review and evidence-based recommendations for future research. *Inflamm Bowel Dis*. 2004;10:245-250.

68. Lawlor G, Moss AC. Cytomegalovirus in inflammatory bowel disease: pathogen or innocent bystander? *Inflamm Bowel Dis*. 2010;16:1620-1627.

69. Krech U. Complement-fixing antibodies against cytomegalovirus in different parts of the world. *Bull World Health Organ.* 1973;49:103-106.

70. Domenech E, Vega R, Ojanguren I, et al. Cytomegalovirus infection in ulcerative colitis: a prospective, comparative study on prevalence and diagnostic strategy. *Inflamm Bowel Dis.* 2008;14:1373-1379.

71. Kandiel A, Lashner B. Cytomegalovirus colitis complicating inflammatory bowel disease. *Am J Gastroenterol.* 2006;101:2857-2865.

72. Kambham N, Vij R, Cartwright CA, Longacre T. Cytomegalovirus infection in steroid-refractory ulcerative colitis: a case-control study. *Am J Surg Pathol.* 2004;28:365-373.

73. Yoshino T, Nakase H, Ueno S, et al. Usefulness of quantitative real-time PCR assay for early detection of cytomegalovirus infection in patients with ulcerative colitis refractory to immunosuppressive therapies. *Inflamm Bowel Dis.* 2007;13:1516-1521.

74. Pfau P, Kochman ML, Furth EE, Lichtenstein GR. Cytomegalovirus colitis complicating ulcerative colitis in the steroid-naive patient. *Am J Gastroenterol.* 2001;96:895-899.

75. Rahbar A, Bostrom L, Lagerstedt U, Magnusson I, Soderberg-Naucler C, Sundqvist VA. Evidence of active cytomegalovirus infection and increased production of IL-6 in tissue specimens obtained from patients with inflammatory bowel diseases. *Inflamm Bowel Dis.* 2003;9:154-161.

76. Maconi G, Colombo E, Zerbi P, et al. Prevalence, detection rate and outcome of cytomegalovirus infection in ulcerative colitis patients requiring colonic resection. *Dig Liver Dis.* 2005;37:418-423.

77. Papadakis KA, Tung JK, Binder SW, et al. Outcome of cytomegalovirus infections in patients with inflammatory bowel disease. *Am J Gastroenterol.* 2001;96:2137-2142.

78. Cottone M, Pietrosi G, Martorana G, et al. Prevalence of cytomegalovirus infection in severe refractory ulcerative and Crohn's colitis. *Am J Gastroenterol.* 2001;96:773-775.

79. Criscuoli V, Casa A, Orlando A, et al. Severe acute colitis associated with CMV: a prevalence study. *Dig Liver Dis.* 2004;36:818-820.

80. Matsuoka K, Iwao Y, Mori T, et al. Cytomegalovirus is frequently reactivated and disappears without antiviral agents in ulcerative colitis patients. *Am J Gastroenterol.* 2007;102:331-337.

81. Maher MM, Nassar MI. Acute cytomegalovirus infection is a risk factor in refractory and complicated inflammatory bowel disease. *Dig Dis Sci.* 2009;54:2456-2462.

82. Wada Y, Matsui T, Matake H, et al. Intractable ulcerative colitis caused by cytomegalovirus infection: a prospective study on prevalence, diagnosis, and treatment. *Dis Colon Rectum.* 2003;46:S59-S65.

83. Cooper HS, Raffensperger EC, Jonas L, Fitts WT Jr. Cytomegalovirus inclusions in patients with ulcerative colitis and toxic dilation requiring colonic resection. *Gastroenterology.* 1977;72:1253-1256.

84. Begos DG, Rappaport R, Jain D. Cytomegalovirus infection masquerading as an ulcerative colitis flare-up: case report and review of the literature. *Yale J Biol Med.* 1996;69:323-328.

85. Suzuki H, Kato J, Kuriyama M, Hiraoka S, Kuwaki K, Yamamoto K. Specific endoscopic features of ulcerative colitis complicated by cytomegalovirus infection. *World J Gastroenterol.* 2010;16:1245-1251.

86. Hinnant KL, Rotterdam HZ, Bell ET, Tapper ML. Cytomegalovirus infection of the alimentary tract: a clinicopathological correlation. *Am J Gastroenterol.* 1986;81:944-950.

87. Ghidini B, Bellaiche M, Berrebi D, et al. Cytomegalovirus colitis in children with inflammatory bowel disease. *Gut.* 2006;55:582-583.

88. Moonka D, Furth EE, MacDermott RP, Lichtenstein GR. Pouchitis associated with primary cytomegalovirus infection. *Am J Gastroenterol.* 1998;93:264-266.

89. Dimitroulia E, Spanakis N, Konstantinidou AE, Legakis NJ, Tsakris A. Frequent detection of cytomegalovirus in the intestine of patients with inflammatory bowel disease. *Inflamm Bowel Dis.* 2006;12:879-884.

90. Rahier JF, Ben-Horin S, Chowers Y, et al. European evidence-based consensus on the prevention, diagnosis and management of opportunistic infections in inflammatory bowel disease. *J Crohns Colitis.* 2009;3:47-91.

91. D'Ovidio V, Vernia P, Gentile G, et al. Cytomegalovirus infection in inflammatory bowel disease patients undergoing anti-TNFalpha therapy. *J Clin Virol*. 2008;43:180-183.
92. Julka K, Surawicz CM. Cytomegalovirus in inflammatory bowel disease: time for another look? *Gastroenterology*. 2009;137:1163-1166.
93. Herfarth HH, Long MD, Rubinas TC, Sandridge M, Miller MB. Evaluation of a non-invasive method to detect cytomegalovirus (CMV)-DNA in stool samples of patients with inflammatory bowel disease (IBD): a pilot study. *Dig Dis Sci*. 2010;55:1053-1058.
94. Criscuoli V, Rizzuto MR, Cottone M. Cytomegalovirus and inflammatory bowel disease: is there a link? *World J Gastroenterol*. 2006;12:4813-4818.
95. Vega R, Bertran X, Menacho M, et al. Cytomegalovirus infection in patients with inflammatory bowel disease. *Am J Gastroenterol*. 1999;94:1053-1056.

SUGGESTED READINGS

Ananthakrishnan AN, Issa M, Binion DG. Clostridium difficile and inflammatory bowel disease. *Gastroenterol Clin North Am*. 2009;38:711-728.

Bartlett JG, Gerding DN. Clinical recognition and diagnosis of *Clostridium difficile* infection. *Clin Infect Dis*. 2008;46(suppl 1):S12-S18.

Hommes DW, Sterringa G, van Deventer SJ, Tytgat GN, Weel J. The pathogenicity of cytomegalovirus in inflammatory bowel disease: a systematic review and evidence-based recommendations for future research. *Inflamm Bowel Dis*. 2004;10:245-250.

Kelly CP. A 76-year-old man with recurrent *Clostridium difficile*-associated diarrhea: review of *C. difficile* infection. *JAMA*. 2009;301:954-962.

Lawlor G, Moss AC. Cytomegalovirus in inflammatory bowel disease: pathogen or innocent bystander? *Inflamm Bowel Dis*. 2010;16:1620-1627.

Pituch H. *Clostridium difficile* is no longer just a nosocomial infection or an infection of adults. *Int J Antimicrob Agents*. 2009;33(suppl 1):S42-S45.

Section **II**

EXTRAINTESTINAL MANIFESTATIONS OF IBD

Chapter 7

Joint Disease

Kim L. Isaacs, MD, PhD

Arthritis is the most common extraintestinal manifestation of inflammatory bowel disease (IBD), occurring in 20% to 50% of patients with IBD.[1] By definition, inflammatory arthritis in patients with IBD is considered a spondyloarthropathy. The other disease entities included under this category are psoriatic arthritis, ankylosing spondylitis, reactive arthritis, and undifferentiated spondylarthritis (SA). These entities are grouped together because they are thought to have a similar genetic predilection and clinical manifestations.[1] Both spondyloarthropathy and SA are used to describe the arthritis associated with IBD to distinguish it from arthritis seen with rheumatoid arthritis and connective tissue diseases.[2] The European Spondylarthropathy Study Group developed criteria for this category of arthritis in 1991 in an attempt to standardize the nomenclature (Table 7-1).[3] The Amor criteria assign point values to various clinical and radiographic findings, with a point score >6 associated with spondyloarthropathy (Table 7-2).[1,4] Both classification schemes lack the sensitivity to make an early diagnosis of SA.[5]

DEFINITIONS AND EPIDEMIOLOGY

Arthritis in IBD may be composed of an axial and/or a peripheral arthritis. Other less common presentations may include enthesitis, which is inflammation at the site of tendon and ligament insertion into bone (plantar fasciitis and Achilles tendonitis), and dactylitis, characterized by inflammatory swelling of the fingers and toes. Arthritis as an extraintestinal manifestation of IBD is more common in Crohn's disease (CD) than in ulcerative colitis (UC).[6] There is a male predominance in ankylosing spondylitis not associated with IBD, whereas in IBD there is an equal gender distribution. There have been multiple epidemiologic studies in IBD populations looking at the prevalence of axial and peripheral arthritis with a wide range in rates of arthritis.[1] In general, in most studies, peripheral arthritis is more common than ankylosing spondylitis. Sacroiliitis is a bit more difficult to track, as it is thought that asymptomatic sacroiliitis may be seen in as many as 50% of patients with IBD—detectable by

Regueiro MD, Swoger JM, eds.
Clinical Challenges and Complications of IBD (pp 127-140).
© 2013 Taylor & Francis Group.

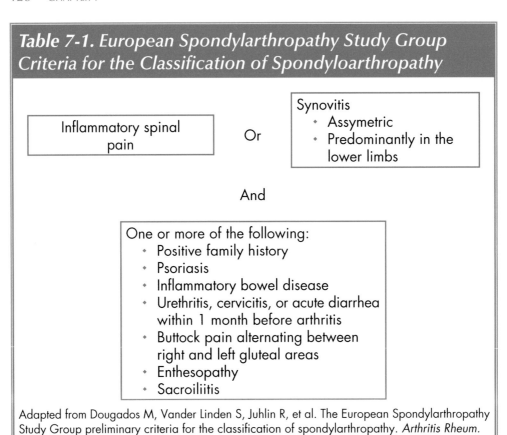

Table 7-1. European Spondylarthropathy Study Group Criteria for the Classification of Spondyloarthropathy

Inflammatory spinal pain	Or	Synovitis • Assymetric • Predominantly in the lower limbs

And

One or more of the following:
  • Positive family history
  • Psoriasis
  • Inflammatory bowel disease
  • Urethritis, cervicitis, or acute diarrhea within 1 month before arthritis
  • Buttock pain alternating between right and left gluteal areas
  • Enthesopathy
  • Sacroiliitis

Adapted from Dougados M, Vander Linden S, Juhlin R, et al. The European Spondylarthropathy Study Group preliminary criteria for the classification of spondylarthropathy. *Arthritis Rheum.* 1991;34:1228-1230.

imaging studies. The figures for axial and peripheral arthritis are similar in both CD and UC, with colonic involvement in CD a key component.

ETIOLOGY AND PATHOPHYSIOLOGY

There has long been an association between certain bacterial gut infections in susceptible patients and the development of reactive arthritis. Twenty percent of the patients who develop this reactive arthritis will develop ankylosing spondylitis.[7] It has also been shown that two-thirds of patients with SA will have evidence of gastrointestinal inflammation at the microscopic level, although most of these patients do not have gastrointestinal symptoms.[7]

ANIMAL MODELS

Animal models have provided some insight into the association of joint and gut inflammation. The HLAB27/human β_2-microglobulin transgenic rat develops an enterocolitis, destructive peripheral arthritis, and sacroiliitis in Lewis or Fisher rats. If the rats are kept in a germ-free environment or if they are athymic, they do not develop disease.[8,9] This suggests that both bacterial

Table 7-2. Amor Criteria for Spondyloarthropathy

CLINICAL SYMPTOMS OR PAST HISTORY OF:

Lumbar or dorsal pain at night, or lumbar or dorsal morning stiffness	1
Asymmetric oligoarthritis	2
Buttock pain (buttock pain = 1, alternating buttock pain = 2)	1 or 2
Sausage-like finger or toe	2
Heel pain	2
Iritis	2
Nongonococcal urethritis or cervicitis accompanying, or within 1 month before, the onset of arthritis	1
Acute diarrhea accompanying, or within 1 month before, the onset of arthritis	1
Presence or history of psoriasis and/or balanitis and/or IBD (UC, CD)	2
Radiographic findings of sacroiliitis (grade >2 if bilateral; grade >3 if unilateral)	3
Genetic background: HLAB27 positive and/or family history of ankylosing spondylitis; triad of uveitis, urethritis, and arthritis; psoriasis; isolated uveitis; or chronic enterocolopathies	3
Response to therapy: clear-cut improvement of rheumatic complaints with NSAIDs in <48 hours, or relapse of pain in <48 hours if NSAIDs are discontinued	3

If the sum of the weighted criteria is ≥6, the patient is considered to have spondyloarthropathy. CD = Crohn's disease; IBD = inflammatory bowel disease; NSAID = nonsteroidal anti-inflammatory drug; UC = ulcerative colitis
Adapted from Salvarani C, Fries W. Clinical features and epidemiology of spondyloarthritides associated with inflammatory bowel disease. *World J Gastroenterol.* 2009;15:2449-2455.

exposure and T cells are required for development of both gut inflammation and arthritis. Recent studies implicate misfolding of the heavy chain of HLAB27, with subsequent accumulation in the endoplasmic reticulum. Addition of β_2-microglobulin leads to less misfolding, amelioration of the colitis, and worsening of the arthritis.[10]

A second animal model that may provide insight into the pathogenesis of the gut and joint inflammation is the tumor necrosis factor (TNF)[ΔARE] mouse. In this model, TNF adenylate-uridylate-rich elements are deleted from the mouse genome and TNF regulation is impaired, with spontaneous TNF protein production in hematopoietic cells and stroma tissue. These animals develop ileitis, sacroiliitis, spondylitis, and enthesitis.[11] If mature T and B cells are absent, there is no gut inflammation; however, there continues to be joint inflammation. Stroma-residing cells are the targets for arthritis.[7] Armaka et al demonstrated that with TNF excess, signaling of synovial fibroblasts and intestinal myofibroblasts through TNFR1 lead to combined gut and joint inflammation.[12]

Genetic Markers

There is a strong genetic link between axial arthritis in IBD and HLAB27, with the prevalence of HLAB27 in IBD patients, with spondylitis or sacroiliitis ranging from 25% to 78%.[7] HLAB27 is normal in IBD patients without ankylosing spondylitis. Studies in the HLAB27/human β_2-microglobulin transgenic rat, as described previously, suggest that the genetic defect that causes misfolding of the HLAB27 gene plays a role in disease pathogenesis. Most patients with IBD and arthritis are not HLAB27 positive, suggesting that other genetic pathways play a role in these diseases.

The CARD15/NOD2 gene is a pattern-recognition receptor of bacteria. When engaged, the NFκB pathway is activated, leading to cell apoptosis. Polymorphisms of this gene are associated with increased risk for CD. Compared to healthy controls there is not an increase in CARD15 polymorphisms in patients with SA; however, in patients with SA, polymorphisms in this gene are associated with chronic intestinal inflammation, suggesting a link between SA and CD.[13]

The gene for the interleukin (IL)-23 receptor may also potentially play a role in the pathogenesis of these diseases. IL-23 is a proinflammatory cytokine that has 2 subunits: p40 and p19. This cytokine appears to play a role in the differentiation of CD4$^+$ T cells into IL-17-producing T helper cells. A unique coding variant of the IL-23 receptor gene (rs11209026, Arg381Gln) gives protection against CD, ankylosing spondylitis, and psoriasis. There are other haplotypes of this gene that are associated with an increased incidence of AS.[14]

Clinical Features

Axial Arthritis

The manifestations of axial involvement include asymptomatic sacroiliitis seen only on imaging studies, inflammatory back pain with or without sacroiliitis, and ankylosing spondylitis, characterized by spine stiffness and pain with characteristic radiographic findings. Patients with inflammatory back pain usually have a subtle onset of pain and stiffness in the lower back. Fatigue is a common complaint, along with stiffness that improves with movement. The pain may initially be unilateral and intermittent. There may be buttock pain as well. Several classification schemes have been developed in attempts to standardize the diagnosis of inflammatory back pain. Sieper et al recently published updated criteria for the clinical diagnosis of inflammatory back pain, including 5 parameters, 4 of which must be positive[15] (Table 7-3). Parameters include pain at night and improvement with exercise. Earlier classification schemes also included morning stiffness.[16] Patients may complain of pain that wakes them from sleep at night and the need to walk around to relieve the pain. The diagnosis of sacroiliitis requires radiographic changes.

Physical examination findings in patients with axial arthritis may include decreased chest mobility and reduced range of motion of the spine. Sacroiliac tenderness may be elicited, and hip flexion may be abnormal.

Table 7-3. *Sieper et al Criteria for Clinical Diagnosis of Inflammatory Back Pain*

Age of onset <40 years
Insidious onset
Improvement with exercise
No improvement with rest
Pain at night (improvement on arising)

Coexistence of 4 out of 5 criteria allows the definition of inflammatory back pain.
Adapted from Sieper J, van der Heijde D, Landewé R, et al. New criteria for inflammatory back pain in patients with chronic back pain: a real patient exercise by experts from the Assessment of SpondyloArthritis international Society (ASAS). *Ann Rheum Dis.* 2009;68:784-788.

Spinal measurements include the following:
◊ Range of motion of the lower back (lumbar flexion): Modified Schober test—With patient standing straight, the examiner marks the back at the 5th lumbar spinous process (dimples of Venus) with a pen. Two additional marks are made 5 cm below and 10 cm above this mark in the midline. The patient should then bend forward fully and the distance between the marks measured. Patients with normal range of motion of the back should have an increase in the measured distance of 5 cm.
◊ Range of motion of the lower back (lateral flexion): The patient stands straight and then leans to the side, sliding the arm/hand down the side. The distance moved by the fingertips is measured and the mean is calculated. The fingertips should move more than 14 cm.
◊ Occiput to wall distance: Flesche test—The patient stands erect, with heels and buttocks against the wall. The patient is asked to extend his or her neck maximally to try to touch the wall with the occiput. The distance between the wall and the occiput is measured. This gives the degree of flexion deformity of the neck in ankylosing spondylitis.
◊ Chest expansion: This is measured at the level of the 4th intercostals space. A tape measure is used and the patient is asked to give a maximum forced expiration followed by a maximal inspiration. The arms are held above the head. Chest expansion should be 5 cm or more.

Sacroiliac Evaluation

1. Sacroiliac tenderness: Apply direct pressure over each sacroiliac joint looking for tenderness of the joint.
2. Supine examination: Patient lies supine on the examination table. The evaluator presses on the anterior-superior iliac spine, forcing the iliac spine in a lateral direction looking for pain.

3. Lateral examination: Patient lies on his or her side on the examination table. The evaluator presses on the patient's side to compress the pelvis. The pressure will cause pain with sacroiliac inflammation.

4. Supine/knee flexion: Patient lies supine on the examination table. He or she is asked to flex one knee, abduct, and externally rotate the hip on the same side. Pressure is applied to the flexed knee that causes pain in the sacroiliac joint on that side.

Hip Joint Evaluation

1. Flexion abnormalities of the hip are tested by having the patient lie supine on the examination table and maximally flex one hip. If there is a flexion deformity in the opposite hip, the knee of the opposite leg will be raised and the angle of the opposite thigh is measured to calculate the degree of flexion deformity.

Peripheral Arthritis

Peripheral arthritis is more common in CD than UC and commonly involves the joints of lower extremities, knees, and ankles. The arthritis tends to be migratory and nonerosive. A small percentage of patients (<20%) will have arthritis that predates recognition of IBD.[17] Peripheral arthritis tends to parallel disease activity. Orchard and colleagues further divide the peripheral arthritis associated with IBD into 2 groups that have different behaviors.[18] Type 1 is a pauciarticular arthritis involving 5 or less joints. The disease is asymmetric and involves joints of the lower limbs. Episodes are self-limited and tend to last less than 10 weeks. They are often associated with IBD relapses and are highly associated with other extraintestinal manifestations, such as erythema nodosum.

Type 2 peripheral arthritis is a polyarticular arthritis involving 5 or more joints. The disease affects large and small joints and tends to be persistent, lasting months or years. It can be either symmetric or asymmetric and joint inflammation does not parallel IBD activity. Type 2 arthritis is associated with uveitis. Patients present with pain and swelling of the affected joints. The affected joints and reachable enthuses are examined on physical examination for swelling, tenderness to palpation and movement, and range of motion.

DIAGNOSTIC TESTING

Routine Blood Work

Common laboratory abnormalities seen in patients with active inflammatory arthritis include anemia, which may be due to the active joint inflammation or to bleeding from active bowel inflammation. There may be leukocytosis and thrombocytosis, also due to active inflammation. Erythrocyte sedimentation rate (ESR) and C-reactive protein (CRP) are elevated in some patients with inflammatory arthritis. The most recent criteria from the Assessment of SpondylArthritis international Society include an elevated CRP in the classification criteria for axial SA.[19] Linear monitoring of CRP or ESR may help define response to therapy. Antinuclear antibodies (ANAs) and rheumatoid factor are usually negative and if positive should raise the question of rheumatoid arthritis or in the case of a positive ANA, systemic lupus erythematosus or drug-induced lupus. Anti-TNF therapy of IBD has been associated with the development of a positive ANA in up to 45% of patients with a minority of patients exhibiting clinically significant systemic lupus erythematosus.[20] HIV testing in appropriate patients may be useful due to the association of reactive arthritis with HIV seroconversion.

GENETIC TESTING

HLAB27

Greater than 90% of patients with primary ankylosing spondylitis and 30% to 70% of patients with IBD-related SA are positive for HLAB27. The prevalence of the gene in the normal population is about 8%.[21] A positive HLAB27 without other clinical features does not confirm a diagnosis of spondyloarthropathy, whereas a negative HLAB27 makes primary ankylosing spondylitis unlikely. HLAB27 testing may be useful for classification in clinical trials but does not have a role at this time in the clinical diagnosis and management of IBD patients with SA.

CARD15 Polymorphisms

Polymorphisms of the CARD15 gene described in patients with CD may be a genetic trigger for arthritis. Comparing CD patients with sacroiliitis to controls with CD and no sacroiliitis, 78% versus 48% of patients carry one or more mutations of the CARD15 gene.[13] Although interesting in terms of disease pathogenesis, this finding does not have clinical application at this time.

Serologic Markers

There are a number of antibodies to microbial antigens that have been described as present more commonly in patients with IBD than in healthy controls. These antibodies include antibodies to *Saccharomyces cerevisiae* mannan (ASCA), perinuculear antineutophil cytoplasmic antibodies (pANCA), antibodies to *Escherichia coli* outer membrane porin (Anti-Omp C), antibodies to a bacteria sequence from *Pseudomonas fluorescens* (Anti-I2), and antibodies to flagellin CBir 1 (Anti-CBir 1).[22] These antibodies may give clues to pathogenesis of these diseases. I2 is elevated compared to controls in patients with ankylosing spondylitis.[23] ASCA positivity is also seen in a higher percentage of patients with AS (20%) versus controls (5.8%).[24] These findings are intriguing but are more useful in the research setting. Serological testing for these antibodies is not part of the routine assessment and management of patients with inflammatory spondyloarthropathy.

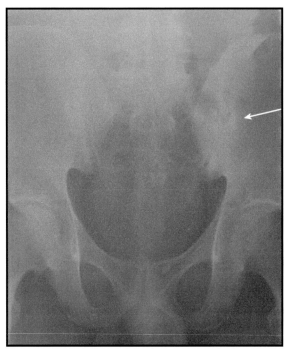

Figure 7-1. Sacroiliitis. Sclerosis of sacroiliac joints (arrow).

IMAGING STUDIES

Sacroiliitis

Initial diagnostic criteria of sacroiliitis are based on conventional x-ray examination of the pelvis. Sclerosis and erosions in the sacroiliac joint may be seen either unilaterally or bilaterally (Figure 7-1). A grading scheme has been developed for these changes (Table 7-4).[1] Changes in the sacroiliac joint seen in plain x-rays occur late in the disease course, whereas magnetic resonance imaging (MRI) identifies changes earlier. T2-weighted signals suppress the signal from bone marrow fat, which allows visualization of a bright signal from free water representing inflammation in the subchondral bone marrow of the sacroiliac joints.[25] Active inflammatory changes that can be seen on MRI include bone marrow edema/osteitis, synovitis, enthesitis, and capsulitis.[26] Inflammation occurs prior to the structural changes of the bone/joint, allowing for earlier diagnosis of sacroiliitis. MRI changes have now been incorporated into the Assessment of SpondyloArthritis international Society classification criteria for axial SA.[26]

Peripheral Arthritis

Plain radiographs of the peripheral joints in IBD are usually normal. The IBD-associated peripheral arthritis is typically a nonerosive process. Radiographs of the affected joints should be done at diagnosis to look for

Table 7-4. Radiographic Grading Criteria for Sacroiliitis	
SACROILIAC JOINTS	
Grade 0	Normal
Grade 1	Suspicious changes
Grade 2	Minimal abnormality: small localized areas with erosions or sclerosis with alternations in joint width
Grade 3	Unequivocal abnormality: moderate or advanced sacroiliitis with one or more of the following—erosions, sclerosis, widening
Grade 4	Severe abnormality: total ankylosis
Adapted from Salvarani C, Fries W. Clinical features and epidemiology of spondyloarthritides associated with inflammatory bowel disease. *World J Gastroenterol.* 2009;15:2449-2455.	

coexisting degenerative joint disease. If there is evidence of erosive joint disease, other erosive forms of inflammatory arthritis, such as rheumatoid arthritis, should be considered in the differential diagnosis.

MANAGEMENT/TREATMENT/OUTCOMES

Goals of Therapy

In patients with IBD-associated arthritis, the main goals of therapy are to treat active inflammation both in the joint and in the gastrointestinal tract and to prevent disease progression. Goals specific to joint involvement include symptomatic relief, leading to improvement of pain and stiffness in the involved joints, restoration of joint function, prevention of structural damage to the joint/spine, and prevention of complications including fracture and vertebral collapse. A combination of lifestyle modification, exercise, and medication therapy is used to achieve these goals.

Smoking Cessation

Cigarette smoking has been associated with a poor outcome in CD, both in terms of relapse and poor response to medications.[27] Smoking has also been shown to be a risk factor for poor long-term outcome in patients with ankylosing spondylitis.[28] In UC, smoking cessation has been associated with disease exacerbation. Despite the potential adverse effect of smoking cessation in patients with UC, the overall health benefits and improvement in disease activity in patients with inflammatory joint disease and CD should be discussed and reinforced with patients. Overall, studies on smoking cessation in patients with CD have shown low success rates (12%) and high relapse rates.[29] In patients with UC, smoking cessation should still be encouraged for the potential improvement in inflammatory arthritis; however, the risk of gastrointestinal disease relapse should be discussed as well.

Physical Therapy

Physical therapy has not been shown to alter disease; however, it is felt to be an essential component of disease management for spondyloarthropathy. Physical therapy as an adjunct to pharmacologic therapy helps to improve symptoms, diminish deformity, and improve function and quality of life.[30,31] Evaluation by a physical therapist with prescribed exercises may be helpful in initiating an exercise program. Methods that have been shown in clinical trials to be effective have included patient education, combined with a home exercise program, supervised group physical therapy, and water therapy.[31] Rarely, inpatient rehabilitation may be necessary. The Spondylitis Association of America (www.spondylitis.org) and the British counterpart, National Ankylosing Spondylitis Society (www.nass.co.uk), have patient educational materials and guidelines for exercises that patients may incorporate into a home exercise program.

Analgesics/Nonsteroidal Anti-Inflammatory Drugs

In idiopathic SA, nonsteroidal anti-inflammatory drugs (NSAIDs) are the drugs of choice. Seventy percent to 80% of patients with ankylosing spondylitis will have a good response to NSAID therapy.[32] In patients with IBD, however, there is some evidence that the use of conventional nonselective NSAIDs may exacerbate disease activity, although other studies do not support this observation.[33] Selective cyclooxygenase-2 NSAIDs (COX-2 inhibitors) may have fewer gastrointestinal adverse effects but have also had mixed results in terms of disease exacerbation in IBD.[33] In those studies that have demonstrated disease exacerbation, the percentage of patients appears to be under 20%.[33] In patients who require active treatment of SA who have active IBD, it is probably best to stay away from NSAIDs as therapy for the arthritic component. In patients with quiescent IBD, if needed, NSAIDs should be used cautiously.

Sulfasalazine

Sulfasalazine is a 5-aminosalicylate medication composed of 5-amino salicylic acid bonded by an azo-bond to sulfapyridine. It is broken down in the colon by bacteria into its components. It has been used in the therapy of arthritis and UC for more than 65 years due to its initial use for "infective" arthritis in the 1940s.[34] As a therapy for arthritis, sulfasalazine is most effective in patients with peripheral arthritis.[35] It is thought that the sulfapyridine component of sulfasalazine is responsible for the antiarthritic effects of the drug, making the newer 5-aminosalicylates (mesalamine-based compounds) not as likely to be effective for joint inflammation. In patients with UC and inflammatory arthritis, sulfasalazine in a dose of 2 to 6 g/day may be beneficial. Patients may have a poor tolerance to the sulfapyridine component that may be overcome with a gradual increase to the target dose. Gastrointestinal side effects are frequent and include nausea, vomiting, and anorexia. Less commonly, hemolytic anemia, renal dysfunction, pancreatitis, and liver abnormalities have been seen with sulfasalazine therapy.

Table 7-5. Methotrexate Laboratory Monitoring Parameters

Baseline, 2 weeks, every 8 to 12 weeks during treatment
• Complete blood count
• Creatinine
• Albumin
• Aspartate aminotransferase (AST)/alanine aminotransferase (ALT)/ alkaline phosphatase
Baseline, annually
• Chest x-ray

Methotrexate

Methotrexate is considered an antimetabolite and acts by inhibiting the enzyme dihydrofolate reductase. It has been used extensively as first-line therapy in rheumatoid arthritis and inflammatory arthritis in doses of 7.5 to 25 mg per week, with marked improvement in joint inflammation.[36] The benefit of methotrexate in patients with ankylosing spondylitis is less clear.[37] Methotrexate has been used effectively in certain patients with IBD both in terms of induction of remission and maintenance of remission. The data are most supportive of a role of methotrexate in patients with CD.[38,39] Available data are lacking for patients with UC. In patients with both inflammatory arthritis and active bowel inflammation requiring immunosuppressive therapy, methotrexate may have an advantage over the thiopurine analogues (azathioprine/6-mercaptopurine), which are less effective for joint disease. Dosing of methotrexate for active CD is usually 25 mg subcutaneously once per week, with a dosage reduction to 15 mg once per week after 16 weeks of therapy or earlier if there is intolerance to the higher dose. Patients will require supplementation with folic acid. There are well-established recommendations for laboratory monitoring for patients on methotrexate (Table 7-5).[40] Routine liver biopsy for detection of methotrexate-induced hepatotoxicity is not part of current monitoring guidelines.

Anti-Tumor Necrosis Factor Therapy

Anti-TNF therapy has been shown to be efficacious in the treatment of IBD-related spondyloarthropathy and undifferentiated SA, with response rates of up to 70%. In 2002, 4 years after approval of infliximab for CD, Van Den Bosch and colleagues reported on a randomized, controlled trial of 40 patients with SA. There was no improvement in disease activity in the placebo group and an approximately 70% improvement in the infliximab-treated group (5 mg/kg).[41] There are 4 anti-TNF agents approved for the treatment of ankylosing spondylitis: infliximab, etanercept, adalimumab, and golimumab.[42] A fifth anti-TNF agent is approved for use in rheumatoid arthritis—certolizumab pegol. For all of the anti-TNF agents approved for ankylosing spondylitis there is significant improvement in spinal inflammation as demonstrated by MRI. There remains some detectable inflammation despite the efficacy of this class of drugs.[42] Long-term follow-up continues to show some radiographic progression of disease. Future goals of therapy will be to eliminate all inflammation detectable on MRI. At this time infliximab, adalimumab, and certolizumab are approved for treatment of CD, and infliximab is approved for therapy in UC. Etanercept was shown to be ineffective in the treatment of CD.[43] Golimumab is currently in clinical trials for IBD. If anti-TNF therapy is indicated for SA, the choice of agent should be one with demonstrated efficacy in IBD. Timing of therapy should be at a point relatively early on in the disease course, where there has not yet been extensive structural damage to the joints or to the gastrointestinal tract. At that point, therapeutic intervention may be able to change the natural course of the disease.

☑ Key Points

☑ Arthritis is the most common extraintestinal manifestation of IBD.

☑ Arthritis may be a central/axial arthritis or a nondestructive peripheral arthritis.

☑ HLAB27 is seen in 25% to 78% of patients with IBD and spondylitis or sacroiliitis.

☑ MRI is the criterion standard imaging technique for diagnosis of early sacroiliac disease.

☑ Treatment includes analgesia, physical therapy, and pharmacotherapy including sulfasalazine, methotrexate, and anti-TNF therapy.

REFERENCES

1. Salvarani C, Fries W. Clinical features and epidemiology of spondyloarthritides associated with inflammatory bowel disease. *World J Gastroenterol*. 2009;15:2449-2455.
2. Braun J, Sieper J. Building consensus on nomenclature and disease classification for ankylosing spondylitis: results and discussion of a questionnaire prepared for the International Workshop on New Treatment Strategies in Ankylosing Spondylitis, Berlin, Germany, 18-19 January 2002. *Ann Rheum Dis*. 2002;61(suppl 3):iii61-iii67.
3. Dougados M, van der Linden S, Juhlin R, et al. The European Spondylarthropathy Study Group preliminary criteria for the classification of spondylarthropathy. *Arthritis Rheum*. 1991;34:1228-1230.
4. Amor B, Dougados M, Mijiyawa M. Criteria of the classification of spondylarthropathies. *Rev Rhum Mal Osteoartic*. 1990;57:85-89.
5. Rostom S, Dougados M, Gossec L. New tools for diagnosing spondyloarthropathy. *Joint Bone Spine*. 2010;77:108-114.

6. Vavricka S, Brun L, Ballabeni P, et al. Frequency and risk factors for extraintestinal manifestations in the Swiss inflammatory bowel disease cohort. *Am J Gastroenterol.* 2011; 106:110-119.

7. Jacques P, Elewaut PD, Meilants H. Interactions between gut inflammation and arthritis/spondylitis. *Curr Opin Rheum.* 2010;22:368-374.

8. Taurog J, Richardson J, Croft J, et al. The germfree state prevents development of gut and joint inflammatory disease in HLA-B27 transgenic rats. *J Exp Med.* 1994;180:2359-2364.

9. Breban M, Fernández-Sueiro J, Richardson J, et al. T cells, but not thymic exposure to HLA-B27, are required for the inflammatory disease of HLA-B27 transgenic rats. *J Immunol.* 1996;156:794-802.

10. Tran T, Dorris M, Satumtira N, et al. Additional human beta2-microglobulin curbs HLA-B27 misfolding and promotes arthritis and spondylitis without colitis in male HLA-B27-transgenic rats. *Arthritis Rheum.* 2006;54:1317-1327.

11. Kontoyiannis D, Pasparakis M, Pizarro T, et al. Impaired on/off regulation of TNF biosynthesis in mice lacking TNF AU-rich elements: implications for joint and gut-associated immunopathologies. *Immunity.* 1999;10:387-398.

12. Armaka M, Apostolaki M, Jacques P, et al. Mesenchymal cell targeting by TNF as a common pathogenic principle in chronic inflammatory joint and intestinal diseases. *J Exp Med.* 2008;205:331-337.

13. Peeters H, Vander Cruyssen B, Laukens D, et al. Radiological sacroiliitis, a hallmark of spondylitis, is linked with CARD15 gene polymorphisms in patients with Crohn's disease. *Ann Rheum Dis.* 2004;63:1131-1134.

14. Sáfrány E, Pazár B, Csöngei V, et al. Variants of the IL23R gene are associated with ankylosing spondylitis but not with Sjögren syndrome in Hungarian population samples. *Scand J Immunol.* 2009;70:68-74.

15. Sieper J, van der Heijde D, Landewé R, et al. New criteria for inflammatory back pain in patients with chronic back pain: a real patient exercise by experts from the Assessment of SpondyloArthritis international Society (ASAS). *Ann Rheum Dis.* 2009;68:784-788.

16. Calin A, Porta J, Fries J, et al. Clinical history as a screening test for ankylosing spondylitis. *JAMA.* 1977;237:2613-2614.

17. Yüksel I, Ataseven H, Başar O, et al. Peripheral arthritis in the course of inflammatory bowel diseases. *Dig Dis Sci.* 2011;56:183-187.

18. Orchard T, Wordsworth B, Jewell D. Peripheral arthropathies in inflammatory bowel disease: their articular distribution and natural history. *Gut.* 1998;42:387-391.

19. Rudwaleit M, van der Heijde D, Landewe R, et al. The development of Assessment of SpondyloArthritis international Society classification criteria for axial spondyloarthritis (part II): validation and final selection. *Ann Rheum Dis.* 2009;68:777-783.

20. Beigel F, Schnitzler F, Paul Laubender R, et al. Formation of antinuclear and double-strand DNA antibodies and frequency of lupus-like syndrome in anti-TNF-α antibody-treated patients with inflammatory bowel disease. *Inflamm Bowel Dis.* 2011;17:91-98.

21. Khan M. Remarkable polymorphism of HLA-B27: an ongoing saga. *Curr Rheum Rep.* 2010; 12:337-341.

22. Arai R. Serologic markers: impact on early diagnosis and disease stratification in inflammatory bowel disease. *Postgrad Med.* 2010;122:177-185.

23. Mundwiler M, Mei L, Landers C, et al. Inflammatory bowel disease serologies in ankylosing spondylitis patients: a pilot study. *Arthritis Res Ther.* 2009;11:R177.

24. Aydin S, Atagunduz P, Temel M, et al. Anti-*Saccharomyces cerevisiae* antibodies (ASCA) in spondyloarthropathies: a reassessment. *Rheumatology.* 2008;47:142-144.

25. van der Heijde D, Maksymowych W. Spondyloarthritis: state of the art and future perspectives. *Ann Rheum Dis.* 2010;69:949-954.

26. Rudwaleit M, Jurik A, Hermann K, et al. Defining active sacroiliitis on magnetic resonance imaging (MRI) for classification of axial spondyloarthritis: a consensual approach by the ASAS/OMERACT MRI group. *Ann Rheum Dis.* 2009;68:1520-1527.

27. Cosnes J. Tobacco and IBD: relevance in the understanding of disease mechanisms and clinical practice. *Best Pract Res Clin Gastroenterol.* 2004;18:481-496.

28. Doran M, Brophy S, MacKay K, et al. Predictors of longterm outcome in ankylosing spondylitis. *J Rheumatol*. 2003;30:316-320.
29. Cosnes J, Beaugerie L, Carbonnel F, et al. Smoking cessation and the course of Crohn's disease: an intervention study. *Gastroenterology*. 2001;120:1093-1099.
30. Elyan M, Khan M. Does physical therapy still have a place in the treatment of ankylosing spondylitis? *Curr Opin Rheumatol*. 2008;20:282-286.
31. Wang C, Chiang P, Lee H, et al. The effectiveness of exercise therapy for ankylosing spondylitis: a review. *Int J Rheum Dis*. 2009;12:207-210.
32. Song I, Poddubnyy D, Rudwaleit M, et al. Benefits and risks of ankylosing spondylitis treatment with nonsteroidal antiinflammatory drugs. *Arthritis Rheum*. 2008;58:929-938.
33. Kefalakes H, Stylianides T, Amanakis G, et al. Exacerbation of inflammatory bowel diseases associated with the use of nonsteroidal anti-inflammatory drugs: myth or reality? *Eur J Clin Pharmacol*. 2009;65:963-970.
34. Watkinson G. Sulphasalazine: a review of 40 years' experience. *Drugs*. 1986;32(suppl 1):1-11.
35. De Vos M. Joint involvement in inflammatory bowel disease: managing inflammation outside the digestive system. *Expert Rev Gastroenterol Hepatol*. 2010;4:81-89.
36. Pincus T, Yazici Y, Sokka T, et al. Methotrexate as the "anchor drug" for the treatment of early rheumatoid arthritis. *Clin Exp Rheumatol*. 2003;21(suppl 31):S179-S185.
37. Chen J, Liu C, Lin J. Methotrexate for ankylosing spondylitis. *Cochrane Database Syst Rev*. 2006;(18):CD004524.
38. Patel V, Macdonald J, McDonald J, et al. Methotrexate for maintenance of remission in Crohn's disease. *Cochrane Database Syst Rev*. 2009;(7):CD006884.
39. Alfadhli A, McDonald J, Feagan B. Methotrexate for induction of remission in refractory Crohn's disease. *Cochrane Database Syst Rev*. 2005;(25):CD003459.
40. American College of Rheumatology Ad Hoc Committee on Clinical Guidelines: guidelines for monitoring drug therapy in rheumatoid arthritis. *Arthritis Rheum*. 1996;39:723-731.
41. Van Den Bosch F, Kruithof E, Baeten D, et al. Randomized double-blind comparison of chimeric monoclonal antibody to tumor necrosis factor alpha (infliximab) versus placebo in active spondylarthropathy. *Arthritis Rheum*. 2002;46:755-765.
42. Heldmann F, Dybowsk iF, Saracbasi-Zender E, et al. Update on biologic therapy in the management of axial spondyloarthritis. *Curr Rheumatol Rep*. 2010;12:325-331.
43. Sandborn W, Hanauer S, Katz S, et al. Etanercept for active Crohn's disease: a randomized, double-blind, placebo-controlled trial. *Gastroenterology*. 2001;121:1088-1094.

Suggested Readings

Brakenhoff LK, van der Heijde DM, Hommes DW, Huizinga TW, Fidder HH. The joint-gut axis in inflammatory bowel diseases. *J Crohns Colitis*. 2010;4:257-268.

De Vos M. Joint involvement associated with inflammatory bowel disease. *Dig Dis*. 2009;27:511-515.

De Vos M, Hindryckx P Laukens D. Novel development in extraintestinal manifestations and spondylarthropathy. *Best Pract Res Clin Gastroenterol*. 2011;25(suppl 1):S19-S26.

Dotson J, Crandall W, Bout-Tabaku S. Exploring the differential diagnosis of joint complaints in pediatric patients with inflammatory bowel disease. *Curr Gastroenterol Rep*. 2011;13:271-278.

Salvarani C, Fries W. Clinical features and epidemiology of spondyloarthritides associated with inflammatory bowel disease. *World J Gastroenterol*. 2009;15:2449-2455.

Chapter 8

Skin and Oral Disease

Lisa M. Grandinetti, MD, FAAD, MMS and
Jason M. Swoger, MD, MPH

EPIDEMIOLOGY

The skin and oral cavity are sites frequently involved with extraintestinal manifestations (EIMs) of inflammatory bowel disease (IBD). Reported frequencies of EIMs in IBD patients are quite variable, with recent reports ranging from 6.2% to as high as 43%.[1,2] It has been hypothesized that the presence of one EIM increases the risk of developing another, suggesting a common pathogenic mechanism.[2] Although this mechanism is not well understood, it is likely due to interplay of genetics, immunologic dysregulation, and environmental exposures. There is evidence that an aberrant immunologic reaction to gut bacterial endotoxin stimulates T-cell activation and autoantibody production, leading to both colonic and extraintestinal injury.[3] Cross reactivity between gut antigens and epitopes in the involved organs further supports this theory.[3]

Mucocutaneous EIMs have traditionally been divided into 3 main categories: disease specific, reactive, and miscellaneous.[4] The first group, disease specific, includes entities such as oral Crohn's disease (CD); cutaneous CD (CCD); and perianal fissures, fistulas, and skin tags. The second group broadly encompasses reactive entities, such as erythema nodosum (EN) and pyoderma gangrenosum (PG), and the last group contains miscellaneous mucocutaneous findings that have been reported in smaller numbers of IBD patients. With the increased armamentarium of both medical and surgical therapies for IBD, we suggest that an additional category, therapy-related dermatoses, should be added to this classification system (Table 8-1). This chapter will highlight the pathophysiology, clinical presentation, diagnostic evaluation, and management options for the most salient mucocutaneous EIMs within each of the above-mentioned categories.

Regueiro MD, Swoger JM, eds.
Clinical Challenges and Complications of IBD (pp 141-164).
© 2013 Taylor & Francis Group.

Table 8-1. Mucocutaneous Lesions Associated With Inflammatory Bowel Disease

DISEASE SPECIFIC
Perianal fissures, fistulas, and skin tags
Oral Crohn's disease
Cutaneous (metastatic) Crohn's disease
REACTIVE
Erythema nodosum
Pyoderma gangrenosum
Aphthous ulcers/stomatitis
Vesiculopustular eruptions
Pyoderma vegetans
Pyostomatitis vegetans
Necrotizing vasculitis
Cutaneous polyarteritis nodosa
Erythema multiforme
Urticaria
Sweet syndrome
Bowel-associated dermatosis arthritis syndrome
MISCELLANEOUS
Epidermolysis bullosa acquisita
Clubbing
Vitiligo
Psoriasis
Secondary amyloidosis
Alopecia areata
Acquired nutritional deficiency dermatoses
THERAPY RELATED
TNF-α-associated psoriasiform dermatoses
Peristomal pyoderma gangrenosum
Nonmelanoma skin cancer

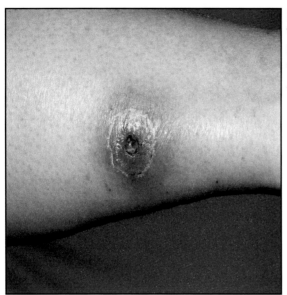

Figure 8-1. A violaceous plaque, with central ulceration, consistent with cutaneous CD. (Reprinted with permission of Joseph C. English III, MD.)

Disease-Specific Extraintestinal Manifestations

Cutaneous Crohn's Disease

Pathophysiology and Clinical Features

CCD is characterized by skin colored to violaceous papules, nodules, and plaques, predominantly located in the genital region, but which can involve any site on the body (Figure 8-1). Other common areas of involvement include the skin folds of the anterior abdominal wall and submammary area.[5] By definition, CCD is separated from the gastrointestinal tract by normal tissue; thus, this does not include classic perianal CD. CCD is the least common dermatologic manifestation of CD.[6] In adults, CCD appears after the initial diagnosis of CD in 70% of cases, whereas in children, it appears at the same time as initial CD diagnosis, approximately 50% of the time.[7] Whether or not the skin lesions of CCD mirror intestinal disease activity is controversial.[5,8] As with many EIMs, the presence of CCD may be more common in patients with colonic involvement.[8]

Diagnostic Evaluation

Tissue biopsy with appropriate staining (Periodic Acid Schiff, Gram, etc) is often necessary to confirm the diagnosis, as the clinical manifestations are nonspecific. Histologically, the lesions of CCD show pseudoepitheliomatous hyperplasia in conjunction with epithelial granulomatous inflammation. The most frequent histologic finding seen in CCD is a sarcoidal nonsuppurative granuloma.[9]

Figure 8-2. Labial mucosa demonstrating common manifestations of OCD, including granulomatous swelling and ulceration. (Reprinted with permission of Robin Gehris, MD.)

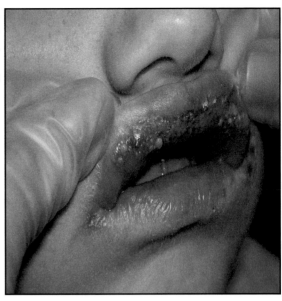

Treatment

Given the infrequent presentation of CCD, evidence-based therapies and treatment guidelines are lacking. There have been a number of reports of the successful use of oral metronidazole therapy for CCD.[10,11] Other reported therapies include oral and topical corticosteroids, azathioprine, and cyclosporine. More recently, infliximab has demonstrated efficacy in the treatment of refractory CCD.[5,12-14] Surgical removal of the CD-involved segments of the gastrointestinal tract does not always improve the lesions of CCD.[7]

Oral Crohn's Disease

Pathophysiology and Clinical Features

Oral cavity lesions are more common in CD than in ulcerative colitis (UC), with estimates ranging from 0.5% to 20% of IBD patients having oral involvement.[4] By far, the more common entities found in the oral cavity are reactive EIMs such as aphthous ulcers (see below). True oral CD (OCD), defined as having known intestinal CD and disease-specific oral manifestations, is uncommon, with a frequency in the range of 6%.[15,16] Nevertheless, recognition of these lesions is important, as they may sometimes precede the diagnosis of IBD by years.[17-19] Clinical manifestations of OCD include oral cobblestoning, granulomatous swelling of the lips and other intraoral sites, hyperplastic buccal mucosa, and deep linear ulcers with hyperplastic margins[15,20] (Figure 8-2). The term *orofacial granulomatosis* (OFG) is used to describe patients with granulomatous oral lesions but without evidence of CD elsewhere in the gastrointestinal tract.[21] OFG has been described in patients with underlying sarcoidosis and with Melkersson-Rosenthal syndrome. At ileocolonoscopy, a large percentage of patients with OFG will have evidence of intestinal inflammation, often in the absence of symptoms. Additionally, a large number of patients who initially present with OFG will go on to develop symptomatic CD.[16,22,23] OFG patients should be followed closely for the possible subsequent development of gastrointestinal symptoms.

Diagnostic Evaluation

Oral tissue biopsy is required to secure a diagnosis of OCD, which may also assist in differentiating CD from UC. Histologic findings are of characteristic granulomas, which are present in a high percentage of cases, up to 100% in some reports.[20,24] As oral lesions may be difficult for a gastroenterologist to accurately identify, involving an oral medical expert (dentist, dermatologist, or oral maxillofacial surgeon) may be beneficial.

Treatment

Many patients with OCD are asymptomatic in terms of their oral lesions, and treatment should be aimed at their underlying intestinal inflammation. Patients who do present with symptoms, or whose intestinal inflammation is not well controlled, may benefit from therapies aimed at the oral lesions. Diet modification, including avoidance of cinnamon and benzoates, has been shown to significantly reduce oral inflammation.[25] Additionally, steroid mouthwashes or gels may lead to symptomatic relief. Intralesional steroid injection has also been reported for granulomatous lip inflammation, which can lead to significant and debilitating lip swelling. Elliott et al reported on the use of infliximab for 14 patients with OFG, 7 of whom had concurrent CD.[26] There was a significant short-term response to infliximab (71%), with a 57% response rate at 1 year. However, longer-term follow-up demonstrated eventual loss of response. A proportion of patients in the study who did lose response were successfully treated with adalimumab.

REACTIVE EXTRAINTESTINAL MANIFESTATIONS

Erythema Nodosum

Pathophysiology and Clinical Features

EN is characterized by painful, indurated, erythematous to violaceous plaques, often located on the anterior surfaces of the lower extremities (Figure 8-3). Although this location is most common, EN can also involve the trunk or upper extremities. EN is the most common cutaneous manifestation of IBD, occurring in 3% to 20% of patients with IBD, and is considered to reside within the realm of IBD-related reactive dermatoses.[2,27-29] A large French cohort study of more than 2400 consecutive IBD patients found an overall prevalence of EN of 4.5%, and it was more commonly present in CD (5.6%) than in UC (1.2%).[30] EN has a female predominance, occurring in women 3 to 6 times more commonly than in men.[31] EN often presents in association with systemic symptoms, including malaise, fatigue, and arthralgias. In terms of associations

Figure 8-3. Indurated, erythematous nodules on the bilateral shins typically seen in a patient with erythema nodosum. (Reprinted with permission of Elizabeth Juhas, MD.)

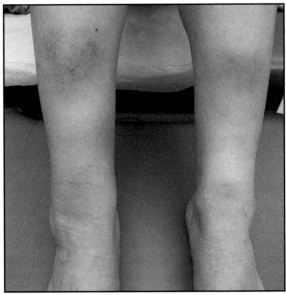

with bowel disease, EN is more common in patients with colonic involvement, and is also seen more commonly in CD than in UC.[8,17,29,30,32]

The pathogenesis of EN is not well understood, and it has been broadly defined as a type IV (delayed type) hypersensitivity reaction, the inciting antigen being identified in approximately 40% of patients.[33] EN is not specific to IBD; rather, it has been associated with numerous infectious causes (eg, streptococcal infections); drug reactions (eg, sulfonamides and oral contraceptives); malignancies such as Hodgkin disease; and other systemic inflammatory conditions, including sarcoidosis, Sjögren syndrome, and Behçet disease. In the typical clinical course of EN, individual nodules are present for approximately 2 weeks, then slowly involute without scarring. New crops of lesions can continue to arise for up to 6 weeks during a disease exacerbation.[34]

Diagnostic Evaluation

In the setting of a patient with known IBD who presents with cutaneous lesions suggestive of EN, the diagnosis is usually made clinically. However, given the broad differential of possible etiologies for EN, a thorough history, physical examination, and laboratory testing, including complete blood count, antistreptolysin O titer, chest x-ray, or stool cultures, may be necessary for patients in whom the underlying history is not clear. Histologically, EN is the prototypic septal panniculitis without evidence of vasculitis (Figure 8-4). EN classically does not ulcerate, and if ulceration is present, additional work-up including deep incisional biopsy of the skin should be performed to rule out an underlying vasculitis or malignancy.

Treatment

Treatment of EN is always aimed at removing the underlying trigger, if possible. In the setting of the IBD patient, EN eruptions are often associated

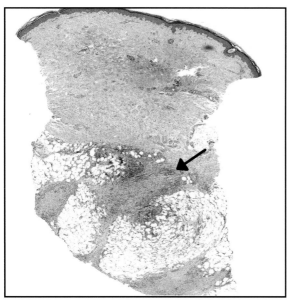

Figure 8-4. A low-power photomicrograph demonstrating a predominantly septal panniculitis (arrow) without evidence of vasculitis. (Reprinted with permission of Jonhan Ho, MD.)

with exacerbations of the bowel disease, but not necessarily with the severity or extent of disease.[31] Thus, therapy aimed at the medical treatment of IBD should be initiated, in addition to symptomatic treatment for EN, if needed. Typically, the first line of therapy for EN is a nonsteroidal anti-inflammatory drug (NSAID). However, in IBD patients, NSAID use may be associated with disease exacerbations and should be used with caution. Other treatment options include rest, elevation, and compression of the affected tissues. One technique involves raising the legs above the level of the heart, to maximize venous return, for at least 30 minutes twice daily, to mitigate discomfort.[34] Support stockings with a 15- to 20-mm Hg pressure gradient may also be helpful.[34] For more severe disease, oral glucocorticoids such as prednisone have been used. Our anecdotal experience suggests that prednisone at a dose of 0.5 to 1.0 mg/kg/day tapered over a 3- to 4-week period, is effective. Biologic agents, including infliximab and adalimumab, have been reported to successfully treat recalcitrant EN.[35] Other less common therapies include colchicine, hydroxychloroquine, and dapsone.

Pyoderma Gangrenosum

Pathophysiology and Clinical Features

Although findings in the literature vary, the prevalence of PG in patients with IBD seems to be between 0.6% and 3%.[8,30,32] PG appears to be more common in patients with UC than in those with CD, and, as with EN, is more common in patients with colonic involvement.[8,36] Most studies have found a prevalence of PG in patients with UC of between 0.5% and 5%.[1,2,17,29,30,37-40] For CD, the prevalence of PG has been reported to be between 0.5% and 2%.[2,17,29,30,32,41,42] A multivariate analysis of a cohort of 2402 patients found PG to be associated with African race, a family history of UC, pancolitis, and the presence of ocular involvement.[30] Co-existing EIMs are often found in patients with IBD-related PG, with arthritis and uveitis being most common.[29] PG can occur prior to, concurrent to, or following the diagnosis of IBD.[31] The most common sites of PG involvement are the lower extremities, although in IBD patients, another important site of involvement is the peristomal skin (see p. 152). Multiple lesions may occur at the same time and can be unilateral or bilateral.[41,43]

Controversy exists regarding the correlation between the development of PG and bowel disease activity.[8,44,45] PG has been described to occur up to 10 years following total proctocolectomy in patients with UC, suggesting that PG is not always linked to disease activity. In some reports, up to 50% to 75% of PG cases were associated with active disease, although this may depend on the PG subtype being reported.[43] For example, the pustular type of PG may be more often associated with active bowel disease, while the ulcerative type may occur independently.[36] PG does have the tendency to recur following successful treatment, in up to 30% of cases, and often does so in the same distribution as the initial episode.[32,46] Recurrence rates have been reported to be as high as 95% at 3 years, and up to 50% of patients may require maintenance therapy.[44,47]

The pathophysiology of PG is not well understood, although it has been hypothesized to involve abnormal neutrophil function and impaired cellular immunity.[48,49] With a clinical response to cyclosporine noted in several studies, T lymphocytes are thought to play a role in the pathogenesis of PG, along with the production of tumor necrosis factor-alpha (TNF-α). Pathergy is a characteristic finding associated with PG, with ulcers developing in response to minor trauma.

Diagnostic Evaluation

PG is classified into 4 distinct subtypes, with the pustular and ulcerative types being most common in IBD patients. Other diseases associated with PG include hepatitis, rheumatoid arthritis, leukemias, multiple myeloma, IgA gammopathy, and hypogammaglobulinemia. PG is usually diagnosed clinically, based on the characteristic appearance of the lesions. Lesions initially present as an erythematous pustule or nodule that then spreads, developing into a burrowing ulcer with violaceous edges and undermined borders (Figure 8-5). The ulcers are often covered in pus or necrotic debris and can contain fistulous tracts. The ulcers are sterile, although they may become superinfected. When the PG lesions heal, there remains typical "web-like" cribriform scarring.[42]

Histologically, early PG shows a perivascular lymphocytic infiltrate and endothelial swelling, with a dense dermal neutrophilic infiltrate.[50] Later in the disease course, lesions show necrosis and ulceration. Skin biopsy is usually not required to make the diagnosis and, with the known pathergy phenomenon, biopsy may theoretically exacerbate the disease. However, biopsy may be helpful in ruling out other diagnoses, such as bacterial pyoderma, fungal infection, necrotizing vasculitis, cutaneous lymphoma, or the halogenodermas.[41] Wound cultures for fungal and bacterial organisms are also an important part of the evaluation of a patient with PG.

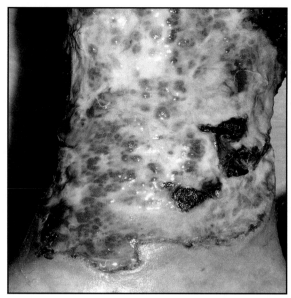

Figure 8-5. A patient with PG affecting the lower extremity. Note the characteristic rolled, violaceous, undermined border. (Reprinted with permission of Joseph C. English III, MD.)

Treatment

The treatment of PG should include treatment of the skin lesions, as well as the underlying IBD, if active. Local therapy, including weekly intralesional corticosteroid injections (triamcinolone acetonide 10 to 40 mg/mL), potent topical corticosteroid ointments, topical tacrolimus ointment, topical dapsone gel, cromolyn sodium, and topical 5-aminosalicylic acid may be successful in healing mild lesions. Local wound care is an important aspect of therapy, including saline lavage, topical antibacterial creams, and hydrocolloid dressings, and trauma should be avoided. For more extensive disease, systemic corticosteroids (prednisone 1.0 to 2.0 mg/kg/day) are the treatment of choice. Other systemic therapies that may be effective include sulfasalazine, dapsone, and immunomodulators such as azathioprine, 6-mercaptopurine, cyclosporine, methotrexate, tacrolimus, and mycophenolate mofetil.[36]

Multiple reports have found oral cyclosporine to be especially effective in healing PG in patients with and without IBD, with complete healing times of approximately 7 months.[51-53] Friedman et al reported that all 11 of their patients experienced healing of their lesions in a mean time of 1.4 months, after being treated with intravenous cyclosporine for a mean of 11.7 days, then continued on oral cyclosporine.[54] The majority of the patients were successfully maintained on immunomodulators and were able to discontinue corticosteroids. A limitation of cyclosporine therapy is its poor oral absorption, as well as the common adverse effects of hypertension, nephrotoxicity, and opportunistic infections.[55]

A retrospective multicenter study reported the effectiveness of infliximab in 13 IBD patients with medically refractory PG. All 13 patients responded to infliximab, with a mean time to response of 11 days and mean time to complete healing of 86 days. Corticosteroid tapering was successful

Figure 8-6. A CD patient with PPG, with a typical ulcerated lesion inferior to the ostomy. (Reprinted with permission of Joseph C. English III, MD.)

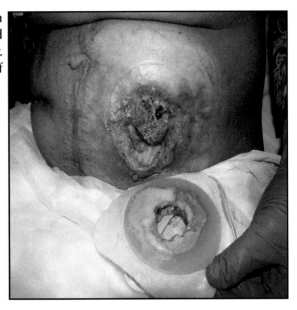

in all subjects. PG recurred in 4 patients, who were then retreated with infliximab with success, and 6 patients were in continued remission with maintenance infliximab.[56] Additionally, Brooklyn et al reported a randomized, placebo-controlled trial of a single dose of infliximab in 30 patients with PG, although only 19 had underlying IBD.[57] Overall, there was significantly greater response in the infliximab group compared to placebo at week 2 (46% versus 6%). After 2 weeks, nonresponders received open-label infliximab, and by week 6, 69% of patients who had received at least one dose of infliximab had a response, with 21% achieving clinical remission. Although associated with rapid healing when treated with infliximab, PG does recur, and maintenance therapy may be required. Other case reports in the literature have shown similar success for treating medically refractory PG with infliximab, with a median response time of 10 days and a median time to complete healing of 45 days.[58]

Peristomal Pyoderma Gangrenosum

Although PG usually occurs on the flexural surfaces of the lower extremities, peristomal PG (PPG) is a special concern in patients with IBD (Figure 8-6). PPG ulcers are exquisitely painful and can be refractory to standard therapies. Several series have reported a female preponderance of PPG.[59,60] An association with active intestinal disease, as with classic PG, is controversial.[59,61] The median time to the appearance of peristomal lesions was 3 months in one study, and 75% of patients had active intestinal disease.[62] A similar case series found the appearance of lesions to occur a median of 6 months following surgery.[59] These lesions often have an adverse effect on stoma adhesion and may adversely affect stoma patency. It is thought that minor trauma associated with the stomal appliance may contribute, at least

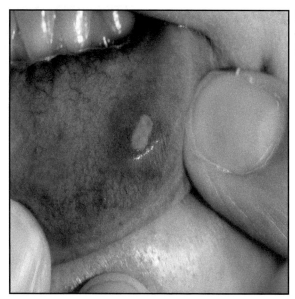

Figure 8-7. Typical appearance of an oral aphthous ulceration. (Reprinted with permission of Rochelle Torgerson, MD, PhD.)

in part, to the development of PPG. Early recognition of PPG is important in ensuring successful treatment, and alternate diagnoses including contact dermatitis, irritation from leaking feces, wound infection, and underlying CD must be ruled out.

Topical therapy for PPG may be difficult, as the medications may interfere with stomal adherence. Wound and stoma care for PPG is critical, in order to improve the likelihood of healing. However, systemic therapy is required in most cases of PPG. Mimouni et al reported a case series demonstrating the efficacy of infliximab in the treatment of refractory PPG ulcerations, similar to the reports of successful treatment of classic PG with infliximab.[63] The most successful method of treating PPG is stomal closure, when possible.[62] Stoma relocation or revision, however, is not as successful, with early recurrence being common at the new stoma site.[59,62]

Aphthous Stomatitis

Pathophysiology and Clinical Features

Aphthous ulcers are the most common oral lesions associated with IBD (Figure 8-7). Aphthae are shallow erythematous ulcers with a central adherent fibrinous exudate and an erythematous halo. The ulcers are often painful and involve nonkeratinized mucosa. The incidence of aphthous stomatitis is 4% to 38% in patients with IBD.[29,64] Ulcers often present during episodes of active intestinal inflammation, mirroring the activity of the underlying IBD.[27] Some additional triggers of aphthous stomatitis have been described in the general population, including emotional stress, food and medication allergies (including 5-aminosalicylates), local trauma, and immunologic disorders. Smoking cessation has been associated with exacerbation of this condition, while pregnancy may be associated with clinical improvement.[65] As with several other EIMs, the pathophysiology of aphthous stomatitis is not well understood. However, it is thought that T lymphocytes infiltrate the oral epithelium in response to an unidentified keratinocyte-associated antigen. Differentiation of cytotoxic T lymphocytes, and the production of TNF-α, leads to keratinocyte death and the clinical manifestation of aphthae.[66]

Diagnostic Evaluation

Oral aphthous ulcers may be seen in association with a variety of systemic illnesses, including celiac disease, systemic lupus erythematosus, herpes simplex virus infection, HIV, and reactive arthritis (formerly Reiter syndrome). Behçet disease, which can also present with oral and intestinal aphthae should be considered in the differential diagnosis. Untreated iron, folic acid, and vitamin B_{12} deficiencies are also associated with aphthous stomatitis, which may be exacerbated by the active intestinal inflammation common in the IBD population and should be corrected if present. Clinical and laboratory evaluation for the above conditions would be appropriate in patients without a known underlying disease association, such as IBD. However, the gastroenterologist must be aware of associations with hematinic deficiencies, infections, and immunosuppression, as IBD patients may be predisposed to these concomitant triggers, which require more specific evaluation and treatment.

In patients with known IBD, a diagnosis of aphthous stomatitis can often be made clinically, as the lesions are often exquisitely painful. Biopsy should be performed in cases of recalcitrant oral lesions that do not heal within 3 to 4 weeks. Biopsy may also be appropriate in patients who smoke cigarettes or use smokeless tobacco products, as oral squamous cell carcinoma may present with similarly appearing, nonhealing oral ulcers.

Treatment

As with several EIMs, treatment of the underlying IBD may be curative. Due to the significant pain often associated with these lesions, symptomatic therapy is often warranted. Viscous lidocaine (2%), topical corticosteroid gels and pastes, or dexamethasone swish and spit (0.5 mg/5 mL) may be effective in providing symptomatic relief. It must be remembered that topical oral corticosteroid use can lead to oral candidiasis, and the patient should be counseled regarding this risk. Amlexanox 5%, a nonsteroidal anti-inflammatory paste, may also promote ulcer healing and reduce pain.[31] Systemic corticosteroids and immunosuppressive medications should be reserved for only the most severe cases, unless appropriate for treatment of the underlying IBD. Other treatment regimens that may be effective for aphthous stomatitis include a combination of dapsone and colchicine, as well as thalidomide, although side effects limit the use of these regimens. Anti-TNF therapy has been successful in the short-term healing of oral aphthae in patients with Behçet disease.[66]

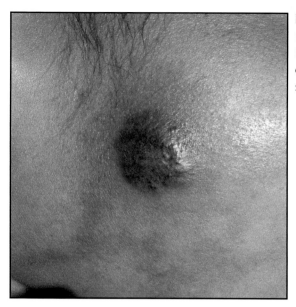

Figure 8-8. A characteristic indurated, violaceous plaque is seen in this patient with Sweet syndrome. (Reprinted with permission of Timothy Patton, DO.)

Pyostomatitis Vegetans

Although rare, pyostomatitis vegetans is highly associated with IBD, most often UC, and is a highly specific marker for underlying IBD.[66] Characteristic findings are of pustules, miliary abscesses, erosions, and vegetative plaques involving the palate and the buccal mucosa. The pustular lesions rupture, leading to ulcerations and fissuring, which has classically been described as a "snail-track" appearance. Pyostomatitis vegetans activity generally mirrors intestinal inflammation and the bowel disease is usually diagnosed months to years prior to the onset of the oral lesions. Controlling intestinal inflammation can lead to healing of the oral lesions. However, topical and systemic corticosteroids are often required in order to resolve the condition, sometimes with the addition of azathioprine or cyclosporine.

Sweet Syndrome

Pathophysiology and Clinical Features

Acute febrile neutrophilic dermatosis, or Sweet syndrome, has been associated with several systemic diseases, including IBD, malignancies, medications, and infections. This condition is rarely associated with IBD, with less than 40 cases of IBD-related Sweet syndrome having been reported in the literature.[27] The typical clinical presentation includes the acute onset of fever and malaise and the development of tender erythematous to violaceous, indurated plaques (Figure 8-8). The most common sites of cutaneous lesions are the head and neck, along with the upper extremities. Associated clinical findings may include arthralgias or arthritis (60%), eye involvement, including conjunctivitis or episcleritis (40%), and increased inflammatory markers on laboratory findings.[67] Colonic involvement by IBD is nearly universal, with no cases of Sweet syndrome being reported in IBD patients with isolated small bowel disease.[67] Females are more often affected than males. Sweet syndrome is usually associated with active intestinal disease.[68,69] The timing between the diagnosis of Sweet syndrome and IBD is variable, and it can occur prior to (20%), concurrent with (28%), or after the diagnosis of IBD (52%).[70] As was described with PG, Sweet syndrome demonstrates pathergy and can be initiated by local trauma such as needle sticks.

The pathogenesis of Sweet syndrome remains unclear, although several different mechanisms have been hypothesized. Potential mechanisms include a type III hypersensitivity reaction, T lymphocyte dysfunction, alteration in neutrophil function, or associations with certain histocompatibility antigens.[67] In addition, certain proinflammatory cytokines and granulocyte colony stimulating factors have been implicated in disease pathogenesis.[67]

Diagnostic Evaluation

When Sweet syndrome is suspected, a lesional skin biopsy should be performed to confirm the diagnosis. Histologic findings are well characterized and include massive edema of the papillary dermis; a dense, diffuse infiltrate of mature neutrophils throughout the dermis; and leukocytoclasia without evidence of vasculitis.[68] In patients without known IBD, a more extensive evaluation is indicated to rule out the other conditions associated with Sweet syndrome, including infection and malignancy. It should also be mentioned that cases of azathioprine-induced Sweet syndrome have been reported in the literature, including in a patient with CD.

Treatment

Systemic corticosteroids are the mainstay of therapy for Sweet syndrome, and the skin lesions rapidly resolve once therapy is commenced. Therapy can be initiated with oral prednisone or intravenous methylprednisolone, followed by a slow tapering course over 2 to 3 months.[68] Other initial therapies may include potassium iodide, given as either tablets or a saturated solution, although this is less frequently used due to concerns about treatment-induced hypothyroidism. Colchicine (0.5 mg 3 times a day) can also be considered first-line therapy for Sweet syndrome, although diarrhea, abdominal pain, and nausea and vomiting can be dose limiting. Other treatments that have been described include dapsone, cyclosporine, indomethacin, and clofazimine. Cases of improvement in Sweet syndrome following treatment with infliximab and tacrolimus have been reported more recently.[71-73]

Bowel-Associated Dermatosis Arthritis Syndrome

Bowel-associated dermatosis arthritis syndrome (BADAS), formerly known as bowel bypass syndrome, was initially described in patients who had undergone intestinal bypass surgery. Subsequently, the syndrome has been reported in patients who have not undergone surgery, but who have other associated conditions including IBD, diverticulitis, and peptic ulcer disease.[74,75] The

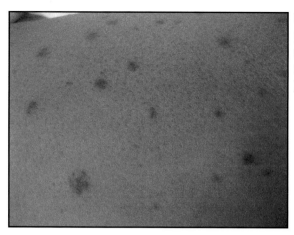

Figure 8-9. Scattered vesiculopustules on the extremity of a patient with CD and BADAS. (Reprinted with permission of Joseph C. English III, MD.)

pathogenesis of BADAS is thought to be due to circulating immune complexes that are deposited in the skin and joints.[75] Ely hypothesized that the immune complexes are formed in response to bacterial peptidoglycans resulting from small bowel bacterial overgrowth.[76] Patients may have a serum sickness-like prodrome consisting of fever, chills, malaise, arthralgias, and myalgias.

The characteristic dermatologic findings in BADAS are of erythematous macules that evolve to papules and purpuric vesiculopustules within 48 hours (Figure 8-9). The skin findings are present for approximately 2 weeks following onset and may recur at 4- to 6-week intervals. The skin lesions typically occur on the proximal extremities and trunk.[77] Histologic findings are of a perivascular, nodular neutrophilic infiltrate, with nuclear dust and dermal edema.[77] Oral antibiotics, including metronidazole, clindamycin, and the tetracycline family, are indicated for the treatment of mild disease. More severe disease necessitates the use of immunomodulatory agents, such as prednisone, azathioprine, cyclosporine, and mycophenolate mofetil. Finally, surgical revision of the bypass or resection of the blind loop of bowel is curative.

Psoriasis

The coexistence of psoriasis and IBD has been well documented. There have been epidemiologic, genetic, and pathogenic similarities documented among these diseases.[78-82] Najarian and Gottleib et al found the presence of psoriasis in 9.6% of CD patients, compared to only 2.2% of controls ($P < 0.02$).[80] In addition, 10% of their CD cohort had a positive family history of psoriasis, compared to only 2.9% of controls having a first-degree relative with psoriasis ($P = 0.02$). Cohen et al found IBD to be present in 0.5% of patients with psoriasis, compared with 0.3% of controls having UC and 0.2% of controls having CD ($P = 0.01$).[83] Finally, Yates et al found psoriasis to be more common among patients with CD (odds ratio 2.49) compared to those with UC (1.64), although other studies have not noted a difference in prevalence among the IBD subtypes.[84]

Genetic similarities among psoriasis and IBD have also begun to be described. There has been significant focus on the Th17 inflammatory pathway in both IBD and psoriasis. Genome-wide studies in CD have found significant associations with a polymorphism in the gene for interleukin (IL)-23R that encodes for a subunit of the IL-23 receptor.[85] This same genetic polymorphism (rs11209026) has also been associated with the development of psoriasis, suggesting a genetic link between psoriasis and IBD.[86] Another genetic locus, 6p21, encompassing the major histocompatibility complex, has been shown to contain susceptibility loci for psoriasis, CD, and UC (IBD3 and PSORS1).[83]

A discussion of the diagnosis and treatment of psoriasis is beyond the scope of this chapter and should be pursued in consultation with a dermatologist. However, a unique psoriasiform reaction to anti-TNF inhibitors has been described in the gastroenterology, rheumatology, and dermatology literature, and this will be the focus of the subsequent discussion.

Anti–Tumor Necrosis Factor-α-Induced Psoriasis

Pathophysiology and Clinical Features

The prevalence of anti-TNF–induced psoriasis in patients with IBD is unknown, and much of the information on this condition is extrapolated from the rheumatology literature. A retrospective literature review, from 2010, attempted to describe all reported cases of anti-TNF–associated psoriasis, which included 207 cases. Of these patients, 41 (20%) had an underlying diagnosis of IBD as the indication for anti-TNF therapy.[87] Infliximab was the medication used in 90% of cases, with 10% of patients receiving adalimumab. The majority of patients had no prior history of psoriasis (95%), although other studies have found up to a 19.7% personal history of psoriasis in patients with these drug reactions.[88] The most common clinical presentations of psoriasis were the plaque type (61%) and the pustular type (49%), with guttate psoriasis occurring in 5% of patients, consistent with findings in other studies.[88,89] Alopecia secondary to TNF-related scalp psoriasis has also been described.[90]

No age or gender differences have been consistently described for anti-TNF–induced psoriasis.[91] The skin lesions can appear at any time during therapy. A literature review found the highest incidence between the third and fourth infliximab infusions (14.3 weeks), while a large French cohort study found a median time of lesion onset of 17 months for infliximab and 12 months for adalimumab.[89,92-94] Wollina et al reported a mean time to appearance of lesions in 9.5 months in their literature review of 127 patients.[88]

Although the exact mechanism of the paraxodical psoriasis reaction associated with anti-TNF therapy is not clear, several hypotheses exist. In psoriasis, plasmacytoid dendritic cells produce interferon (IFN)-α, which stimulates the activation of pathogenic T-cells. Normally, TNF-α suppresses the development of plasmacytoid dendritic cells and their production of IFN-α. However, when a TNF-α antibody is present, TNF-α downregulation of the PDCs is removed, leading to unopposed IFN-α production. This IFN-α overproduction leads to the release of proinflammatory cytokines, which ultimately leads to the development of Th17 cells. Th17 cells, which release IL-17, have been associated with the development of de novo psoriasis, both in animal models, and in patients undergoing treatment for hepatitis with IFN-α.[95] Increased levels of IFN-α have

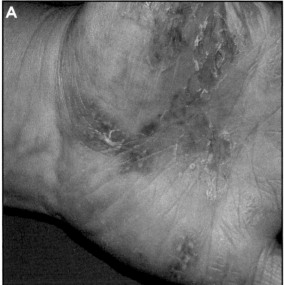

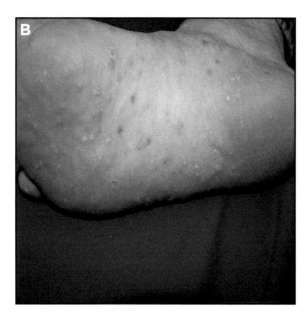

Figure 8-10. (A) Palm of hand and (B) sole of foot demonstrating firm, intraepidermal pustules, on a background of scaly, erythematous plaques. These findings are characteristic of palmoplantar pustulosis. (Reprinted with permission of Joseph C. English III, MD.)

also been found in skin biopsies of patients with TNF-α-associated psoriasis.[96] In addition, IFN-α leads to increased expression of the CXCR3 receptor on T-cells, which induces the recruitment of these lymphocytes to the skin.[97]

The majority of cases of reported TNF-α-associated psoriasis have presented as either palmoplantar pustulosis (pustular psoriasis) or plaque psoriasis. Palmoplantar pustulosis is characterized by small, firm pustules on a background of erythematous, scaly plaques (Figure 8-10). Although this classically occurs on the palms and soles, it can occur anywhere on the body. Prototypic plaque psoriasis presents with pink to erythematous plaques, with micaceous scale, which favors the flexural surfaces of the body but can occur anywhere. The scalp and nails are also common sites of psoriatic involvement.

Diagnostic Evaluation

Although the clinical presentation of psoriasis can be characteristic, a skin biopsy is often helpful in differentiating psoriasis from other clinical mimickers, including pustular drug eruptions, such as acute generalized exanthematous pustulosis, or conditions such as pityriasis rubra pilaris. Systemic atopic dermatitis, cutaneous T-cell lymphoma, and allergic contact dermatitis can all present with erythroderma (erythema > 80% of body surface area) and must be ruled out. Bacterial and viral infection should also be excluded.

The histologic findings of anti-TNF–induced psoriasis are identical to findings in conventional plaque and pustular psoriasis, as opposed to the findings associated with pustular drug eruptions.[87] These include epidermal hyperplasia, parakeratosis, dilated capillaries, intraepidermal pustulosis, and epidermal lymphocytic infiltrates.

Treatment

A review of TNF-induced psoriasis found that almost half of patients (46%) had resolution of their skin lesions following discontinuation of the TNF therapy, with only 10% having partial or no resolution.[93] In this descriptive study, 34% of patients had either complete or partial resolution of their skin lesions while continuing the TNF therapy.

Although there is disagreement in the literature, the majority of treatment approaches do not recommend withdrawal of the anti-TNF antibody upon initial presentation. Patients may respond to topical therapies, such as corticosteroids, keratolytics, and vitamin D analogues, without interrupting their biologic therapy.[87,93] Ultraviolet light therapy may also be useful should patients not respond to topical therapies.[99] Rahier et al noted a 40% response to topical therapy, with 5 of 10 (50%) patients who received ultraviolet therapy responding.[93] Other systemic therapies for psoriasis, including methotrexate and cyclosporine, have also been used to treat these lesions while allowing patients to continue their biologic therapy. Reassuringly, almost all patients will experience resolution of their skin lesions following withdrawal of the anti-TNF agent. Patients with more aggressive presentations, including severe lesions, erythroderma, or lesions significantly affecting their quality of life, should discontinue the offending medication. Wollina et al, in their series of 127 patients, did not find significantly different response rates between patients who continued or discontinued anti-TNF therapy.[88]

If patients do not respond to the above therapies, switching to an alternative anti-TNF agent may be considered, as can a drug holiday, with subsequent rechallenge with the same anti-TNF agent.[87] Rahier et al reported a cohort study of 62 IBD patients with TNF-associated psoriasis.[93] In their cohort, 16 patients (25.8%) with skin lesions discontinued their initial TNF therapy due to dermatological reasons. Of the 26 patients who were switched to a second TNF agent, only one patient experienced improvement of his or her skin lesions, suggesting a possible class effect. However, the second agent was continued in 14 patients due to manageable dermatologic symptoms or to a risk-benefit analysis favoring continued TNF therapy for their underlying IBD. Overall, 25 of 62 (40%) discontinued TNF therapy due to their skin lesions. Controversy remains as to the best approach to the IBD patient who develops TNF-induced psoriasis; while various reports in the literature have demonstrated success with the withdrawl of the biologic agent, initiation of topical or skin-directed therapies to control the psoriasis, and the subsequent reintroduction of biologic therapy, treatment must be tailored to the individual needs of the patient.

Conclusion

Many dermatologic manifestations of IBD have been described, making the skin and oral cavity 2 of the most common target organs for EIMs of IBD. Skin manifestations have been classified into several categories, including disease specific, reactive, miscellaneous, and, more recently, therapy related. Association with particular IBD subtypes and disease activity differ among the specific skin disorders. There are symptomatic therapies that can ameliorate discomfort, pruritus, or skin lesions, although resolution of these skin disorders often requires treatment of the underlying IBD. A good working relationship with a medical dermatologist or oral disease specialist knowledgeable in the varying presentations of these complex diseases is integral to the successful management of affected IBD patients.

☑ Key Points

☑ Dermatologic manifestations of IBD have been well described and are diverse in their clinical presentation.

☑ Dermatologic conditions associated with IBD can be disease related, reactive, miscellaneous, or therapy related.

☑ Several of the dermatologic conditions associated with IBD mirror intestinal disease activity, and definitive treatment is often aimed at the underlying bowel disease.

☑ EN is the most common cutaneous manifestation of IBD. Patients typically present with tender, erythematous nodules on the extensor surfaces of their lower extremities.

☑ PG does not necessarily parallel intestinal disease activity and is associated with pathergy. Treatment can be challenging, and often requires either immunomodulator or biologic therapy.

☑ Close collaboration with a dermatologist or oral medicine specialist is important to ensure optimal management of these complex syndromes.

REFERENCES

1. Bernstein CN, Blanchard JF, Rawsthorne P, et al. The prevalence of extraintestinal diseases in inflammatory bowel disease: a population-based study. *Am J Gastroenterol*. 2001;96: 1116-1122.

2. Vavricka SR, Brun L, Ballabeni P, et al. Frequency and risk factors for extraintestinal manifestations in the Swiss Inflammatory Bowel Disease Cohort. *Am J Gastroentrol*. 2011;106:110-119.

3. Das KM. Relationship of extraintestinal involvements in inflammatory bowel disease: new insights into autoimmune pathogenesis. *Dig Dis Sci*. 1999;44:1-13.

4. Gregory B, Ho VC. Cutaneous manifestations of gastrointestinal disorders. Part II. *J Am Acad Dermatol*. 1992;26:371-383.

5. Hoffmann RM, Kruis W. Rare extraintestinal manifestations of inflammatory bowel disease. *Inflamm Bowel Dis*. 2004;10:140-147.

6. Peltz S, Vestey J, Ferguson A, Hunter J, McLaren K. Disseminated metastatic cutaneous Crohn's disease. *Clin Exp Dermatol*. 1993;18:55-59.

7. Palamaras I, El-Jabbour J, Pietropaolo N, et al. Metastatic Crohn's disease: a review. *J Eur Acad Dermatol Venereol*. 2008;22:1033-1043.

8. Veloso FT. Review article: skin complications associated with inflammatory bowel disease. *Aliment Pharmaol Ther*. 2004;20(suppl 4):50-53.

9. Magro C, Crowson AN, Mihm M. Cutaneous manifestations of nutritional deficiency states and gastrointestinal disease. In: Elder DE, Elenitsas R, Johnson BL Jr, Murphy GF, eds. *Lever's Histopathology of the Skin*. 9th ed. Philadelphia, PA: Lippincott Williams & Wilkins; 2005:426-428.

10. Boerr LA, Bai JC, Olivares L, et al. Cutaneous metastatic Crohn's disease: treatment with metronidazole. *Am J Gastroenterol*. 1987;82:1326-1327.

11. Brandt LJ, Bernstein LH, Boley SJ, Frank MS. Metronidazole therapy for perineal Crohn's disease: a follow up study. *Gastroenterology*. 1982;83:383-387.

12. Carranza DC, Young L. Successful treatment of metastatic Crohn's disease with cyclosporine. *J Drugs Dermatol*. 2008;7:789-791.

13. Miller AM, Elliott PR, Fink R, Connell W. Rapid response of severe refractory metastatic Crohn's disease to infliximab. *J Gastroenterol Hepatol*. 2001;16:940-942.

14. Escher JC, Stoof TJ, van Deventer SJ, van Furth AM. Successful treatment of metastatic Crohn's disease with infliximab. *J Pediatr Gastroenterol Nutr*. 2002;34:420-423.

15. Basu MK, Asquith P. Oral manifestations of inflammatory bowel disease. *Clin Gastroenterol*. 1980;9:307-321.

16. Williams AJK, Wray D, Ferguson A. The clinical entity of orofacial Crohn's disease. *Q J Med*. 1991;79:451-458.

17. Greenstein AJ, Janowitz HD, Sachar DB. The extraintestinal manifestations of Crohn's disease and ulcerative colitis: a study of 700 patients. *Medicine*. 1976;55:401-412.

18. Lisciandrano D, Ranzi T, Carrassi A, et al. Prevalence of oral lesions in inflammatory bowel disease. *Am J Gastroenterol*. 1996;91:7-10.

19. Ekbom A, Helmick C, Zack M, Adami HO. The epidemiology of inflammatory bowel disease: a large, population-based study in Sweden. *Gastroenterology*. 1991;100:350-358.

20. Plauth M, Jenss H, Meyle J. Oral manifestations of Crohn's disease. An analysis of 79 cases. *J Clin Gastroenterol*. 1991;13:29-37.

21. Rowland M, Felming P, Bourke B. Looking in the mouth for Crohn's disease. *Inflamm Bowel Dis*. 2010;16:332-337.

22. Girlich C, Bogenrieder T, Palitzsch KD, et al. Orofacial granulomatosis as initial manifestation of Crohn's disease: a report of two cases. *Eur J Gastroenterol Hepatol*. 202;14:873-876.

23. Field EA, Tyldesley WR. Oral Crohn's disease revisited—a 10 year review. *Br J Oral Maxillofac Surg*. 1989;27:114-123.

24. Harty S. Fleming P, Rowland M, et al. A prospective study of the oral manifestations of Crohn's disease. *Clin Gastroenterol Hepatol*. 2005;3:886-891.

25. White A, Nunes C, Escudier M, et al. Improvement in orofacial granulomatosis on a cinnamon- and benzoate-free diet. *Inflamm Bowel Dis.* 2006;12:508-514.

26. Elliott T, Campbell H, Escudier M, Poate T, et al. Experience with anti-TNF-α therapy for orofacial granulomatosis. *J Oral Pathol Med.* 2011;40:14-19.

27. Larsen S, Bendtzen K, Nielsen OH. Extraintestinal manifestations of inflammatory bowel disease: epidemiology, diagnosis, and management. *Ann Med.* 2010;42:97-114.

28. Barrie A, Regueiro M. Biologic therapy in the management of extraintestinal manifestations of inflammatory bowel disease. *Inflamm Bowel Dis.* 2008;13:1424-1429.

29. Yuksel I, Basar O, Ataseven H, et al. Mucocutaneous manifestations in inflammatory bowel disease. *Inflamm Bowel Dis.* 2009;15:546-550.

30. Farhi D, Cosnes J, Zizi N, et al. Significance of erythema nodosum and pyoderma gangrenosum in inflammatory bowel diseases: a cohort study of 2402 patients. *Medicine.* 2008;87:281-293.

31. Trost LB, McDonnell JK. Important cutaneous manifestations of inflammatory bowel disease. *Postgrad Med J.* 2005;81:580-585.

32. Tromm A, May D, Almus E, et al. Cutaneous manifestations in inflammatory bowel disease. *Z Gastroenterol.* 2001;39:137-144.

33. Timani S, Mutasim DF. Skin manifestations of inflammatory bowel disease. *Clin Dermatol.* 2008;26:265-273.

34. Gilchrist H, Patterson JW. Erythema nodosum and erythema induratum (nodular vasculitis): diagnosis and management. *Dermatol Ther.* 2010;23:320-327.

35. Agrawal D. Rukkannagari S, Kethu S. Pathogenesis and clinical approach to extraintestinal manifestations of inflammatory bowel disease. *Minerva Gastroenterol Dietol.* 2007;53:233-248.

36. Su CG, Judge TA, Lichtenstein GR. Extraintestinal manifestations of inflammatory bowel disease. *Gastroenterol Clin North Am.* 2002;31:307-327.

37. Johnson ML, Wilson HTH. Skin lesions in ulcerative colitis. *Gut.* 1969;10:255.

38. Moschella SL. Pyoderma gangrenosum. *Arch Dermatol.* 1967;95:121.

39. McCallum DI, Kinmont PDC. Dermatological manifestations of Crohn's disease. *Br J Dermatol.* 1968;80:1.

40. Basler RSW. Ulcerative colitis and the skin. *Med Clin North Am.* 1980;64:941-954.

41. Lebwohl M, Lebwohl O. Cutaneous manifestations of inflammatory bowel disease. *Inflamm Bowel Dis.* 1998;4:142-148.

42. Ruhl AP, Ganz JE, Bickston SJ. Neutrophilic folliculitis and the spectrum of pyoderma gangrenosum in inflammatory bowel disease. *Dig Dis Sci.* 2007;52:18-24.

43. Levitt MD, Ritchie JK, Lennard-Jones JE, Phillips RK. Pyoderma gangrenosum in inflammatory bowel disease. *Br J Surg.* 1991;78:676-678.

44. Bennett ML, Jackson JM, Jorizzo JL, et al. Pyoderma gangrenosum. A comparison of typical and atypical forms with an emphasis on time to remission. Case review of 86 patients from 2 institutions. *Medicine.* 2000;79:37-46.

45. Wollina V. Clinical management of pyoderma gangrenosum. *Am J Clin Dermatol.* 2002;3:14-58.

46. Freeman HJ. Erythema nodosum and pyoderma gangrenosum in 50 patients with Crohn's disease. *Can J Gastroenterol.* 2005;19:603-606.

47. Van den Driesch P. Pyoderma gangrenosum: a report of 44 cases with follow-up. *Br J Dermatol.* 1997;137:1000-1005.

48. Jorizzo J, Soloman AR, Leshin B, et al. Neutrophilic vascular reactions. *J Am Acad Dermatol.* 1988;19:983-1005.

49. Huang W, McNeely MC. Neutrophilic tissue reactions. *Adv Dermatol.* 1998;13:33-63.

50. Boh EE, al-Smadi RMF. Cutaneous manifestations of gastrointestinal diseases. *Dermatol Clin.* 2002;20:533-546.

51. Shelley ED, Shelley WB. Cyclosporine therapy for pyoderma gangrenosum associated with sclerosing cholangitis and ulcerative colitis. *J Am Acad Dermatol.* 1988;18:1084-1088.

52. Matis WL, Ellis CN, Griffiths CE, et al. Treatment of pyoderma gangrenosum with cyclosporine. *Arch Dermatol.* 1992;128:1060-1064.

53. Gupta AK, Ellis CN, Nickoloff BJ, et al. Oral cyclosporine in the treatment of inflammatory and noninflammatory dermatoses. *Arch Dermatol.* 1990;126:339-350.

54. Friedman S, Marion J, Scherl E, Rubin PH, Present DH. Intravenous cyclosporine in refractory pyoderma gangrenosum complicating inflammatory bowel disease. *Inflamm Bowel Dis.* 2001;7:1-7.

55. Baumgart DC, Wiedenmann B, Dignass AU. Successful therapy of refractory pyoderma gangrenosum and periorbital phlegmona with tacrolimus (FK506) in ulcerative colitis. *Inflamm Bowel Dis.* 2004;10:421-424.

56. Regueiro M, Valentine J, Plevy S, Fleisher MR, Lichtenstein GR. Infliximab for the treatment of pyoderma gangrenosum associated with inflammatory bowel disease. *Am J Gastroenterol.* 2003;98:1821-1826.

57. Brooklyn TN, Dunnill MGS, Shetty A, et al. Infliximab for the treatment of pyoderma gangrenosum: a randomized, double-blind, placebo controlled trial. *Gut.* 2006;55:505-509.

58. Reguiai Z, Grange F. The role of anti-tumor necrosis factor-α therapy in pyoderma gangrenosum associated with inflammatory bowel disease. *Am J Clin Dermatol.* 2007;8:67-77.

59. Kiran RP, O'Brien-Ermlich B, Achkar JP, Fazio VW, Delaney CP. Management of peristomal pyoderma gangrenosum. *Dis Colon Rectum.* 2005;48:1397-1403.

60. Cairns BA, Herbst CA, Sartor BR, Briggman RA, Koruda MJ. Peristomal pyoderma gangrenosum and inflammatory bowel disease. *Arch Surg.* 1994;129:769-772.

61. Funayama Y, Kumagai E, Takahashi KI, Fukushima K, Sasaki I. Early diagnosis and early corticosteroid administration improves healing of peristomal pyoderma gangrenosum in inflammatory bowel disease. *Dis Colon Rectum.* 2009;52:311-314.

62. Poritz LS, Lebo MA, Bobb AD, Ardell CM, Koltun WA. Management of peristomal pyoderma gangrenosum. *J Am Coll Surg.* 2008;206:311-315.

63. Mimouni D, Anhalt GJ, Kouba DJ, Nousari HC. Infliximab for peristomal pyoderma gangrenosum. *Br J Dermatol.* 2003;148:813-816.

64. Veloso FT, Carvalho J, Magro F. Immune-related systemic manifestations of inflammatory bowel disease. A prospective study of 792 patients. *J Clin Gastroenterol.* 1996;23:29-34.

65. Mirowski GW, Parker ER. Disorders of the oral and genital integument. In: Wolff K, Goldsmith LA, Katz SI, et al, eds. *Dermatology in General Medicine.* 7th ed. New York, NY: McGraw Hill Medical; 2008:645-646.

66. Field EA, Allan RB. Review article; oral ulceration—aetiopathogenesis, clinical diagnosis and management in the gastrointestinal clinic. *Aliment Phramacol Ther.* 2003;18:949-962.

67. Catalan-Serra I, Martin-Moraleda L, Navarro-Lopez L, et al. Crohn's disease and Sweet's syndrome: an uncommon association. *Rev Esp Enferm Dig* (*Madrid*). 2010;102:331-336.

68. Moschella S, Davis MDP. Neutrophilic dermatoses. In: Bolognia JL, Jorizzo JL, Rapini RP, et al, eds. *Dermatology.* 2nd ed. Philadelphia, PA: Elsevier Mosby; 2008:380-383.

69. Ytting H, Vind I, Bang D, Munkholm P. Sweet's syndrome—an extraintestinal manifestation in inflammatory bowel disease. *Digestion.* 2005;72:195-200.

70. Travis S, Innes N, Davies MG, Daneshmend T, Hughes S. Sweet's syndrome: an unusual cutaneous feature of Crohn's disease or ulcerative colitis. The South West Gastroenterology Group. *Eur J Gastroenterol Hepatol.* 1997;9:715-720.

71. Fellerman K, Rudolph B, Witthof T, et al. Sweet syndrome and erythema nodosum in ulcerative colitis, refractory to steroids: successful treatment with tacrolimus. *Med Klin* (*Munich*). 2001;96:105-108.

72. Vanbiervleit G, Anty R, Schneider S, et al. Sweet syndrome and erythema nodosum associated with Crohn's disease treated by infliximab. *Gastroenterol Clin Biol.* 2002;26:295-297.

73. Rahier JF, Lion L, Dewit O, Lambeert M. Regression of Sweet's syndrome associated with Crohn's disease after anti-tumor necrosis factor therapy. *Acta Gastroenterol Belg.* 2005;68:376-379.

74. Fenske NA, Gern JE, Pierce D, et al. Vesiculopustular eruption of ulcerative colitis. *Arch Dermatol.* 1983;119:664-669.

75. Jorizzo JL, Apisarnthanarax P, Subrt P, et al. Bowel bypass syndrome without bowel bypass; bowel associated dermatosis-arthritis syndrome. *Arch Intern Med.* 1983;143:457-461.

76. Ely PH. The bowel bypass syndrome: a response to bacterial peptidoglycans. *J Am Acad Dermatol*. 1980;2:473-487.

77. Moschella S, Davis MDP. Neutrophilic dermatoses. In: Bolognia JL, Jorizzo JL, Rapini RP, et al, eds. *Dermatology*. 2nd ed. Philadelphia, PA: Elsevier Mosby; 2008:390-391.

78. Hoffmann R, Schieferstein G, Schunter F, Janss H. Increased occurrence of psoriasis in patients with Crohn's disease and their relatives. *Am J Gastroenterol*. 1991;86:787-788.

79. Hughes S, Williams SE, Turnberg LA. Crohn's disease and psoriasis. *N Engl J Med*. 1983;308:101.

80. Najarian DJ, Gottleib AN. Connections between psoriasis and Crohn's disease. *J Am Acad Dermatol*. 2003;48:805-821.

81. Rudikoff D. Baral J, Lebwohl M. Psoriasis and Crohn's disease. *Mt Sinai J Med*. 1999;66:206.

82. Lee F, Bellary S, Francis C. Increased occurrence of psoriasis in patients with Crohn's disease and their relatives. *Am J Gastroenterol*. 1990;85:962-963.

83. Cohen AD, Dreiher J, Birkenfeld S. Psoriasis associated with ulcerative colitis and Crohn's disease. *J Eur Acad Dermatol Venerol*. 2009;23:561-565.

84. Yates VM, Watkinson G, Kelman A. Further evidence for an association between psoriasis, Crohn's disease and ulcerative colitis. *Br J Dermatol*. 1982;106:323-330.

85. Lees CW, Satsangi J. Genetics of inflammatory bowel disease: implications for disease pathogenesis and natural history. *Expert Rev Gastroenterol Hepatol*. 2009;3:513-534.

86. Duerr RH, Taylor KD, Brant DR, et al. A genome-wide association study identifies IL23R as an inflammatory bowel disease gene. *Science*. 2006;314:1461-1463.

87. Collamer AN, Battafarano DF. Psoriatic skin lesions induced by tumor necrosis factor antagonist therapy: clinical features and possible immunopathogenesis. *Semin Arthritis Rheum*. 2010;40:233-240.

88. Wollina Y, Hansel G, Koch A, et al. Tumor necrosis factor-α inhibitor-induced psoriasis or psoriasiform exanthemata: first 120 cases from the literature including a series of six new patients. *Am J Clin Dermatol*. 2008;9:1-14.

89. Fiorino G, Allez M, Malesci A, and Danese S. Review article: anti TNF-α induced psoriasis in patients with inflammatory bowel disease. *Aliment Pharmacol Ther*. 2009;29:921-927.

90. El Shabrawi-Caelen L, La Placa M, Vincenzi C, et al. Adalimumab-induced psoriasis of the scalp with diffuse alopecia: a severe potentially irreversible cutaneous side effect of TNF-alpha blockers. *Inflamm Bowel Dis*. 2010;16:182-183.

91. Borras-Blasco J, Navarro-Ruiz A, Borras C, Castera E. Adverse cutaneous reactions induced by TNF-α antagonist therapy. *South Med J*. 2009;102:1133-1140.

92. Dereure O, Guillot B, Jorgensen C, et al. Psoriatic lesions induced by antitumor necrosis factor-α treatment: two cases. *Br J Dermatol*. 2004;150:506-507.

93. Rahier J-F, Buche S, Peyrin-Biroulet L, et al. Severe skin lesions cause patients with inflammatory bowel disease to discontinue anti-tumor necrosis factor therapy. *Clin Gastroenterol Hepatol*. 2010;8:1048-55.

94. Passarini B, Infusino SD, Barbieri E, et al. Cutaneous manifestations in inflammatory bowel diseases: Eight cases of psoriasis induced by anti-tumor-necrosis-factor antibody therapy. *Dermatology*. 2007;215:295-300.

95. Ketikoglou I, Karatapanis S, Elefsiniotis I, et al. Extensive psoriasis induced by pegylated interferon-alpha-2b treatment for chronic hepatitis B. *Eur J Dermatol*. 2005;15:107-109.

96. De Gannes G, Ghoreishi M, Pope J, et al. Psoriasis and pustular dermatitis triggered by TNF-α inhibitors in patients with rheumatologic conditions. *Arch Dermatol*. 2007;143:223-231.

97. Aeberli D, Seitz M, Juni P. Increase of peripheral CXCR3 positive T lymphocytes upon treatment of RA patients with TNF-α inhibitors. *Rheumatology*. 2005;44:172-175.

98. Sladden MJ, Clarke PJ, Wettenhall J. Infliximab-induced palmoplantar pustolosis in a patient with Crohn's disease. *Arch Dermatol*. 2007;143:1449.

99. Peramiquel L, Puig L, Dalmau J, Ricart E, Roe E, Alomar A. Onset of flexural psoriasis during infliximab treatment for Crohn's disease. *Clin Exp Dermatol*. 2005;30:713-714.

Suggested Readings

Boh EE, al-Smadi RMF. Cutaneous manifestations of gastrointestinal diseases. *Dermatol Clin.* 2002;20:533-546.

Larsen S, Bendtzen K, Nielsen OH. Extraintestinal manifestations of inflammatory bowel disease: epidemiology, diagnosis, and management. *Ann Med.* 2010;42:97-114.

Lebwohl M, Lebwohl O. Cutaneous manifestations of inflammatory bowel disease. *Inflamm Bowel Dis.* 1998;4:142-148.

Regueiro M, Valentine J, Plevy S, Fleisher MR, Lichtenstein GR. Infliximab for the treatment of pyoderma gangrenosum associated with inflammatory bowel disease. *Am J Gastroenterol.* 2003;98:1821-1826.

Rowland M, Felming P, Bourke B. Looking in the mouth for Crohn's disease. *Inflamm Bowel Dis.* 2010;16:332-337.

Wollina Y, Hansel G, Koch A, et al. Tumor necrosis factor-α inhibitor-induced psoriasis or psoriasiform exanthemata: first 120 cases from the literature including a series of six new patients. *Am J Clin Dermatol.* 2008;9:1-14.

Chapter 9

Eye Disease

Aaron S. Bancil, BSc (Hons);
David G. Walker, BSc (Hons), MBBS, MD (Res), MRCP;
and Timothy R. Orchard, MA, MD, DM, FRCP

Eye disease has been associated with inflammatory bowel disease (IBD) ever since Crohn recorded 2 ulcerative colitis (UC) patients suffering from corneal inflammation with conjunctivitis that resembled a "xerophthalmia."[1] They now include uveitis (limited to the anterior chamber of the eye), episcleritis (inflammation of the outermost layer of the collagenous shell surrounding the eye), scleritis (deeper inflammation of the collagenous shell), and conjunctivitis. Ocular complications can also be related to exposure to drugs such as corticosteroids, resulting in cataracts or glaucoma. They are a significant cause of morbidity in IBD patients and can be distressing, debilitating, and occasionally irreversible. Thus, quick detection and referral to an ophthalmologist are essential.

EPIDEMIOLOGY

Extraintestinal manifestations (EIMs) occur frequently in IBD, with ocular disease incidence ranging from 3.5% to 12%.[2-5] There is no reported overall difference in ocular EIMs in terms of age or gender.[6,7]

The most common ocular manifestations are uveitis (17%), episcleritis (29%), and scleritis (18%).[2,8] Inflammation of the posterior segment of the eye in Crohn's disease (CD) and UC is rare, with a prevalence of less than 0.1% of cases.[9] This is in contrast to other systemic conditions, such as Behçet disease, where posterior chamber inflammation is the norm.[10] Other rarer manifestations include optic neuritis (4%), keratitis, retinitis, blepharitis, and vaso-occlusive disease.[2] Cataracts have also been reported, but they are primarily associated with the long-term use of steroids, and scleritis is associated with peripheral corneal infiltrates or limbal guttering.[11-13]

Eye manifestations rarely precede IBD diagnosis.[2] They are more often associated with colitis than small bowel disease and are generally associated with active intestinal disease.[1,12,14] Ocular EIMs appear to be more common in CD colitis than in UC, with pediatric research suggesting that the prevalence of

Regueiro MD, Swoger JM, eds.
Clinical Challenges and Complications of IBD (pp 165-174).
© 2013 Taylor & Francis Group.

anterior uveitis may be as high as 6.2% in CD.[15] Most studies of the prevalence of eye complications have been small and have often not included ophthalmic examinations, which makes defining the prevalence of the different subtypes difficult. However, uveitis seems to be more common in UC, while episcleritis and scleritis appear more commonly in CD.[16] Episcleritis appears to be more common in females.[12]

Uveitis activity may run parallel with IBD activity—ocular manifestations are rare during remission of IBD, but the risk increases 2-fold with intermittent activity and doubles again in gut disease with continuous activity.[7] In addition, colectomy induces remission of the eye disease in about half of uveitis cases.[11]

Up to 68% of patients with ocular manifestations have at least one other extraintestinal complication.[11] Hopkins et al found that nearly half of their 332 CD patient cohort had a coexisting arthritic manifestation alongside their ocular disease.[7] Wright et al found a strong association in UC patients with anterior uveitis and sacroiliac joint abnormalities, while another study has shown that uveitis, erythema nodosum, and arthritic manifestations commonly occur together.[14,17] These findings suggest some degree of association and a possible systemic pathogenesis behind EIMs.

Other rare ocular pathology in IBD includes keratitis, retinitis, pars planitis, orbital inflammatory disease, scleromalacia perforans, and central artery and vein occlusion.

UC may also rarely give rise to necrotizing scleritis, which may present as blurry vision, discomfort, and redness. On examination, there may be patches of avascularity and uvea, seen with surrounding inflammation, as well as evidence of scleral necrosis.[18]

A study by Satchi et al reported 9 patients (7 female, 2 male) with lacrimal obstruction associated with IBD who reported symptoms of sinonasal disease, suggesting the lacrimal outflow system may be another site for extraintestinal inflammation.[19]

Etiology and Pathophysiology

Although the existence of EIMs has been known for years, the exact pathogenesis behind them remains unclear. Eye disease can be caused by the IBD itself or may be due to secondary factors such as protein, vitamin, or mineral deficiencies and drug adverse effects. It is possible that the mechanism behind EIMs is an autoimmune process. A number of mechanisms may be involved (Table 9-1).[20]

There are numerous theories as to how these factors may operate. There may exist an immune-complex hypersensitivity reaction to a colonic antigen, which could potentially explain why eye disease is more common in those suffering with colitis and ileocolitis.[21] Additionally, a delayed hypersensitivity reaction or cytotoxic antibody reaction may cause ocular inflammation.[21]

Ocular disease often coexists with other EIMs, such as erythema nodosum or arthritic manifestations. This may be due to the similarity between the

Table 9-1. *Putative Mechanisms Underlying Extraintestinal Manifestations in Inflammatory Bowel Disease*

Genetic susceptibility
Antigenic display of autoantigen
Aberrant self-recognition
Immunopathogenetic auto-antibodies
Immune complexes
Cytokine imbalances
Bacterial antigens/toxins
Adapted from Das KM. Relationship of extraintestinal involvements in inflammatory bowel disease: new insights into autoimmune pathogenesis. *Dig Dis Sci.* 1999;44(1):1-13.

vasculature of the uvea and the synovium, which both have the capacity for leukocyte migration, cytokine activity, and antigen presentation.[21]

It is thought that ocular disease occurs due to an abnormal T-cell response to antigens in the eye, leading to T-cell and macrophage-mediated damage to the eye.[22] Tumor necrosis factor (TNF)-α has been implicated as an important proinflammatory cytokine in the pathogenesis of ocular EIMs. It upregulates other proinflammatory cytokines and cellular adhesion molecules such as intercellular adhesion molecule-1 (ICAM-1) and vascular adhesion molecule-1 (VCAM-1), thus enhancing leukocyte recruitment to inflammation sites.[23] In a murine model, interleukin-1 and TNF-α knockout mice showed reduced inflammation in immune-complex-induced uveitis, thus displaying their important role.[24] The importance of TNF-α in the pathogenesis of eye disease in IBD is further supported by the efficacy of anti-TNF antibodies in treating it.

It has also been suggested that a particular type of novel colonic epithelial cell that has a unique cross-reactivity with the eyes, joints, bile ducts, and skin may cause eye, skin, and joint inflammation.[20,25,26] This was an antigenic form of tropomyosin expressed both in the eye and the gut.[27,28] However, the proposed antigen was found in the ciliary body of the eye, which is rarely affected by inflammation in IBD, and other studies have failed to replicate these findings.

Another suggestion is that the development of inflammatory cell infiltrates in extraintestinal areas may be due to the adhesion of mucosal immune cells with endothelial cells.[29] It remains unclear as to why all patients do not thus suffer from EIMs in IBD or why only certain sites are affected.

One explanation for why not all patients or extraintestinal sites are affected may be genetic involvement, as EIMs have a familial predisposition. Up to an 83% concordance between siblings has been reported.[30] Phenotypic analysis of Blacks versus Whites with UC found that the former were significantly more likely to suffer from EIMs such as uveitis (8.1% versus 1.6%, $P < 0.005$), further supporting a genetic component to the disease phenotype.[31]

The role of specific genes is supported by a study looking at human leukocyte antigen (HLA) associations with ocular inflammation in IBD, which found that uveitis is strongly associated with HLA-B*27, B*58, and HLA-DRB1*0103, and that uveitis commonly occurs with erythema nodosum and arthritic manifestations. It was suggested that the reason for overlapping but independent clinical manifestations may be due to linkage disequilibrium among the HLA genes. This is the phenomenon whereby genes coding for different conditions are inherited together more often than expected by chance because they are located close by on the same chromosome.[14] Thus the HLA region, which contains a number of important genes involved in the immune response, may be an important area in the pathogenesis of extraintestinal IBD.

It thus seems likely that the pathogenesis of ocular inflammation occurs in genetically susceptible individuals who encounter some environmental trigger that provokes ocular inflammation, and despite the large number of theories detailed above, there is little firm evidence to support one over the remainder.

CLINICAL FEATURES

The wide variance in the clinical manifestations of eye disease include tearing, burning, itching, ocular pain, photophobia, conjunctival hyperemia, sclera hyperemia, blurred vision, loss of visual acuity, and potentially blindness.[21]

Patients with uveitis often present with a painful eye, blurred vision, and photophobia. This may progress to a miotic eye and potential papillary defects, such as an abnormal response to light. Patients with uveitis also exhibit a ciliary flush, where the redness extends from the limbus, fading outward, involving the circumlimbal vessels. If visual acuity is compromised, posterior uveitis or retinal involvement should be suspected.[21]

It is important to distinguish episcleritis from scleritis, as this can predict the likelihood of long-term ocular complications, and thus guide therapy. Episcleritis can be diffuse or nodular and presents unilaterally or bilaterally as acute redness with irritation or burning (Figure 9-1). The eyes are commonly tender to palpation. It is usually associated with active intestinal disease. On examination, focal or diffuse patches of redness can be seen.[21] Scleritis is a more severe and destructive ocular process, as it may cause severe visual impairment. It presents with severe eye pain, which is tender upon palpation. It can be distinguished from episcleritis as the sclera viewed on examination is pinkish in color rather than white between the dilated vessels on the surface (Figure 9-2). It may also present with subconjunctival hemorrhages.[21] The posterior part of the eye can also be involved in scleritis, presenting with moderate to severe eye pain, along with mild redness in the anterior chamber, distributed either focally or diffusely.

Corneal involvement is rare, but presents with eye pain, irritation, or the sensation of the presence of a foreign body. This may also be associated with decreased vision. Conjunctivitis can also not be ruled out, as this is the most common cause of eye redness in the general population. This presents with itchiness, redness, and a watery or purulent discharge, with an underlying

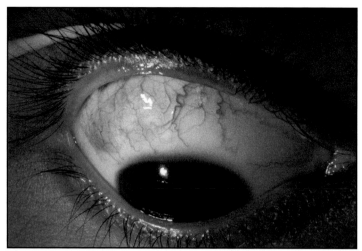

Figure 9-1. A patient presenting with the acute eye redness consistent with episcleritis. (Reprinted with permission from Kara Cavuoto, MD.)

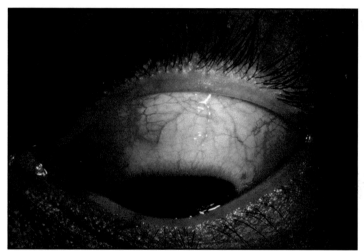

Figure 9-2. A patient with scleritis. Note the pink sclera in between the dilated surface vessels. (Reprinted with permission from Kara Cavuoto, MD.)

allergic, bacterial, or viral etiology. The degree to which conjunctivitis is associated with IBD remains unclear.[21]

Optic neuritis is the most common neuropathy in IBD. A number of IBD cases have been diagnosed with optic neuritis, giving symptoms of abnormal color vision, a relative afferent papillary defect, and visual field defects. Ocular deterioration may lead to vision of only a "counting fingers" level.[2,9,13,32-35]

DIAGNOSTIC EVALUATION

Basic blood tests including a full blood count, erythrocyte sedimentation rate, and blood biochemistry may be helpful, potentially showing results of anemia due to iron, vitamin B_{12}, or folate deficiency and also a thrombocytosis. Blood coagulation studies may be performed if one suspects vaso-occlusive disease, and it may be warranted to perform tests for rheumatoid factor and antinuclear antibody.[11]

However, definitive diagnosis is performed by slit-lamp examination with dilated pupils. Visual acuity and intraocular pressure should be tested using Snellen optotypes and a Goldmann tonometer.[36] It is vital to exclude infective causes of an acute red eye, such as herpetic infection; otherwise, incorrect therapeutic interventions (eg, corticosteroids) may exacerbate the condition.

Uveitis can be diagnosed by its characteristic "ciliary flush," while episcleritis and scleritis can be distinguished from each other as the sclera are white in episcleritis and pinkish in scleritis.[37]

Fluorescein angiography may be able to detect optic neuritis by showing capillary dilation, plus venous stasis on the optic disc.[2] Disc swelling may be accompanied by splinter hemorrhages and venous engorgement, showing similarities to the presentation of papillophlebitis.[38,39]

An orbital ultrasound may be useful in the diagnosis of scleritis and choroidopathies, while computed tomography scans may play a role in orbital inflammation.[2]

MANAGEMENT/TREATMENT/OUTCOMES

The exact treatment of ocular inflammation in IBD depends on the area of the eye involved. With the exception of simple conjunctivitis, all patients presenting with acute ocular inflammation should have a full ophthalmologic evaluation to make the diagnosis and to exclude other causes such as infection with herpes viruses. Treatment will normally consist of topical steroid treatment, initially hourly, and subsequently tapering. A 6- to 8-week course is usual. A cycloplegic agent such as atropine may be added to prevent the formation of posterior synechiae.

For uveitis, it is essential to treat the inflammation thoroughly, as long-term complications can include intraocular adhesions that may lead to secondary cataracts or glaucoma. Macular dysfunction and papillary defects may also occur.[21] The primary treatment for uveitis is topical corticosteroids to prevent blindness and corneal perforation. Occasionally periocular injection or oral steroids are required.

Infliximab (a chimeric monoclonal antibody to TNF-α) is another treatment that works effectively. It is clear that TNF-α has a role in the pathogenesis of ocular EIMs, and there is growing evidence to suggest that infliximab maintains remission in refractory CD uveitis patients.[40] It has been shown to be a powerful therapy in the treatment of HLA-B27-positive acute anterior uveitis, and a retrospective study found that infliximab was a safe and effective treatment for patients with uveitis or scleritis who did not respond to conventional immunosuppression.[23,41]

Adalimumab, a completely humanized anti-TNF-α antibody, has been shown to be effective in treating uveitis in children with juvenile idiopathic arthritis, effectively treating 88% of cases.[42] More research needs to be conducted specifically with this drug and ocular disease in IBD, but given the efficacy in other forms of uveitis, it is likely to be effective. Azathioprine, methotrexate, and cyclosporin may be used, but each of these is associated with important side effects.[43] Azathioprine specifically may not fully control uveitis, but nonetheless it has been shown to decrease severity and duration of acute anterior uveitis.[11]

Episcleritis should be treated with cool compresses and/or topical glucocorticoids, alongside treatment for underlying IBD. A minority of patients do not require treatment.[44] Nonsteroidal anti-inflammatory drugs (NSAIDs) may be useful in selected cases but should be used with caution, as they may result in a flaring of underlying IBD.[21]

Scleritis is a more severe form of ocular inflammation. It is important to treat it expeditiously, as it has the potential to develop into scleromalacia, retinal detachment, or optic nerve swelling. Aggressive treatment with corticosteroids or other immunosuppressants is thus necessary.[11,21,44] Periocular injection of corticosteroid or oral steroids is often effective in scleritis. NSAIDs may be useful in anterior scleritis also.

Infliximab was also found to be a safe and effective treatment for scleritis, but repeated administration may be required to keep the ocular inflammation under control.[23]

Posterior segment inflammation, although uncommon, warrants more aggressive treatment, as there is a lack of penetration from topical agents. Intraocular injection of corticosteroid may be effective, but oral steroids are usually required. These may need to be continued for up to 4 weeks. However, if there is poor response, patients can be started on azathioprine, methotrexate, or cyclosporin, in addition to corticosteroids.

If scleromalacia does develop, treatment with 0.5% ethylenediaminetetraacetate was beneficial in one particular CD-associated case.[13]

Those patients with optic neuritis respond well to systemic steroids, and vision is usually restored, although some cases may require steroid-sparing cytotoxics.[2]

Necrotizing scleritis, although only rarely associated with UC, can be managed with prednisolone, and adding other immunosuppressants may be helpful. An eye can be salvaged using a surgical technique that combines an amniotic membrane material and processed pericardium.[18]

Lacrimal obstruction can be treated surgically by a dacryocystorhinostomy.[19]

Treatment for steroid-induced cataracts is surgical removal, but this should be deferred until control of ocular inflammation occurs. Patients may also need anti-inflammatory support perioperatively.[11]

Although these treatments may be effective, it is necessary for patients to be closely monitored and for all physicians to be cooperative, including the gastroenterologist, the ophthalmologist, and the rheumatologist.

☑ Key Points

☑ On suspicion of acute ocular inflammation in IBD, refer to an ophthalmologist immediately for diagnosis and management.

☑ Ocular manifestations are a significant cause of morbidity in IBD patients.

☑ The most common ocular complications of IBD are uveitis, episcleritis, and scleritis.

☑ Ocular manifestations occur early in the pathogenesis of IBD and during active disease.

☑ It is important to diagnose ocular disease early to prevent significant complications such as scleromalacia and to help guide the patient's therapy.

☑ Biologic therapies such as infliximab are being used more commonly in the treatment of ocular disease in IBD, and there is growing evidence to support this.

References

1. Billson FA, De Dombal FT, Watkinson G, Goligher JC. Ocular complications of ulcerative colitis. *Gut.* 1967;8(2):102-106.
2. Ghanchi FD, Rembacken BJ. Inflammatory bowel disease and the eye. *Surv Ophthalmol.* 2003;48(6):663-676.
3. Knox DL, Schachat AP, Mustonen E. Primary, secondary and coincidental ocular complications of Crohn's disease. *Ophthalmology.* 1984;91(2):163-173.
4. Rankin GB, Watts HD, Melnyk CS, Kelley ML Jr. National Cooperative Crohn's Disease Study: extraintestinal manifestations and perianal complications. *Gastroenterology.* 1979;77(4 pt 2):914-920.
5. Greenstein AJ, Janowitz HD, Sachar DB. The extra-intestinal complications of Crohn's disease and ulcerative colitis: a study of 700 patients. *Medicine.* 1976;55(5):401-412.
6. Yilmaz S, Aydemir E, Maden A, Unsal B. The prevalence of ocular involvement in patients with inflammatory bowel disease. *Int J Colorectal Dis.* 2007;22(9):1027-1030.
7. Hopkins DJ, Horan E, Burton IL, Clamp SE, de Dombal FT, Goligher JC. Ocular disorders in a series of 332 patients with Crohn's disease. *Br J Ophthalmol.* 1974;58(8):732-737.

8. Banares A, Jover JA, Fernandez-Gutierrez B, et al. Patterns of uveitis as a guide in making rheumatologic and immunologic diagnoses. *Arthritis Rheum.* 1997;40(2):358-370.

9. Ernst BB, Lowder CY, Meisler DM, Gutman FA. Posterior segment manifestations of inflammatory bowel disease. *Ophthalmology.* 1991;98(8):1272-1280.

10. Ozdal PC, Ortac S, Taskintuna I, Firat E. Posterior segment involvement in ocular Behcet's disease. *Eur J Ophthalmol.* 2002;12(5):424-431.

11. Soukiasian SH, Foster CS, Raizman MB. Treatment strategies for scleritis and uveitis associated with inflammatory bowel disease. *Am J Ophthalmol.* 1994;118(5):601-611.

12. Salmon JF, Wright JP, Murray AD. Ocular inflammation in Crohn's disease. *Ophthalmology.* 1991;98(4):480-484.

13. Evans PJ, Eustace P. Scleromalacia perforans associated with Crohn's disease. Treated with sodium versenate (EDTA). *Br J Ophthalmol.* 1973;57(5):330-335.

14. Orchard TR, Chua CN, Ahmad T, Cheng H, Welsh KI, Jewell DP. Uveitis and erythema nodosum in inflammatory bowel disease: clinical features and the role of HLA genes. *Gastroenterology.* 2002;123(3):714-718.

15. Hofley P, Roarty J, McGinnity G, et al. Asymptomatic uveitis in children with chronic inflammatory bowel diseases. *J Pediatr Gastroenterol Nutr.* 1993;17(4):397-400.

16. Ardizzone S, Puttini PS, Cassinotti A, Porro GB. Extraintestinal manifestations of inflammatory bowel disease. *Dig Liver Dis.* 2008;40(suppl 2):S253-S259.

17. Wright R, Lumsden K, Luntz MH, Sevel D, Truelove SC. Abnormalities of the sacro-iliac joints and uveitis in ulcerative colitis. *Q J Med.* 1965;34:229-236.

18. Lazzaro DR. Repair of necrotizing scleritis in ulcerative colitis with processed pericardium and a Prokera amniotic membrane graft. *Eye Contact Lens.* 2010;36(1):60-61.

19. Satchi K, McNab AA. Lacrimal obstruction in inflammatory bowel disease. *Ophthal Plast Reconstr Surg.* 2009;25(5):346-349.

20. Das KM. Relationship of extraintestinal involvements in inflammatory bowel disease: new insights into autoimmune pathogenesis. *Dig Dis Sci.* 1999;44(1):1-13.

21. Mintz R, Feller ER, Bahr RL, Shah SA. Ocular manifestations of inflammatory bowel disease. *Inflamm Bowel Dis.* 2004;10(2):135-139.

22. Forrester JV. Duke-Elder Lecture: new concepts on the role of autoimmunity in the pathogenesis of uveitis. *Eye.* 1992;6(pt 5):433-446.

23. Murphy CC, Ayliffe WH, Booth A, Makanjuola D, Andrews PA, Jayne D. Tumor necrosis factor alpha blockade with infliximab for refractory uveitis and scleritis. *Ophthalmology.* 2004;111(2):352-356.

24. Brito BE, O'Rourke LM, Pan Y, Anglin J, Planck SR, Rosenbaum JT. IL-1 and TNF receptor-deficient mice show decreased inflammation in an immune complex model of uveitis. *Invest Ophthalmol Vis Sci.* 1999;40(11):2583-2589.

25. Salmi M, Jalkanen S. Endothelial ligands and homing of mucosal leukocytes in extraintestinal manifestations of IBD. *Inflamm Bowel Dis.* 1998;4(2):149-156.

26. Das KM, Vecchi M, Sakamaki S. A shared and unique epitope(s) on human colon, skin, and biliary epithelium detected by a monoclonal antibody. *Gastroenterology.* 1990;98(2):464-469.

27. Das KM, Sakamaki S, Vecchi M, Diamond B. The production and characterization of monoclonal antibodies to a human colonic antigen associated with ulcerative colitis: cellular localization of the antigen by using the monoclonal antibody. *J Immunol.* 1987;139(1):77-84.

28. Bhagat S, Das KM. A shared and unique peptide in the human colon, eye, and joint detected by a monoclonal antibody. *Gastroenterology.* 1994;107(1):103-108.

29. Jalkanen S. Lymphocyte traffic to mucosa-associated lymphatic tissues. *Immunol Res.* 1991;10(3-4):268-270.

30. Satsangi J, Grootscholten C, Holt H, Jewell DP. Clinical patterns of familial inflammatory bowel disease. *Gut.* 1996;38(5):738-741.

31. Nguyen GC, Torres EA, Regueiro M, et al. Inflammatory bowel disease characteristics among African Americans, Hispanics, and non-Hispanic Whites: characterization of a large North American cohort. *Am J Gastroenterol.* 2006;101(5):1012-1023.

32. Campieri M, Ferguson A, Doe W, Persson T, Nilsson LG. Oral budesonide is as effective as oral prednisolone in active Crohn's disease. The Global Budesonide Study Group. *Gut.* 1997;41(2):209-214.

33. Edwards RL, Levine JB, Green R, et al. Activation of blood coagulation in Crohn's disease. Increased plasma fibrinopeptide A levels and enhanced generation of monocyte tissue factor activity. *Gastroenterology.* 1987;92(2):329-337.

34. Farmer RG, Whelan G, Fazio VW. Long-term follow-up of patients with Crohn's disease. Relationship between the clinical pattern and prognosis. *Gastroenterology.* 1985;88(6): 1818-1825.

35. Sedwick LA, Klingele TG, Burde RM, Behrens MM. Optic neuritis in inflammatory bowel disease. *J Clin Neuroophthalmol.* 1984;4(1):3-6.

36. Felekis T, Katsanos K, Kitsanou M, et al. Spectrum and frequency of ophthalmologic manifestations in patients with inflammatory bowel disease: a prospective single-center study. *Inflamm Bowel Dis.* 2009;15(1):29-34.

37. Larsen S, Bendtzen K, Nielsen OH. Extraintestinal manifestations of inflammatory bowel disease: epidemiology, diagnosis, and management. *Ann Med.* 2010;42(2):97-114.

38. Heuer DK, Gager WE, Reeser FH. Ischemic optic neuropathy associated with Crohn's disease. *J Clin Neuroophthamol.* 1982;2(3):175-181.

39. Macoul KL. Ocular changes in granulomatous ileocolitis. *Arch Ophthalmol.* 1970;84(1):95-97.

40. Ally MR, Veerappan GR, Koff JM. Treatment of recurrent Crohn's uveitis with infliximab. *Am J Gastroenterol.* 2008;103(8):2150-2151.

41. El-Shabrawi Y, Hermann J. Anti-tumor necrosis factor-alpha therapy with infliximab as an alternative to corticosteroids in the treatment of human leukocyte antigen B27-associated acute anterior uveitis. *Ophthalmology.* 2002;109(12):2342-2346.

42. Biester S, Deuter C, Michels H, et al. Adalimumab in the therapy of uveitis in childhood. *Br J Ophthalmol.* 2007;91(3):319-324.

43. Shah SS, Lowder CY, Schmitt MA, Wilke WS, Kosmorsky GS, Meisler DM. Low-dose methotrexate therapy for ocular inflammatory disease. *Ophthalmology.* 1992;99(9):1419-1423.

44. Jabs DA, Mudun A, Dunn JP, Marsh MJ. Episcleritis and scleritis: clinical features and treatment results. *Am J Ophthalmol.* 2000;130(4):469-476.

SUGGESTED READINGS

Billson FA, De Dombal FT, Watkinson G, Goligher JC. Ocular complications of ulcerative colitis. *Gut.* 1967;8(2):102-106.

Ghanchi FD, Rembacken BJ. Inflammatory bowel disease and the eye. *Surv Ophthalmol.* 2003;48(6):663-676.

Mintz R, Feller ER, Bahr RL, Shah SA. Ocular manifestations of inflammatory bowel disease. *Inflamm Bowel Dis.* 2004;10(2):135-139.

Orchard TR, Chua CN, Ahmad T, Cheng H, Welsh KI, Jewell DP. Uveitis and erythema nodosum in inflammatory bowel disease: clinical features and the role of HLA genes. *Gastroenterology.* 2002;123(3):714-718.

Soukiasian SH, Foster CS, Raizman MB. Treatment strategies for scleritis and uveitis associated with inflammatory bowel disease. *Am J Ophthalmol.* 1994;118(5):601-611.

Chapter 10

Hepatobiliary Disease

Mark E. Gerich, MD and Edward V. Loftus Jr, MD

The interaction between inflammatory bowel disease (IBD) and liver disease was first described more than 100 years ago.[1] Although previously believed to be rare, hepatobiliary disease in IBD is now recognized as one of the more common extraintestinal manifestations of IBD.[2-4] The exact prevalence of hepatobiliary disease in IBD is difficult to assess because of variability across studies in the definition of hepatobiliary dysfunction, diagnostic aggressiveness, and the patient cohorts that were studied.[3] For instance, when transient elevation of hepatic biochemistries is considered to indicate hepatobiliary disease associated with IBD, the prevalence may be greater than 50%. Yet, reports of persistently elevated hepatic biochemistries from population-based IBD cohorts, which theoretically better represent the true prevalence of disease, range from 5% to 16%.[2,5-8] Estimates from referral centers and patients undergoing intestinal resection are higher but are likely confounded by selection bias.[9-15]

While transient hepatic biochemistry elevations are commonly attributed to IBD activity and thought to have no impact on long-term prognosis, there is recent evidence to suggest that these abnormalities may be independent of IBD activity and, although transient, may be associated with poorer long-term survival.[16] Persistent hepatic biochemical abnormalities in patients with IBD should definitely raise suspicion for hepatobiliary complications of IBD, which include primary sclerosing cholangitis (PSC), small-duct PSC (or "pericholangitis"), cholangiocarcinoma (CCA), autoimmune hepatitis (AIH), cholelithiasis, and fatty liver.

PRIMARY SCLEROSING CHOLANGITIS

PSC is the best described hepatobiliary manifestation of IBD.[4] It is a chronic, progressive cholestatic liver disease characterized by inflammation and fibrosis of both the intrahepatic and extrahepatic bile ducts, which leads to multifocal biliary strictures and the eventual development of cirrhosis and its attendant complications[17-20] Liver transplantation is the only effective treatment at present.[19]

Regueiro MD, Swoger JM, eds.
Clinical Challenges and Complications of IBD (pp 175-194).
© 2013 Taylor & Francis Group.

Epidemiology

PSC typically affects men in their third to fourth decade of life, although the first onset of hepatic biochemical abnormalities may occur years earlier.[2,17,21] In Western countries, between 60% and 80% of PSC cases are associated with IBD, particularly ulcerative colitis (UC).[3] In population-based studies of UC patients, the prevalence of PSC ranges from 2% to 8%, whereas the prevalence among Crohn's disease (CD) patients is generally lower (approximately 1%).[3,4] PSC occurs much less frequently in patients with isolated small bowel CD.[22,23] Owing to the rarity of PSC, only a few population-based measurements of disease prevalence have been performed. In Scandinavia, the estimated prevalence has been reported to be between 5 and 16.2 cases per 100,000 persons.[6,24,25] In Olmsted County, Minnesota, the estimated prevalence was 13.6 cases per 100,000 persons in 2000, which results in a crude estimate of at least 29,000 US residents with PSC.[26] Although earlier studies in the United States and the United Kingdom did not show a statistically significant increase in the incidence of PSC, a very large population-based Swedish study recently reported a 35% (95% confidence interval [CI] 0.06 to 82.5) increase in PSC incidence over a 10-year period prior to 2005; however, it is unclear if this is related to a concomitant increase in the incidence of IBD or some other cause.[25-27]

Etiology

The cause of PSC is unclear but, given its increased risk among first-degree relatives as well as its association with other autoimmune diseases such as UC and AIH, it is generally felt to be the result of a combination of genetic and immunologic factors.[28-30] In patients with autoimmune disorders, certain human leukocyte antigens (HLAs) are more frequently expressed. HLAs are major histocompatibility antigens important in immune regulation. PSC appears to be strongly associated with the alleles HLA-B8, DR3, and DRw52A.[9,31,32] The association of these genetic susceptibility factors with PSC supports the notion that both genetic and immunologic processes are important in its pathogenesis.

PSC patients produce a variety of autoantibodies; however, none of these have been shown to be disease specific or have been clearly implicated in disease pathogenesis.[33] Nevertheless, they may provide insight into the link between PSC and UC. Most PSC and UC patients have detectable levels of circulating antineutrophil cytoplasmic antibodies (ANCAs). These are called atypical pANCA because they stain fixed neutrophils in a perinuclear and nuclear pattern that is distinct from the perinuclear staining pattern of classical pANCA that target myeloperoxidase in microscopic polyangiitis.[34] Approximately 70% of PSC patients (with or without UC) will have detectable atypical pANCA.[35-37] Recently, it was shown that atypical pANCA in autoimmune liver disorders react with the autoantigen b-tubulin isotype 5 (TBB5) as well as its evolutionary precursor, the bacterial cell division protein FtsZ, which is highly conserved across bacterial species in the intestinal microflora.[38] Although the specific role of atypical pANCA in disease pathogenesis is still unclear, their presence

Table 10-1. Secondary Causes of Sclerosing Cholangitis

AIDS cholangiopathy

Cholangiocarcinoma

Choledocholithiasis

Diffuse intrahepatic metastasis

Eosinophilic cholangitis

Fascioliasis

Hepatic inflammatory pseudotumor

Histocytosis X

IgG4-associated cholangiopathy

Intra-arterial chemotherapy

Ischemic cholangitis

Mast cell cholangiopathy

Portal hypertensive biliopathy

Recurrent pancreatitis

Recurrent pyogenic cholangitis

Surgical biliary trauma

Adapted from Chapman R, Fevery J, Kalloo A, et al. Diagnosis and management of primary sclerosing cholangitis. *Hepatology.* 2010;51(2):660-678.

supports theories regarding the combined pathogenesis of PSC and UC based on a loss of tolerance to human immune cell antigens resulting from primary altered immune response to bacterial antigens in the gut lumen.[39,40]

Clinical Features and Diagnostic Evaluation

The diagnosis of PSC typically requires the presence of a cholestatic biochemistry profile in a patient with the characteristic cholangiographic findings of multifocal strictures and segmental dilations that are not attributable to disorders causing secondary sclerosing cholangitis (Table 10-1).[19]

The clinical presentation of patients with PSC varies greatly. Most patients are asymptomatic with no physical examination findings at the time of diagnosis, which is often the result of an investigation of a persistently elevated hepatic panel.[17,19] Nonspecific symptoms such as fatigue and weight loss are common, as are right upper quadrant pain and pruritus, all of which generally indicate more advanced disease.[17,41,42] In symptomatic patients, abnormal physical examination findings are more common and include jaundice, icterus, hepatomegaly, and splenomegaly.[19,21,43] It is uncommon for patients to present with acute cholangitis.

Figure 10-1. "Onionskin" lesion of sclerosing cholangitis. Periductal concentric fibrosis is a classic but infrequent histologic finding of PSC, which can also be seen in secondary sclerosing cholangitis.

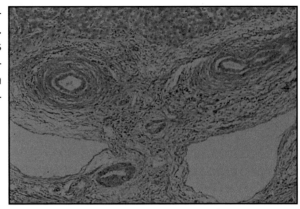

Hepatic biochemistries usually indicate cholestasis. Elevation of serum alkaline phosphatase is very common but can be absent.[17,18,41,44] Serum aminotransferase levels are often 2 to 3 times the upper limit of normal but, again, may not be elevated. Most patients have normal serum bilirubin levels at the time of presentation but, as the disease progresses, these will rise.[17] Prolongation in prothrombin time and diminished serum albumin level often are present in the later course of the disease and suggest progression to hepatic failure. Likewise, a platelet count less than 150×10^3/dL has been shown to be predictive of esophageal varices in PSC patients.[45]

Multiple autoantibodies are often present in patients with PSC, including antinuclear antibody (ANA), rheumatoid factor, and pANCA; however, they are not specific for PSC and have no role in its routine diagnosis.[19] Although atypical pANCA is often present in PSC and is suggestive of a colonic interaction, it is nonspecific and is also present in patients with AIH, primary biliary cirrhosis, and UC who do not have PSC.[33] There is no difference in autoantibody profiles between patients with PSC and those with PSC-associated IBD (PSC-IBD).[46]

Liver biopsy findings may support a diagnosis of PSC but generally show nonspecific findings of biliary disease. The classic finding of periductal concentric fibrosis (the "onionskin lesion") is pathognomonic of sclerosing cholangitis but rare[19] (Figure 10-1). Although liver biopsy can be essential in diagnosing small-duct PSC or PSC overlap syndromes (eg, PSC-AIH), it has been shown to rarely add useful information in the setting of cholangiographic abnormalities and is not required for the diagnosis of large-duct PSC.[19,47]

Endoscopic retrograde cholangiopancreatography (ERCP) has traditionally been the diagnostic criterion standard for PSC.[17] More recently, magnetic resonance cholangiopancreatography (MRCP) has emerged as a viable noninvasive, radiation-free alternative to ERCP for the diagnosis of suspected PSC.[19] MRCP and ERCP have been shown to have similar sensitivity (≥80%) and specificity (≥87%), although ERCP may still be preferable in patients for whom MRCP visualization is suboptimal or who are suspected of having early changes of PSC.[48-50]

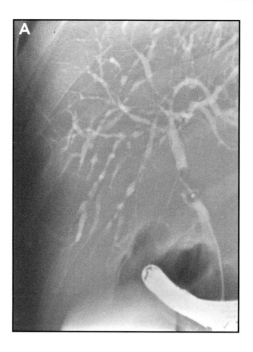

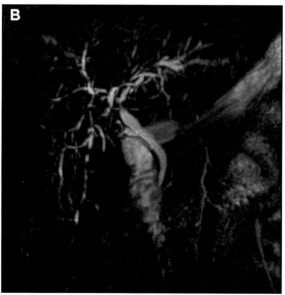

Figure 10-2. (A) ERCP and (B) MRCP images of PSC.

Regardless of the modality, the characteristic cholangiographic find-ings consist of multifocal, short biliary strictures alternating with normal or slightly dilated ducts to produce a "beaded" pattern[51] (Figure 10-2). Both the intra- and extrahepatic ductal systems are typically involved; how-ever, findings can be solely intrahepatic in a minority of patients and long,

Figure 10-3. ERCP image of dominant stricture in the setting of PSC. ERCP demonstrating typical findings of PSC, including diffuse dilation, irregularity, and strictures. There is a dominant stricture in the common hepatic duct (arrow).

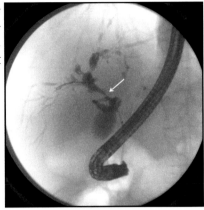

confluent strictures may be present and should raise concern for superimposed CCA[19] (Figure 10-3).

Management/Treatment/Outcomes

Patients with PSC are subject to increased mortality, with overall 10-year survival of approximately 65% and a median survival of 10 to 12 years.[21,26,41,43] Asymptomatic patients have a significantly better survival than those who are symptomatic at the time of diagnosis.[41] Multiple prognostic models have been developed in an attempt to predict outcomes. Age, serum bilirubin, serum aspartate aminotransferase (AST), the presence of esophageal varices, histologic stage of PSC, and cholangiographic findings have been reported as predictors of survival in different studies.[52-54] While the Mayo Model appears to be superior to the Child-Pugh score in assessing the risk of death in a cohort of PSC patients, agreement does not exist about an optimal model and the use of prognostic models is not recommended for predicting clinical outcomes in an individual patient.[19,55,56]

Therapies for PSC are aimed at treating the complications of PSC and slowing the progression of the disease. Chronic cholestasis in the setting of PSC can result in pruritus and malabsorption. The etiology of pruritus in cholestatic liver disease is unclear, but it is believed that pruritogenic substances normally excreted in bile accumulate in tissue as a result of cholestasis. Cholestyramine, a bile acid-sequestering resin, is considered the first line of therapy for cholestasis-related pruritus.[57] The enzyme inducer rifampicin, the opioid anatagonist naltrexone, and the antidepressant sertraline have all demonstrated antipruritic effects.[58-60] Decreased luminal bile acid concentrations are the most common cause for fat malabsorption in PSC, although chronic pancreatitis and celiac disease can also contribute. Together, these can commonly result in fat-soluble vitamin deficiencies that require supplementation.[61] As with other chronic liver diseases, PSC can also result in metabolic bone disease. The incidence of osteoporosis in PSC is between 4% and 10%.[62] Current recommendations are to perform bone density examinations at diagnosis and every 2 to 3 years thereafter. Calcium and vitamin D should be prescribed for patients with osteopenia, and bisphosphonates should be added for patients with osteoporosis.[19]

Other complications of PSC include gallstone and gallbladder disease, acute bacterial cholangitis, dominant biliary strictures, and CCA. Up to one-third of PSC patients develop cholelithiasis or choledocholithiasis.[61,62] A high rate of malignancy has been reported to be associated with gallbladder polyps in the setting of PSC, leading to the recommendation to perform annual gall-bladder surveillance and a cholecystectomy if a polyp is identified.[19,62-64] Most PSC patients do not develop bacterial cholangitis unless they have undergone instrumentation of the biliary tree or have developed a dominant stricture. When this occurs, therapeutic drainage of the obstruction and antibiotics are usually required.[63] Recurrent cholangitis may hasten the progression of PSC, so long-term antibiotic prophylaxis may be necessary.

Dominant strictures are benign, high-grade strictures that can present with worsening pruritus, ductal dilation on imaging, and/or cholangitis. They occur in approximately 50% of PSC patients and can be very difficult to differentiate from CCA, which is much less common.[65,66] Dominant strictures can lead to biliary obstruction and may reduce survival free of liver transplantation.[62] After evaluation for CCA (discussed below), patients with symptoms of obstruction are generally treated with endoscopic biliary sphincterotomy, stone extraction, and balloon dilation; a percutaneous approach may also be used but is associated with increased morbidity. Biliary stenting is reserved for strictures refractory to balloon dilation due to increased risk for complications with stenting.[64] Although the existing evidence is retrospective, endoscopic therapy of dominant biliary strictures appears to improve survival.[64,67] Surgical management, either by biliary bypass or by extrahepatic biliary resection with Roux Y hepaticojejunostomy, is controversial and should generally be avoided in order not to interfere with potential future liver transplantation.[67]

CCA is the most feared complication of PSC, with a 10-year cumulative incidence of 7% to 9%.[65,66] It can occur at any stage of disease and is found at the time of PSC diagnosis in 20% to 30% of patients and within 1 year of diagnosis in 50%.[68] CCA typically presents as an intraductal tumor that can be very difficult to distinguish from a benign PSC stricture by cross-sectional imaging or cholangiography. Serum carbohydrate antigen (CA) 19-9 measurement alone has not shown benefit for screening asymptomatic PSC patients for CCA because it is somewhat nonspecific; however, a highly elevated level may suggest CCA in symptomatic patients suspected of having CCA.[69] The combination of CA 19-9 measurement with cross-sectional liver imaging significantly improves sensitivity but is still relatively nonspecific.[70] Conversely, ERCP with brush cytology of strictures is highly specific for CCA but lacks sensitivity.[71] Application of fluorescence in situ hybridization to cytological specimens to assess for chromosomal gains (polysomy) appears to improve sensitivity significantly but not sufficiently and still requires further validation (Figure 10-4).[19,72]

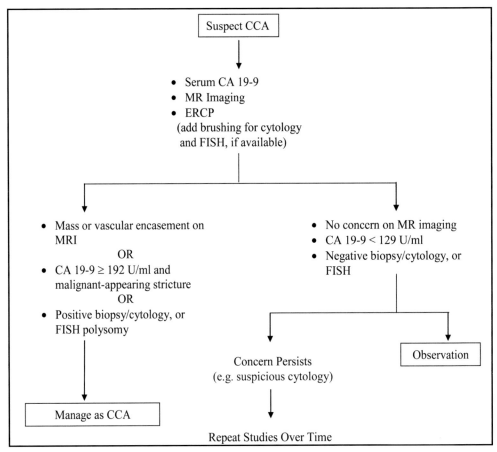

Figure 10-4. Suggested diagnostic algorithm for suspected CCA. (Adapted from Chapman R, Fevery J, Kalloo A, et al. Diagnosis and management of primary sclerosing cholangitis. *Hepatology.* 2010;51[2]:660-678.) CCA = cholangiocarcinoma; CA = carbohydrate antigen; MRI = magnetic resonance imaging; ERCP = endoscopic retrograde cholangiopancreatography; FISH = fluorescence in situ hybridization

Treatment options for CCA are severely limited. Liver transplantation following neoadjuvant chemoradiation therapy has achieved 70% 5-year survival rates in highly selected patients with early stage CCA, but this is not currently recommended for practice beyond experienced transplant centers.[19,73,74] Moreover, due to the difficulty in diagnosis and the common presence of multifocal lesions, patients often present with advanced disease.[75] Chemotherapy may provide a small benefit for locally advanced or metastatic CCA, but surgical resection is the only potential curative therapy, resulting in 5-year survival rates of 9% to 50% and median survival of 15 to 40 months.[76-78] That said, chemotherapeutic or surgical therapy for CCA is often limited by the presence of cholestasis or the sequelae of cirrhosis, and the median survival for patients with unresectable CCA is less than 1 year.[79]

No medical therapy has been clearly successful in slowing the progression of PSC. Ursodeoxycholic acid (UDCA), a hydrophilic bile acid, has been investigated at a variety of doses as a potential therapy for PSC due to its efficacy in primary biliary cirrhosis. Low-dose UDCA improved liver biochemical values but did not impact symptoms or hard endpoints such as progression to liver transplantation or mortality.[80] Although initial studies suggested a survival benefit with higher dose UDCA, a recent multicenter study was aborted early because a higher risk of transplantation or death was noted in the treatment group.[81-84] Neither steroids nor other immunosuppressants, including agents targeting tumor necrosis factor-alpha, have been effective for PSC.[85-87] Antifibrotic agents such as d-penicillamine, pirfenidone, and colchicine have also been ineffective.[88-90]

Currently, liver transplantation, either orthotopic (OLT) or from a living donor, is the only curative therapy available for PSC. Timing of OLT is dependent primarily on the degree of liver dysfunction, as measured by the Model for End-Stage Liver Disease score; however, patients with PSC can receive prioritization for OLT based on the presence of disease-specific complications such as intractable pruritus, recurrent bacterial cholangitis, and CCA. The outcomes of OLT for PSC are favorable with 5- and 10-year survival rates of up to 85% and 70%, respectively.[91,92] However, approximately 20% to 25% of transplanted patients develop recurrent PSC after 5 to 10 years.[93-95]

PERICHOLANGITIS OR SMALL-DUCT PRIMARY SCLEROSING CHOLANGITIS

Pericholangitis was the term originally used to describe the chronic cholestatic hepatitis seen in IBD patients; however, as diagnostic techniques improved, it became clear that many pericholangitis patients actually had the classical cholangiographic features of PSC.[96] Now, small-duct PSC refers to patients with biochemical and histologic features of PSC but with a normal cholangiogram.[97] Approximately 80% of patients with small-duct PSC have IBD, of whom a larger proportion than usual may have CD colitis.[23,98] Compared to classical or large-duct PSC, patients with small-duct PSC have a relatively favorable prognosis with longer transplant-free survival. About one-fourth of patients with small-duct PSC progress to large-duct PSC. Unless they progress to large-duct PSC, patients with small-duct PSC do not appear to develop CCA.[98]

Primary Sclerosing Cholangitis-Associated Inflammatory Bowel Disease

In the majority of patients with concomitant PSC and IBD, the diagnosis of IBD is made before that of PSC, which can be diagnosed after a long interval, even following proctocolectomy; however, PSC diagnosis can sometimes precede IBD diagnosis or occur simultaneously.[21,22,41,43,99-103] The clinical features of PSC-IBD are distinct from those of IBD in the absence of PSC, suggesting that PSC-IBD is a unique phenotype of pediatric and adult IBD. The colitis in PSC-IBD is often extensive with rectal sparing and backwash ileitis.[99,104]

Although this may suggest a diagnosis of CD and may be variably categorized as indeterminate colitis due to ileal involvement and/or lack of rectal involvement, other findings characteristic of CD, such as perianal involvement, transmural inflammation, or skip lesions, are lacking.[99] Although the colitis in PSC-IBD is extensive, it is often mild and may be present only histologically.[105] Patients with PSC-IBD appear to have a more quiescent clinical course in terms of their colitis, often requiring less steroids and hospitalization.[106,107] The presence of PSC in IBD patients does not seem to influence their disease-specific quality of life, but it is associated with increased work disability.[108] Additionally, up to one-third of PSC-IBD patients will ultimately undergo colectomy, usually either for chronic symptoms or for the prevention or treatment of colorectal neoplasia.[109]

PSC-IBD patients who undergo restorative proctocolectomy are more likely to develop pouchitis.[110,111] Pouchitis in this patient population does not appear to be related to liver disease severity and does not change after liver transplantation.[110,112] Of note, de novo pouchitis appears to occur less frequently if ileal pouch-anal anastomosis (IPAA) is performed after liver transplantation and the initiation of immunosuppression (58.3%) than if IPAA precedes transplantation (100%; $P = 0.047$).[113]

As liver disease progresses to the point of portal hypertension, patients with ileostomies can develop peristomal varices.[111,114] Bleeding from these can be extremely difficult to control.[115] Stomal revision is usually unsuccessful and interventions to address portal hypertension, such as transjugular intrahepatic portosystemic shunt or liver transplantation, may be necessary. As a consequence, IPAA is the favored procedure for patients requiring colectomy. IPAA appears to have minimal effect on the disease course of PSC[14,102,116]; however, colectomy may confer protection against recurrent PSC post-transplant in patients with UC.[95] Liver transplant outcomes do not appear to be affected by the performance of colectomy, either with or without IPAA, prior to transplant.[117] Outcomes from proctocolectomy in PSC-IBD patients appear dependent upon the degree of hepatic dysfunction. For patients with poor hepatic reserve, concomitant OLT with total colectomy followed subsequently by IPAA appears to be the optimal course.[118]

Risk of Colorectal Neoplasia

The presence of PSC in patients with IBD may increase the risk of developing colorectal neoplasia; however, the published results are often conflicting. For instance, a 2002 meta-analysis of 11 studies showed a 4- to 5-fold increased risk of colorectal neoplasia in PSC-UC patients compared to patients with UC.[119] There are reports of early development of colorectal neoplasm in patients with PSC-IBD following liver transplant.[120,121] Moreover, there may even be an increased risk of pouch dysplasia in patients with PSC after IPAA.[122] On the other hand, in a matched case-control cohort study of 71 PSC IBD and 142 UC patients, no increase in the risk of neoplasia or death was detected in the matched analysis.[99] At this time, the most recently published society guidelines recommend starting colonoscopic surveillance with random biopsies once the coexistence of PSC and UC is established and continuing every 1 to 2 years.[19,123]

Treatment

In general, the treatment of IBD in the setting of PSC is the same as that for isolated IBD, consisting primarily of sulfasalazine or 5-aminosalicylates for mild disease, tapering courses of corticosteroids for exacerbations, and immunosuppressants for steroid-dependent or -refractory disease.[123] Immunosuppressive regimens following liver transplantation have been reported to have variable effects on the activity of IBD, with some reports suggesting symptomatic improvement[124,125] and others reporting worsening of symptoms.[103,126,127]

Given concern for an increased incidence of colorectal neoplasia in PSC-IBD patients, chemoprevention with UDCA has been evaluated by several retrospective studies. A cross-sectional study of 59 PSC-IBD patients showed that patients receiving UDCA had an adjusted odds ratio of 0.14 (95% CI 0.03 to 0.64; $P = 0.01$) for the development of colonic dysplasia.[128] In a secondary analysis of 52 UC patients in a previous trial of UDCA for PSC, those assigned to receive UDCA had a relative risk of 0.26 (95% CI 0.06 to 0.92; $P = 0.034$) for the development of colorectal dysplasia or cancer.[129] Twenty-eight PSC-IBD patients in a historical cohort study who received UDCA for at least 6 months did not show a significant reduction in the incidence of dysplasia or cancer but were at less risk for death.[130] Despite these findings, the lack of certainty regarding the risk of colorectal neoplasia in PSC-IBD makes the benefit of UDCA unclear. As a result, guidelines recommend against the standard use of UDCA for chemoprevention in PSC-IBD.[19]

AUTOIMMUNE HEPATITIS

AIH is an idiopathic chronic inflammatory condition of the liver characterized by periportal hepatitis with interface hepatitis, hypergammaglobulinemia, and the presence of serum autoantibodies, such as antinuclear and antismooth muscle antibody.[131] Although AIH is rare overall in patients with IBD, UC may occur in up to 16% of AIH patients. Of those patients with both UC and AIH, up to 42% have abnormal cholangiographic findings that indicate the concomitant presence, or "overlap," of PSC.[132] Patients with AIH/PSC overlap and colitis respond relatively poorly to immunosuppression and progress more rapidly to cirrhosis when compared to patients with colitis and AIH.[132] Cholangiography should be performed in patients with AIH and concomitant UC to evaluate for the presence of PSC if they have cholestatic features, evidence of cholangitis on liver biopsy, or a poor response of their hepatitis to immunosuppression.[133] Among patients with PSC, the presence of an AIH/(PSC) overlap syndrome is indicated by an elevation of aminotransferases and should prompt performance of a liver biopsy as these patients appear to receive some benefit from immunosuppression when compared to patients with PSC alone.[19,134]

CHOLELITHIASIS

Patients with CD are at increased risk for cholelithiasis. There is a 2-fold increase in the incidence of gallstones in patients with CD, whereas patients with UC and intact colons have no increased risk of gallstones.[135-138] In CD, the terminal ileum is often diseased or resected, leading to decreased bile salt resabsorption and presumably causing cholelithiasis as a consequence of cholesterol supersaturation.[139-141] Increased enterohepatic circulation of bilirubin may also play a role in pigment stone formation in ileal CD.[142] A recent multivariate analysis suggested the following factors contribute to the formation of gallstones in patients with CD: ileocolonic disease, disease duration over 15 years, multiple recurrences, over 30-cm ileal resection, over 3 hospitalizations, multiple total parenteral nutrition treatments, and long hospital stays.[137]

FATTY LIVER

Abnormal hepatic ultrasound findings other than gallstones are common in patients with IBD, even those without abnormal hepatic biochemistries. Most often, these consist of hepatomegaly and a dysechoic pattern consistent with fatty liver.[143] Estimates of the population prevalence of hepatic steatosis range between 5% and 40% in adults, but are typically in the mid-teens, and depend primarily on the diagnostic method used and the population studied.[144] Many early reports of liver disease in IBD patients describe fatty infiltration of the liver.[145] Older autopsy-based series report a prevalence of fatty liver in IBD of up to 80% of cases.[146,147] In a more recent population-based study of liver disease among UC patients in Stockholm, 15% of patients with persistently abnormal hepatic biochemistries were felt to have fatty liver disease, although this was confirmed histologically in only half of the group.[2] In a large Spanish series of IBD patients with at least one abnormal hepatic panel, 41% were found to have sonographic evidence of fatty liver.[148] In an Italian study of more than 500 nonobese IBD patients without metabolic disorders, 38% had sonographic evidence of fatty liver compared to 17% of controls ($P < 0.001$).[138] Given the lack of clarity about the population prevalence of fatty liver disease, it remains unclear if the prevalence of hepatic steatosis is higher in the IBD population than in the general population, but it appears likely. Furthermore, the severity of fatty liver may correlate with disease duration and/or severity of IBD.[149]

☑Key Points

☑ Hepatobiliary disease is one of the more common extraintestinal manifestations of IBD.

☑ Pruritus, fat-soluble vitamin deficiencies, and osteoporosis are important, treatable complications of PSC.

☑ Currently, liver transplantation is the only curative therapy available for PSC. No medical therapy has been clearly successful in slowing the progression of PSC.

☑ PSC-IBD is a unique phenotype of pediatric and adult IBD. The colitis in PSC-IBD is often mild and extensive, with rectal sparing and backwash ileitis.

☑ The presence of PSC in patients with IBD may increase the risk of developing colorectal neoplasia. Guidelines recommend initiating colonoscopic surveillance with random biopsies once the coexistence of PSC and UC is established and continuing every 1 to 2 years.

☑ There is a 2-fold increase in the incidence of gallstones in patients with CD, whereas patients with UC and intact colons have no increased risk of gallstones.

REFERENCES

1. Thomas CH. Ulceration of the colon with a much enlarged fatty liver. *Trans Pathol Sci Phila.* 1873;4:87-88.
2. Broome U, Glaumann H, Hellers G, Nilsson B, Sorstad J, Hultcrantz R. Liver disease in ulcerative colitis: an epidemiological and follow up study in the county of Stockholm. *Gut.* 1994;35(1):84-89.
3. Loftus EV, Sandborn WJ, Lindor KD, et al. Interactions between chronic liver disease and inflammatory bowel disease. *Inflamm Bowel Dis.* 1997;3:288-302.
4. Bernstein CN, Blanchard JF, Rawsthorne P, Yu N. The prevalence of extraintestinal diseases in inflammatory bowel disease: a population-based study. *Am J Gastroenterol.* 2001;96(4):1116-1122.
5. Tobias R, Wright JP, Kottler RE, et al. Primary sclerosing cholangitis associated with inflammatory bowel disease in Cape Town, 1975-1981. *S Afr Med J.* 1983;63(7):229-235.
6. Olsson R, Danielsson A, Jarnerot G, et al. Prevalence of primary sclerosing cholangitis in patients with ulcerative colitis. *Gastroenterology.* 1991;100(5 pt 1):1319-1323.
7. Rasmussen HH, Fallingborg J, Mortensen PB, et al. Primary sclerosing cholangitis in patients with ulcerative colitis. *Scand J Gastroenterol.* 1992;27(9):732-736.
8. Aitola P, Karvonen AL, Matikainen M. Prevalence of hepatobiliary dysfunction in patients with ulcerative colitis. *Ann Chir Gynaecol.* 1994;83(4):275-278.
9. Schrumpf E, Fausa O, Kolmannskog F, Elgjo K, Ritland S, Gjone E. Sclerosing cholangitis in ulcerative colitis. A follow-up study. *Scand J Gastroenterol.* 1982;17(1):33-39.

10. Shepherd HA, Selby WS, Chapman RW, et al. Ulcerative colitis and persistent liver dysfunction. *Q J Med.* 1983;52(208):503-513.

11. Hashimoto E, Ideta M, Taniai M, et al. Prevalence of primary sclerosing cholangitis and other liver diseases in Japanese patients with chronic ulcerative colitis. *J Gastroenterol Hepatol.* 1993;8(2):146-149.

12. Purrmann J, Modder U, Cleveland S, et al. Association of primary sclerosing cholangitis with inflammatory bowel diseases: a prospective study. *Z Gastroenterol.* 1993;31(suppl 5): 56-59.

13. Mattila J, Aitola P, Matikainen M. Liver lesions found at colectomy in ulcerative colitis: correlation between histological findings and biochemical parameters. *J Clin Pathol.* 1994;47(11):1019-1021.

14. Mikkola K, Kiviluoto T, Riihela M, Taavitsainen M, Jarvinen HJ. Liver involvement and its course in patients operated on for ulcerative colitis. *Hepatogastroenterology.* 1995;42(1): 68-72.

15. Navaneethan U, Remzi FH, Nutter B, Fazio VW, Shen B. Risk factors for abnormal liver function tests in patients with ileal pouch-anal anastomosis for underlying inflammatory bowel disease. *Am J Gastroenterol.* 2009;104(10):2467-2475.

16. Mendes FD, Levy C, Enders FB, Loftus EV Jr, Angulo P, Lindor KD. Abnormal hepatic biochemistries in patients with inflammatory bowel disease. *Am J Gastroenterol.* 2007;102(2):344-350.

17. Lee YM, Kaplan MM. Primary sclerosing cholangitis. *N Engl J Med.* 1995;332(14):924-933.

18. Chapman RW, Arborgh BA, Rhodes JM, et al. Primary sclerosing cholangitis: a review of its clinical features, cholangiography, and hepatic histology. *Gut.* 1980;21(10):870-877.

19. Chapman R, Fevery J, Kalloo A, et al. Diagnosis and management of primary sclerosing cholangitis. *Hepatology.* 2010;51(2):660-678.

20. Tischendorf JJ, Hecker H, Kruger M, Manns MP, Meier PN. Characterization, outcome, and prognosis in 273 patients with primary sclerosing cholangitis: a single center study. *Am J Gastroenterol.* 2007;102(1):107-114.

21. Wiesner RH, Grambsch PM, Dickson ER, et al. Primary sclerosing cholangitis: natural history, prognostic factors and survival analysis. *Hepatology.* 1989;10(4):430-436.

22. Fausa O, Schrumpf E, Elgjo K. Relationship of inflammatory bowel disease and primary sclerosing cholangitis. *Semin Liver Dis.* 1991;11(1):31-39.

23. Rasmussen HH, Fallingborg JF, Mortensen PB, Vyberg M, Tage-Jensen U, Rasmussen SN. Hepatobiliary dysfunction and primary sclerosing cholangitis in patients with Crohn's disease. *Scand J Gastroenterol.* 1997;32(6):604-610.

24. Boberg KM, Aadland E, Jahnsen J, Raknerud N, Stiris M, Bell H. Incidence and prevalence of primary biliary cirrhosis, primary sclerosing cholangitis, and autoimmune hepatitis in a Norwegian population. *Scand J Gastroenterol.* 1998;33(1):99-103.

25. Lindkvist B, Benito de Valle M, Gullberg B, Bjornsson E. Incidence and prevalence of primary sclerosing cholangitis in a defined adult population in Sweden. *Hepatology.* 2010;52(2):571-577.

26. Bambha K, Kim WR, Talwalkar J, et al. Incidence, clinical spectrum, and outcomes of primary sclerosing cholangitis in a United States community. *Gastroenterology.* 2003;125(5):1364-1369.

27. Card TR, Solaymani-Dodaran M, West J. Incidence and mortality of primary sclerosing cholangitis in the UK: a population-based cohort study. *J Hepatol.* 2008;48(6):939-944.

28. Bergquist A, Montgomery SM, Bahmanyar S, et al. Increased risk of primary sclerosing cholangitis and ulcerative colitis in first-degree relatives of patients with primary sclerosing cholangitis. *Clin Gastroenterol Hepatol.* 2008;6(8):939-943.

29. Karlsen TH, Schrumpf E, Boberg KM. Genetic epidemiology of primary sclerosing cholangitis. *World J Gastroenterol.* 2007;13(41):5421-5431.

30. Saarinen S, Olerup O, Broome U. Increased frequency of autoimmune diseases in patients with primary sclerosing cholangitis. *Am J Gastroenterol.* 2000;95(11):3195-3199.

31. Chapman RW, Varghese Z, Gaul R, Patel G, Kokinon N, Sherlock S. Association of primary sclerosing cholangitis with HLA-B8. *Gut.* 1983;24(1):38-41.

32. Prochazka EJ, Terasaki PI, Park MS, Goldstein LI, Busuttil RW. Association of primary sclerosing cholangitis with HLA-DRw52a. *N Engl J Med.* 1990;322(26):1842-1844.

33. Terjung B, Spengler U. Role of auto-antibodies for the diagnosis of chronic cholestatic liver diseases. *Clin Rev Allergy Immunol.* 2005;28(2):115-133.

34. Falk RJ, Jennette JC. Anti-neutrophil cytoplasmic autoantibodies with specificity for myeloperoxidase in patients with systemic vasculitis and idiopathic necrotizing and crescentic glomerulonephritis. *N Engl J Med.* 1988;318(25):1651-1657.

35. Duerr RH, Targan SR, Landers CJ, et al. Neutrophil cytoplasmic antibodies: a link between primary sclerosing cholangitis and ulcerative colitis. *Gastroenterology.* 1991;100(5 pt 1):1385-1391.

36. Duerr RH, Targan SR, Landers CJ, Sutherland LR, Shanahan F. Anti-neutrophil cytoplasmic antibodies in ulcerative colitis. Comparison with other colitides/diarrheal illnesses. *Gastroenterology.* 1991;100(6):1590-1596.

37. Saxon A, Shanahan F, Landers C, Ganz T, Targan S. A distinct subset of anti-neutrophil cytoplasmic antibodies is associated with inflammatory bowel disease. *J Allergy Clin Immunol.* 1990;86(2):202-210.

38. Terjung B, Sohne J, Lechtenberg B, et al. p-ANCAs in autoimmune liver disorders recognise human beta-tubulin isotype 5 and cross-react with microbial protein FtsZ. *Gut.* 2010;59(6):808-816.

39. Terjung B, Spengler U. Atypical p-ANCA in PSC and AIH: a hint toward a "leaky gut"? *Clin Rev Allergy Immunol.* 2009;36(1):40-51.

40. Selmi C, Gershwin ME. Autoantibodies in autoimmune liver disease: biomarkers versus epiphenomena. *Gut.* 2010;59(6):712-713.

41. Broome U, Olsson R, Loof L, et al. Natural history and prognostic factors in 305 Swedish patients with primary sclerosing cholangitis. *Gut.* 1996;38(4):610-615.

42. Olsson R, Broome U, Danielsson A, et al. Spontaneous course of symptoms in primary sclerosing cholangitis: relationships with biochemical and histological features. *Hepatogastroenterology.* 1999;46(25):136-141.

43. Farrant JM, Hayllar KM, Wilkinson ML, et al. Natural history and prognostic variables in primary sclerosing cholangitis. *Gastroenterology.* 1991;100(6):1710-1717.

44. Balasubramaniam K, Wiesner RH, LaRusso NF. Primary sclerosing cholangitis with normal serum alkaline phosphatase activity. *Gastroenterology.* 1988;95(5):1395-1398.

45. Zein CO, Lindor KD, Angulo P. Prevalence and predictors of esophageal varices in patients with primary sclerosing cholangitis. *Hepatology.* 2004;39(1):204-210.

46. Angulo P, Peter JB, Gershwin ME, et al. Serum autoantibodies in patients with primary sclerosing cholangitis. *J Hepatol.* 2000;32(2):182-187.

47. Burak KW, Angulo P, Lindor KD. Is there a role for liver biopsy in primary sclerosing cholangitis? *Am J Gastroenterol.* 2003;98(5):1155-1158.

48. Moff SL, Kamel IR, Eustace J, et al. Diagnosis of primary sclerosing cholangitis: a blinded comparative study using magnetic resonance cholangiography and endoscopic retrograde cholangiography. *Gastrointest Endosc.* 2006;64(2):219-223.

49. Berstad AE, Aabakken L, Smith HJ, Aasen S, Boberg KM, Schrumpf E. Diagnostic accuracy of magnetic resonance and endoscopic retrograde cholangiography in primary sclerosing cholangitis. *Clin Gastroenterol Hepatol.* 2006;4(4):514-520.

50. Angulo P, Pearce DH, Johnson CD, et al. Magnetic resonance cholangiography in patients with biliary disease: its role in primary sclerosing cholangitis. *J Hepatol.* 2000;33(4):520-527.

51. MacCarty RL, LaRusso NF, Wiesner RH, Ludwig J. Primary sclerosing cholangitis: findings on cholangiography and pancreatography. *Radiology.* 1983;149(1):39-44.

52. Boberg KM, Rocca G, Egeland T, et al. Time-dependent Cox regression model is superior in prediction of prognosis in primary sclerosing cholangitis. *Hepatology.* 2002;35(3):652-657.

53. Majoie CB, Reeders JW, Sanders JB, Huibregtse K, Jansen PL. Primary sclerosing cholangitis: a modified classification of cholangiographic findings. *AJR Am J Roentgenol.* 1991;157(3):495-497.

54. Ponsioen CY, Vrouenraets SM, Prawirodirdjo W, et al. Natural history of primary sclerosing cholangitis and prognostic value of cholangiography in a Dutch population. *Gut.* 2002;51(4):562-566.

55. Kim WR, Poterucha JJ, Wiesner RH, et al. The relative role of the Child-Pugh classification and the Mayo natural history model in the assessment of survival in patients with primary sclerosing cholangitis. *Hepatology.* 1999;29(6):1643-1648.

56. Kim WR, Therneau TM, Wiesner RH, et al. A revised natural history model for primary sclerosing cholangitis. *Mayo Clin Proc.* 2000;75(7):688-694.

57. Lindor KD, Gershwin ME, Poupon R, Kaplan M, Bergasa NV, Heathcote EJ. Primary biliary cirrhosis. *Hepatology.* 2009;50(1):291-308.

58. Tandon P, Rowe BH, Vandermeer B, Bain VG. The efficacy and safety of bile acid binding agents, opioid antagonists, or rifampin in the treatment of cholestasis-associated pruritus. *Am J Gastroenterol.* 2007;102(7):1528-1536.

59. Khurana S, Singh P. Rifampin is safe for treatment of pruritus due to chronic cholestasis: a meta-analysis of prospective randomized-controlled trials. *Liver Int.* 2006;26(8):943-948.

60. Mayo MJ, Handem I, Saldana S, Jacobe H, Getachew Y, Rush AJ. Sertraline as a first-line treatment for cholestatic pruritus. *Hepatology.* 2007;45(3):666-674.

61. Jorgensen RA, Lindor KD, Sartin JS, LaRusso NF, Wiesner RH. Serum lipid and fat-soluble vitamin levels in primary sclerosing cholangitis. *J Clin Gastroenterol.* 1995;20(3):215-219.

62. Collier J. Bone disorders in chronic liver disease. *Hepatology.* 2007;46(4):1271-1278.

63. Pohl J, Ring A, Stremmel W, Stiehl A. The role of dominant stenoses in bacterial infections of bile ducts in primary sclerosing cholangitis. *Eur J Gastroenterol Hepatol.* 2006;18(1):69-74.

64. Kaya M, Petersen BT, Angulo P, et al. Balloon dilation compared to stenting of dominant strictures in primary sclerosing cholangitis. *Am J Gastroenterol.* 2001;96(4):1059-1066.

65. Burak K, Angulo P, Pasha TM, Egan K, Petz J, Lindor KD. Incidence and risk factors for cholangiocarcinoma in primary sclerosing cholangitis. *Am J Gastroenterol.* 2004;99(3):523-526.

66. Claessen MM, Vleggaar FP, Tytgat KM, Siersema PD, van Buuren HR. High lifetime risk of cancer in primary sclerosing cholangitis. *J Hepatol.* 2009;50(1):158-164.

67. Ahrendt SA, Pitt HA, Kalloo AN, et al. Primary sclerosing cholangitis: resect, dilate, or transplant? *Ann Surg.* 1998;227(3):412-423.

68. Fevery J, Verslype C, Lai G, Aerts R, Van Steenbergen W. Incidence, diagnosis, and therapy of cholangiocarcinoma in patients with primary sclerosing cholangitis. *Dig Dis Sci.* 2007;52(11):3123-3135.

69. Levy C, Lymp J, Angulo P, Gores GJ, Larusso N, Lindor KD. The value of serum CA 19-9 in predicting cholangiocarcinomas in patients with primary sclerosing cholangitis. *Dig Dis Sci.* 2005;50(9):1734-1740.

70. Charatcharoenwitthaya P, Enders FB, Halling KC, Lindor KD. Utility of serum tumor markers, imaging, and biliary cytology for detecting cholangiocarcinoma in primary sclerosing cholangitis. *Hepatology.* 2008;48(4):1106-1117.

71. Boberg KM, Jebsen P, Clausen OP, Foss A, Aabakken L, Schrumpf E. Diagnostic benefit of biliary brush cytology in cholangiocarcinoma in primary sclerosing cholangitis. *J Hepatol.* 2006;45(4):568-574.

72. Moreno Luna LE, Kipp B, Halling KC, et al. Advanced cytologic techniques for the detection of malignant pancreatobiliary strictures. *Gastroenterology.* 2006;131(4):1064-1072.

73. Gores GJ, Nagorney DM, Rosen CB. Cholangiocarcinoma: is transplantation an option? For whom? *J Hepatol.* 2007;47(4):455-459.

74. Rea DJ, Heimbach JK, Rosen CB, et al. Liver transplantation with neoadjuvant chemoradiation is more effective than resection for hilar cholangiocarcinoma. *Ann Surg.* 2005;242(3):451-458; discussion 458-461.

75. Khan SA, Miras A, Pelling M, Taylor-Robinson SD. Cholangiocarcinoma and its management. *Gut.* 2007;56(12):1755-1756.

76. Hemming AW, Reed AI, Fujita S, Foley DP, Howard RJ. Surgical management of hilar cholangiocarcinoma. *Ann Surg.* 2005;241(5):693-699; discussion 699-702.

77. Jarnagin WR, Fong Y, DeMatteo RP, et al. Staging, resectability, and outcome in 225 patients with hilar cholangiocarcinoma. *Ann Surg.* 2001;234(4):507-517; discussion 517-509.

78. Valle J, Wasan H, Palmer DH, et al. Cisplatin plus gemcitabine versus gemcitabine for biliary tract cancer. *N Engl J Med.* 2010;362(14):1273-1281.

79. Cheng JL, Bruno MJ, Bergman JJ, Rauws EA, Tytgat GN, Huibregtse K. Endoscopic pal-liation of patients with biliary obstruction caused by nonresectable hilar cholangiocarci-noma: efficacy of self-expandable metallic wallstents. *Gastrointest Endosc.* 2002;56(1):33-39.

80. Lindor KD. Ursodiol for primary sclerosing cholangitis. Mayo Primary Sclerosing Cholangitis-Ursodeoxycholic Acid Study Group. *N Engl J Med.* 1997;336(10):691-695.

81. Lindor KD, Kowdley KV, Luketic VA, et al. High-dose ursodeoxycholic acid for the treat-ment of primary sclerosing cholangitis. *Hepatology.* 2009;50(3):808-814.

82. Mitchell SA, Bansi DS, Hunt N, Von Bergmann K, Fleming KA, Chapman RW. A pre-liminary trial of high-dose ursodeoxycholic acid in primary sclerosing cholangitis. *Gastroenterology.* 2001;121(4):900-907.

83. Olsson R, Boberg KM, de Muckadell OS, et al. High-dose ursodeoxycholic acid in primary sclerosing cholangitis: a 5-year multicenter, randomized, controlled study. *Gastroenterology.* 2005;129(5):1464-1472.

84. Chen W, Gluud C. Bile acids for primary sclerosing cholangitis. *Cochrane Database Syst Rev.* 2003;2(2):CD003626.

85. Giljaca V, Poropat G, Stimac D, Gluud C. Glucocorticosteroids for primary sclerosing chol-angitis. *Cochrane Database Syst Rev.* 2010;20(1):CD004036.

86. Bharucha AE, Jorgensen R, Lichtman SN, LaRusso NF, Lindor KD. A pilot study of pentoxifylline for the treatment of primary sclerosing cholangitis. *Am J Gastroenterol.* 2000;95(9):2338-2342.

87. Hommes DW, Erkelens W, Ponsioen C, et al. A double-blind, placebo-controlled, randomized study of infliximab in primary sclerosing cholangitis. *J Clin Gastroenterol.* 2008;42(5):522-526.

88. Klingenberg SL, Chen W. D-penicillamine for primary sclerosing cholangitis. *Cochrane Database Syst Rev.* 2006;25(1):CD004182.

89. Angulo P, MacCarty RL, Sylvestre PB, et al. Pirfenidone in the treatment of primary scle-rosing cholangitis. *Dig Dis Sci.* 2002;47(1):157-161.

90. Olsson R, Broome U, Danielsson A, et al. Colchicine treatment of primary sclerosing cholangitis. *Gastroenterology.* 1995;108(4):1199-1203.

91. Graziadei IW, Wiesner RH, Marotta PJ, et al. Long-term results of patients undergoing liver transplantation for primary sclerosing cholangitis. *Hepatology.* 1999;30(5):1121-1127.

92. Brandsaeter B, Friman S, Broome U, et al. Outcome following liver transplantation for prima-ry sclerosing cholangitis in the Nordic countries. *Scand J Gastroenterol.* 2003;38(11):1176-1183.

93. Graziadei IW, Wiesner RH, Batts KP, et al. Recurrence of primary sclerosing cholangitis following liver transplantation. *Hepatology.* 1999;29(4):1050-1056.

94. Campsen J, Zimmerman MA, Trotter JF, et al. Clinically recurrent primary sclerosing cholangitis following liver transplantation: a time course. *Liver Transpl.* 2008;14(2):181-185.

95. Alabraba E, Nightingale P, Gunson B, et al. A re-evaluation of the risk factors for the recurrence of primary sclerosing cholangitis in liver allografts. *Liver Transpl.* 2009;15(3): 330-340.

96. Ludwig J, Barham SS, LaRusso NF, Elveback LR, Wiesner RH, McCall JT. Morphologic features of chronic hepatitis associated with primary sclerosing cholangitis and chronic ulcerative colitis. *Hepatology.* 1981;1(6):632-640.

97. Wee A, Ludwig J, Coffey RJ, Jr, LaRusso NF, Wiesner RH. Hepatobiliary carcinoma asso-ciated with primary sclerosing cholangitis and chronic ulcerative colitis. *Hum Pathol.* 1985;16(7):719-726.

98. Bjornsson E, Olsson R, Bergquist A, et al. The natural history of small-duct primary sclerosing cholangitis. *Gastroenterology.* 2008;134(4):975-980.

99. Loftus EV Jr, Harewood GC, Loftus CG, et al. PSC-IBD: a unique form of inflammatory bowel disease associated with primary sclerosing cholangitis. *Gut.* 2005;54(1):91-96.

100. Broome U, Lofberg R, Veress B, Eriksson LS. Primary sclerosing cholangitis and ulcerative colitis: evidence for increased neoplastic potential. *Hepatology.* 1995;22(5):1404-1408.

101. Kornfeld D, Ekbom A, Ihre T. Is there an excess risk for colorectal cancer in patients with ulcerative colitis and concomitant primary sclerosing cholangitis? A population based study. *Gut.* 1997;41(4):522-525.

102. Cangemi JR, Wiesner RH, Beaver SJ, et al. Effect of proctocolectomy for chronic ulcerative colitis on the natural history of primary sclerosing cholangitis. *Gastroenterology.* 1989;96(3):790-794.

103. Verdonk RC, Dijkstra G, Haagsma EB, et al. Inflammatory bowel disease after liver transplantation: risk factors for recurrence and de novo disease. *Am J Transplant.* 2006;6(6):1422-1429.

104. Faubion WA Jr, Loftus EV, Sandborn WJ, Freese DK, Perrault J. Pediatric "PSC-IBD": a descriptive report of associated inflammatory bowel disease among pediatric patients with PSC. *J Pediatr Gastroenterol Nutr.* 2001;33(3):296-300.

105. Joo M, Abreu-e-Lima P, Farraye F, et al. Pathologic features of ulcerative colitis in patients with primary sclerosing cholangitis: a case-control study. *Am J Surg Pathol.* 2009;33(6):854-862.

106. Lundqvist K, Broome U. Differences in colonic disease activity in patients with ulcerative colitis with and without primary sclerosing cholangitis: a case control study. *Dis Colon Rectum.* 1997;40(4):451-456.

107. Broome U, Bergquist A. Primary sclerosing cholangitis, inflammatory bowel disease, and colon cancer. *Semin Liver Dis.* 2006;26(1):31-41.

108. Ananthakrishnan AN, Beaulieu DB, Ulitsky A, et al. Does primary sclerosing cholangitis impact quality of life in patients with inflammatory bowel disease? *Inflamm Bowel Dis.* 2010;16(3):494-500.

109. Loftus EV Jr, Sandborn WJ, Tremaine WJ, et al. Risk of colorectal neoplasia in patients with primary sclerosing cholangitis. *Gastroenterology.* 1996;110(2):432-440.

110. Penna C, Dozois R, Tremaine W, et al. Pouchitis after ileal pouch-anal anastomosis for ulcerative colitis occurs with increased frequency in patients with associated primary sclerosing cholangitis. *Gut.* 1996;38(2):234-239.

111. Kartheuser AH, Dozois RR, LaRusso NF, Wiesner RH, Ilstrup DM, Schleck CD. Comparison of surgical treatment of ulcerative colitis associated with primary sclerosing cholangitis: ileal pouch-anal anastomosis versus Brooke ileostomy. *Mayo Clin Proc.* 1996;71(8):748-756.

112. Zins BJ, Sandborn WJ, Penna CR, et al. Pouchitis disease course after orthotopic liver transplantation in patients with primary sclerosing cholangitis and an ileal pouch-anal anastomosis. *Am J Gastroenterol.* 1995;90(12):2177-2181.

113. Freeman K, Shao Z, Remzi FH, Lopez R, Fazio VW, Shen B. Impact of orthotopic liver transplant for primary sclerosing cholangitis on chronic antibiotic refractory pouchitis. *Clin Gastroenterol Hepatol.* 2008;6(1):62-68.

114. Wiesner RH, LaRusso NF, Dozois RR, Beaver SJ. Peristomal varices after proctocolectomy in patients with primary sclerosing cholangitis. *Gastroenterology.* 1986;90(2):316-322.

115. Peck JJ, Boyden AM. Exigent ileostomy hemorrhage. A complication of proctocolectomy in patients with chronic ulcerative colitis and primary sclerosing cholangitis. *Am J Surg.* 1985;150(1):153-158.

116. Lepisto A, Kivisto S, Kivisaari L, Arola J, Jarvinen HJ. Primary sclerosing cholangitis: outcome of patients undergoing restorative proctocolecetomy for ulcerative colitis. *Int J Colorectal Dis.* 2009;24(10):1169-1174.

117. Mathis KL, Dozois EJ, Larson DW, et al. Ileal pouch-anal anastomosis and liver transplantation for ulcerative colitis complicated by primary sclerosing cholangitis. *Br J Surg.* 2008;95(7):882-886.

118. Poritz LS, Koltun WA. Surgical management of ulcerative colitis in the presence of primary sclerosing cholangitis. *Dis Colon Rectum.* 2003;46(2):173-178.

119. Soetikno RM, Lin OS, Heidenreich PA, Young HS, Blackstone MO. Increased risk of colorectal neoplasia in patients with primary sclerosing cholangitis and ulcerative colitis: a meta-analysis. *Gastrointest Endosc.* 2002;56(1):48-54.

120. Higashi H, Yanaga K, Marsh JW, Tzakis A, Kakizoe S, Starzl TE. Development of colon cancer after liver transplantation for primary sclerosing cholangitis associated with ulcerative colitis. *Hepatology.* 1990;11(3):477-480.

121. Bleday R, Lee E, Jessurun J, Heine J, Wong WD. Increased risk of early colorectal neoplasms after hepatic transplant in patients with inflammatory bowel disease. *Dis Colon Rectum.* 1993;36(10):908-912.

122. Stahlberg D, Veress B, Tribukait B, Broome U. Atrophy and neoplastic transformation of the ileal pouch mucosa in patients with ulcerative colitis and primary sclerosing cholangitis: a case control study. *Dis Colon Rectum.* 2003;46(6):770-778.

123. Kornbluth A, Sachar DB. Ulcerative colitis practice guidelines in adults: American College of Gastroenterology, Practice Parameters Committee. *Am J Gastroenterol.* 2010;105(3):501-523; quiz 524.

124. Befeler AS, Lissoos TW, Schiano TD, et al. Clinical course and management of inflammatory bowel disease after liver transplantation. *Transplantation.* 1998;65(3):393-396.

125. Saldeen K, Friman S, Olausson M, Olsson R. Follow-up after liver transplantation for primary sclerosing cholangitis: effects on survival, quality of life, and colitis. *Scand J Gastroenterol.* 1999;34(5):535-540.

126. Riley TR, Schoen RE, Lee RG, Rakela J. A case series of transplant recipients who despite immunosuppression developed inflammatory bowel disease. *Am J Gastroenterol.* 1997;92(2):279-282.

127. Papatheodoridis GV, Hamilton M, Mistry PK, Davidson B, Rolles K, Burroughs AK. Ulcerative colitis has an aggressive course after orthotopic liver transplantation for primary sclerosing cholangitis. *Gut.* 1998;43(5):639-644.

128. Tung BY, Emond MJ, Haggitt RC, et al. Ursodiol use is associated with lower prevalence of colonic neoplasia in patients with ulcerative colitis and primary sclerosing cholangitis. *Ann Intern Med.* 2001;134(2):89-95.

129. Pardi DS, Loftus EV, Jr, Kremers WK, Keach J, Lindor KD. Ursodeoxycholic acid as a chemopreventive agent in patients with ulcerative colitis and primary sclerosing cholangitis. *Gastroenterology.* 2003;124(4):889-893.

130. Wolf JM, Rybicki LA, Lashner BA. The impact of ursodeoxycholic acid on cancer, dysplasia and mortality in ulcerative colitis patients with primary sclerosing cholangitis. *Aliment Pharmacol Ther.* 2005;22(9):783-788.

131. Alvarez F, Berg PA, Bianchi FB, et al. International Autoimmune Hepatitis Group Report: review of criteria for diagnosis of autoimmune hepatitis. *J Hepatol.* 1999;31(5):929-938.

132. Perdigoto R, Carpenter HA, Czaja AJ. Frequency and significance of chronic ulcerative colitis in severe corticosteroid-treated autoimmune hepatitis. *J Hepatol.* 1992;14(2-3):325-331.

133. Czaja AJ. The variant forms of autoimmune hepatitis. *Ann Intern Med.* 1996;125(7):588-598.

134. Floreani A, Rizzotto ER, Ferrara F, et al. Clinical course and outcome of autoimmune hepatitis/primary sclerosing cholangitis overlap syndrome. *Am J Gastroenterol.* 2005;100(7):1516-1522.

135. Fraquelli M, Losco A, Visentin S, et al. Gallstone disease and related risk factors in patients with Crohn's disease: analysis of 330 consecutive cases. *Arch Intern Med.* 2001;161(18):2201-2204.

136. Lapidus A, Bangstad M, Astrom M, Muhrbeck O. The prevalence of gallstone disease in a defined cohort of patients with Crohn's disease. *Am J Gastroenterol.* 1999;94(5):1261-1266.

137. Parente F, Pastore L, Bargiggia S, et al. Incidence and risk factors for gallstones in patients with inflammatory bowel disease: a large case-control study. *Hepatology.* 2007;45(5):1267-1274.

138. Bargiggia S, Maconi G, Elli M, et al. Sonographic prevalence of liver steatosis and biliary tract stones in patients with inflammatory bowel disease: study of 511 subjects at a single center. *J Clin Gastroenterol.* 2003;36(5):417-420.

139. Whorwell PJ, Hawkins R, Dewbury K, Wright R. Ultrasound survey of gallstones and other hepatobiliary disorders in patients with Crohn's disease. *Dig Dis Sci.* 1984;29(10):930-933.

140. Heaton KW, Read AE. Gall stones in patients with disorders of the terminal ileum and disturbed bile salt metabolism. *Br Med J.* 1969;3(5669):494-496.

141. Dowling RH, Bell GD, White J. Lithogenic bile in patients with ileal dysfunction. *Gut.* 1972;13(6):415-420.

142. Brink MA, Slors JF, Keulemans YC, et al. Enterohepatic cycling of bilirubin: a putative mechanism for pigment gallstone formation in ileal Crohn's disease. *Gastroenterology.* 1999;116(6):1420-1427.

143. de Fazio C, Torgano G, de Franchis R, Meucci G, Arrigoni M, Vecchi M. Detection of liver involvement in inflammatory bowel disease by abdominal ultrasound scan. *Int J Clin Lab Res.* 1992;21(4):314-317.

144. Lazo M, Clark JM. The epidemiology of nonalcoholic fatty liver disease: a global perspective. *Semin Liver Dis.* 2008;28(4):339-350.

145. De Dombal FT, Goldie W, Watts JM, Goligher JC. Hepatic histological changes in ulcerative colitis. A series of 58 consecutive operative liver biopsies. *Scand J Gastroenterol.* 1966;1(3):220-227.

146. Perrett AD, Higgins G, Johnston HH, Massarella GR, Truelove SC, Wright R. The liver in ulcerative colitis. *Q J Med.* 1971;40(158):211-238.

147. Perrett AD, Higgins G, Johnston HH, Massarella GR, Truelove SC, Wright R. The liver in Crohn's disease. *Q J Med.* 1971;40(158):187-209.

148. Gisbert JP, Luna M, Gonzalez-Lama Y, et al. Liver injury in inflammatory bowel disease: long-term follow-up study of 786 patients. *Inflamm Bowel Dis.* 2007;13(9):1106-1114.

149. Riegler G, D'Inca R, Sturniolo GC, et al. Hepatobiliary alterations in patients with inflammatory bowel disease: a multicenter study. Caprilli & Gruppo Italiano Studio Colon-Retto. *Scand J Gastroenterol.* 1998;33(1):93-98.

Suggested Readings

Bambha K, Kim WR, Talwalkar J, et al. Incidence, clinical spectrum, and outcomes of primary sclerosing cholangitis in a United States community. *Gastroenterology.* 2003;125(5):1364-1369.

Chapman R, Fevery J, Kalloo A, et al. Diagnosis and management of primary sclerosing cholangitis. *Hepatology.* 2010;51(2):660-678.

Faubion WA Jr, Loftus EV, Sandborn WJ, Freese DK, Perrault J. Pediatric "PSC-IBD": a descriptive report of associated inflammatory bowel disease among pediatric patients with PSC. *J Pediatr Gastroenterol Nutr.* 2001;33(3):296-300.

Loftus EV Jr, Harewood GC, Loftus CG, et al. PSC-IBD: a unique form of inflammatory bowel disease associated with primary sclerosing cholangitis. *Gut.* 2005;54(1):91-96.

Terjung B, Spengler U. Atypical p-ANCA in PSC and AIH: a hint toward a "leaky gut"? *Clin Rev Allergy Immunol.* 2009;36(1):40-51.

Section III

GENERAL HEALTH AND METABOLIC COMPLICATIONS OF IBD

Chapter 11

Women's Health
Pregnancy, Fertility, and Cervical Cancer

Monika Fischer, MD, MSCR and Sunanda Kane, MD, MSPH

The majority of female patients with Crohn's disease (CD) and ulcerative colitis (UC) are diagnosed either before or during their childbearing years. There are many issues that arise for the female patient with inflammatory bowel disease (IBD) who is pregnant or contemplating pregnancy. Inheritance in the offspring, fertility, the effect of the gestational period on IBD, and conversely, the effect of IBD on the pregnancy, as well as the safety of drugs on the developing fetus and nursing newborn are all important clinical considerations. In addition, certain health maintenance issues such as cervical cancer screening become more important in women with chronic inflammatory disease who are treated with long-term immunosuppressive medications. This chapter will review those key issues regarding fertility, pregnancy, and cervical cancer.

FERTILITY, FECUNDITY, AND FAMILY PLANNING AMONG WOMEN WITH IBD

Fecundity describes the biologic capacity to conceive. It is expressed as the probability of becoming pregnant per month with unprotected intercourse. This can be interpreted to patients as the probable waiting time until conception. Fertility, on the other hand, is defined and measured by the actual production of live offspring and alone does not convey any information regarding etiology (Figure 11-1). Infertility defined as the absence of offspring is often the result of active decision making and contraceptive use. These terms are frequently confused.

Although fecundity is under genetic and environmental control, it is a major indicator of physical and psychological fitness. Fecundity may be

Regueiro MD, Swoger JM, eds.
Clinical Challenges and Complications of IBD (pp 197-230).
© 2013 Taylor & Francis Group.

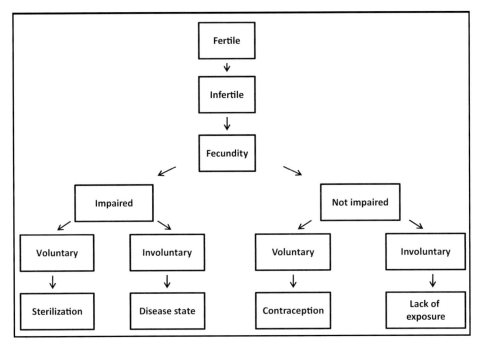

Figure 11-1. Fertility and fecundity. (Adapted from Moody GA, Mayberry JF. Perceived sexual dysfunction amongst patients with inflammatory bowel disease. *Digestion*. 1993;54[4]:256-260.)

compromised by a variety of voluntary and involuntary factors in patients with IBD. Sexual dysfunction is reported in up to 75% of women.[1] It is commonly underestimated and insufficiently addressed by physicians. A German cross-sectional study demonstrated low sexual activity in the majority of the 336 women with IBD interviewed: 17% reported none at all, 63% low activity, and only 20% moderate or high activity.[2] Depression was the strongest predictor of low sexual function. Disease activity had moderate negative impact on desire, while disease severity was inversely associated with intercourse frequency. Smokers had vaginal lubrication problems more often than nonsmokers. Libido may be also diminished due to IBD-related distortion of body image and fear of sexual rejection[3] or the systemic effects of active disease such as fatigue, diarrhea, or pain. Dyspareunia is reported by 60% of CD patients, and it is even more common in the presence of perianal, rectovaginal fistulizing disease[1] or restorative proctocolectomy.[4]

In general, fecundity and fertility rates in both UC and CD patients are comparable to non-IBD controls. A Scandinavian study by Olsen comparing 290 women with UC to 661 healthy controls showed no impairment of fecundability rates (the probability of conception per month of unprotected intercourse).[5] In the same study, however, fecundability decreased severely to 20% compared to healthy controls after restorative proctocolectomy with ileal pouch-anal anastomosis (IPAA) formation. A more recent study confirmed reduced fecundability, but to a much lesser degree (81%), which was attributed to improved surgical techniques.[6] This finding was also observed in patients with familial adenomatous polyposis undergoing IPAA whose fecundity rate decreased to 54% after surgery. Notably, the fecundity rate remained completely normal in those familial adenomatous polyposis (FAP) patients who only underwent subtotal colectomy with ileorectal anastomosis.[7] The reduced postoperative fecundability from IPAA is attributed to the deranged pelvic anatomy and postoperative adhesions causing fallopian tube occlusion.[8]

Olsen and colleagues also demonstrated severe impairment of fertility (measuring the actual number of births) after IPAA in women with UC, with the fertility ratio dropping from 0.91 to 0.35.[9] A meta-analysis of 7 studies found a 3.2-fold increased relative risk of infertility, defined as failure to become pregnant during 12 months of unprotected intercourse, in UC patients after IPAA. The weighted average infertility rate increased from 15% to 48% postoperatively.[10] In a systematic review, analyzing the results from 7 studies, the infertility rate increased from 12% to 26% after IPAA.[11] After IPAA, more women require infertility investigations and treatments. Although both fecundity and fertility decreased after IPAA, one Scandinavian study concluded that the lifetime chance of having at least one live birth is still 80%.[6] Women who still wish to conceive but are facing surgery for UC should consider having a subtotal colectomy with ileostomy to avoid pelvic dissection and delay the creation of an internal pouch until after desired pregnancies are complete.

An earlier large case-control study performed in 5 European countries in the 1980s reported decreased fertility rates in CD patient (58% versus 72%) despite less frequent use of contraception suggestive of diminished fecundity.[12] The rate of spontaneous abortion increased (6.5% versus 13%) after IBD was diagnosed in a large European cohort.[13] CD complicated with pelvic adhesions involving the fallopian tubes and ovaries negatively impacts fecundity.[14] Prior surgery for CD is associated with increased risk for infertility.[15]

More recent studies emphasize voluntary childlessness rather than decreased ability to conceive among women with CD as well as with UC.[16,17] A survey by means of anonymous questionnaire found high prevalence of voluntary childlessness among IBD patients compared to the general population: 18% in CD, 14% in UC versus 6.2%.[17] Similarly, in an Australian study, 14% of IBD patients reported making this decision as a direct result of IBD.[16] Nonvoluntary childlessness or infertility rates were similar to the background population in both studies. IBD patients often express fear as the source of their voluntary childlessness. Fear of IBD-related congenital abnormalities, genetic transmission of IBD to the child, medication teratogenicity, and disease flare as a result of pregnancy were most commonly cited. In addition, a surprisingly high portion of patients (35%) with voluntary childlessness were advised against pregnancy by their physician in the same study.[16]

None of the medications used to treat IBD appear to affect fecundity and fertility in women[18] but can be an area of concern in men, specifically the use of sulfasalazine, which is associated with reversible decreased sperm count and motility.[19]

Table 11-1. Lifetime Risk of IBD in Offspring				
TYPE OF IBD IN THE PARENT	CROHN'S DISEASE		ULCERATIVE COLITIS	
Ethnicity	Jewish	Non-Jewish	Jewish	Non-Jewish
Lifetime risk of IBD to the child (%)	7.8	5.2	4.5	1.6

PREGNANCY

Inheritance

One of the most commonly asked questions when contemplating pregnancy is, "What is the likelihood that my baby will have IBD?" A large population-based study from Denmark found that the risk of developing IBD is increased by 2- to 13-fold compared to the background population if one parent is affected by the disease.[20] The progeny was more likely to inherit the same disorder as the parent, but he or she was also at higher risk to develop the opposite disease compared to the general population. Specifically, if the parent had UC, the offspring had a 5.1-fold increased risk to develop UC and a 2.6-fold increased risk to develop CD (Table 11-1). On the other hand, if the parent had CD, the risk of inheriting CD was 12.8-fold higher and the risk of inheriting UC was 4.0-fold higher than the general population. A study from Belgium found that if one parent is affected with CD, the child's lifetime risk to develop IBD was 10.4% with a relative risk of 4.5. Interestingly, the parents with IBD had a higher chance to have a daughter with IBD (12.6%) than a son with IBD (7.9%).[21] If both parents have IBD, the lifetime risk of developing IBD is 36%.[22] Jewish ethnicity is associated with increased empirical genetic risk for IBD. If the proband has CD, the first-degree relative's lifetime risk to develop IBD was 5.2% in non-Jewish Whites and 7.8% in Jewish families. In first-degree relatives of UC probands, the lifetime risk of IBD is 1.6% in non-Jews and 4.5% in Jews.[23,24]

In summary, the magnitude of the genetic risk to develop IBD depends on the genealogical proximity of the affected family member, ethnicity, and the type of disease. Although the single most important risk factor in developing IBD is positive family history, we have to keep in mind that IBD is a non-mendelian polygenic disorder with multiple environmental factors leading to its development.

Effect of Pregnancy on IBD

Overall, pregnancy does not affect the rate of disease exacerbation. Early studies from the 1980s reported an exacerbation rate of 34% per year during pregnancy versus 32% per year in nonpregnant UC patients,[25] with comparable numbers in CD patients.[26] However, later data suggest that the best predictor of disease activity during pregnancy is the disease activity at the time of conception. Patients with quiescent IBD at conception have a 70% to 80% chance of staying in remission, and when relapse occurs, it is likely to happen in the first trimester.[27] By contrast, the clinical course of patients with active disease at conception will usually fall into thirds: one-third will improve, one-third remains unchanged, and one-third will worsen during pregnancy. Disease flare during pregnancy is often associated with discontinuation of maintenance therapy.[28] Cessation of smoking also occurs often during pregnancy and may have a positive effect on disease activity in CD. Agret et al[29] found significantly lower clinical activity scores (Harvey-Bradshaw index) during the gestation period in women with CD who smoked before pregnancy and most of whom reduced cigarette use during pregnancy. Disease flare during the first pregnancy predicts IBD course during the subsequent pregnancies: women were 4 times more likely to flare (odds ratio 4.0, 95% confidence interval 1.19 to 13.63) in the second pregnancy, regardless of breastfeeding history.[30]

A cohort study from the UK demonstrated inverse correlation between the number of pregnancies and number of surgical resections in women with ileal and colonic CD during a mean 15-year follow-up.[31] This protective effect could not be replicated in a recent study by Riis at al.[13] Disease phenotype does not appear to change during or after pregnancy.[13]

Patients with IPAA, in general, do well during pregnancy. Anal sphincter and pouch function may be altered, leading to mild incontinence and increased stool frequency in 20% to 30% of the patients, usually in the third trimester.[32,33] In most cases, baseline pouch function returns within 3 months of childbirth.

Mode of Delivery

There is no general consensus as to the optimal delivery mode in IBD patients due to paucity of data. Potential risk of perineal CD flare and injury to the anal sphincter is an area of major concern. Clinicians commonly recommend cesarean section (C-section) in women with IBD due to fears of perianal disease development or reactivation and fecal incontinence due to occult trauma to the sphincter during vaginal delivery. Elective C-section is more commonly performed in the IBD population than in the general population, 9% in both CD and UC versus 5.4% ($P < 0.01$ for each).[34] The use of C-section increased from 8.1% to 28.7% after IBD diagnosis was made in a large European cohort of women.[13]

It is currently disputed whether vaginal delivery and episiotomy increases the risk for de novo perineal involvement of CD. Brandt and colleagues surveyed 80 women with CD without history of perineal disease who had a total of 140 vaginal deliveries and 123 episiotomies: 18% reported development of perineal disease sometime after giving birth with a majority of these occurring within 2 months of the delivery and episiotomy.[35] These data may be skewed by selection bias and/or lack of data verification because subsequent studies did not corroborate these findings. In a Canadian survey, only 1 of 39 women with vaginal deliveries and no history of perineal disease, of whom 27 had an episiotomy, developed perineal disease within 1 year of the delivery.[34] In the same study, those with inactive perineal disease (n = 11) had no relapse of the perineal disease within 1-year postpartum. A small case series by Rogers and Katz[36] of 17 CD women showed no relationship between the mode of delivery and development of perineal disease. A retrospective small French study reported that vaginal delivery in 20 patients did not lead to development or exacerbation of perineal CD.[37]

Women with active perineal disease consistently tend to do worse after vaginal delivery.[34,36] C-section should be recommended to avoid trauma to the perineum and to protect the integrity of the anal sphincter in women with active perineal disease.[34] On the other hand, there is absence of clear evidence to recommend C-section from the gastroenterologist's perspective to women without a history of perineal CD to avoid de novo development of perineal CD. Furthermore, based upon limited retrospective data, women with quiescent perineal disease can also be considered for vaginal delivery. The mode of delivery should be determined on a case-by-case basis considering the pregestational anal continence and the condition of the perineum and should be a joint decision between the patient, the gastroenterologist, the obstetrician, and the colorectal surgeon if needed.[38]

There is no consensus regarding the recommended route of delivery for patients with IPAA. Several retrospective studies demonstrated that uncomplicated vaginal delivery does not affect pouch function, anal continence, or quality of life on short term, but there are no data on pouch function with aging several decades following vaginal delivery. A recent study warned that vaginal delivery may increase the risk of sphincter muscle injury that could compromise pouch function on the long run.[39] Currently, most colorectal surgeons would recommend C-section for patients with IPAA to avoid fecal incontinence in the future.[40] It is also debated whether patients with UC should avoid vaginal delivery to minimize trauma to the anal sphincter in anticipation of future IPAA. Further research is needed to elucidate this question as well.

Postpartum Course

Disease flare due to hormonal and physical changes in postpartum period is a concern for many patients. However, the data in the IBD literature are rather reassuring on this topic. The odds of disease exacerbation in the postpartum year were similar to those nonpregnant controls in a large Canadian cohort study.[30] In a survey in the 1980s of 324 patients, only 13% with quiescent to mild disease and 53% of those with active disease at term developed flare within 3 months of the delivery.[27] Moreover, a small Italian cohort study demonstrated that both UC and CD women had actually significantly reduced number of flares for the first 3 years after pregnancy compared to the 3 years before pregnancy and to the incidence in nonpregnant-matched controls.[41] Riis et al observed in a large European cohort of 177 UC and 77 CD postpartum women that the exacerbation rate per year decreased from 0.35 to 0.18 in UC and from 0.76 to 0.12 in CD during a 10-year follow-up.[13] The favorable effect of pregnancy on the disease course during gestation and the postpartum period positively correlates with the degree of human leukocyte antigens-disparity between mother and fetus (disparity in 0, 1, versus 2 DRB1 and DQ loci). This positive effect is due to gestation-induced immunosuppression that enables the successful reproductive outcome and downregulates maternal autoimmune disease.[42] The exact mechanism is currently unknown; however, one proposed mechanism is the inhibition of maternal T-cells in the pregnant uterus.[43] The Th1 immune response is downregulated with shift toward Th2 response, which may explain why more CD patients seem to experience symptomatic improvement than UC patients.[13,42] Another proposed mechanism for the pregnancy-induced maternal immunosuppression is the inhibition of the maternal decidual natural killer cells by HLA-G to protect the fetus from rejection.[44] Kane et al pointed to the fact that disease activity before delivery predicts postpartum disease activity.[42]

Breastfeeding

Kane and Lemieux[45] found that only 44% of women with IBD breast-fed their infants. History of breastfeeding had no impact on the risk of IBD flare in the postpartum period after medication cessation was accounted for. A significant number (75%) of women discontinued the maintenance IBD medication after delivery. Gastroenterologists should play an active role in counseling their patients to adhere to their maintenance therapy. A more recent survey in Manitoba, Canada, suggested that women with IBD are just as likely to breast-feed (83%) as their healthy counterparts.[30] Breastfeeding in this study was not a risk factor for disease flare; rather, it was found to be protective up to 1-year postpartum.

A large number of women with IBD choose not to breast-feed mainly due to fear of medication passage into the breast milk. The benefits of breastfeeding to the infant are well established, including a decreased chance to develop IBD later in life.[46,47] Clinicians should keep these facts in mind when counseling IBD patients on the advantages of nursing. Risks and benefits of IBD therapy to the mother and the neonates in the case of breastfeeding should be carefully considered on an individual basis in the postpartum period.

Effect of Inflammatory Bowel Disease on Pregnancy and Birth Outcome

In general, women with IBD appear to have a slightly increased risk for pregnancy-related complications and adverse birth outcomes even when in remission. Several population-based cohort and case-control studies have described an association between IBD and preterm birth and low birth weight (LBW). The strongest risk factor for adverse pregnancy outcome is active disease at the time of conception. The data on congenital anomalies are discordant and the IBD associated risk is questionable.

The diagnosis of IBD itself was found to be an independent risk factor for preterm birth, LBW, and small for gestational age (SGA) in a large Swedish population-based cohort study, but disease type (CD versus UC), disease activity, and medical treatment were not taken into account.[48] Mahadevan reported similar findings in the Northern California Kaiser Permanente population examining the outcomes of 461 pregnancies by women with UC or CD. IBD diagnosis was an independent predictor of an adverse conception outcome such as spontaneous abortion, adverse pregnancy outcome such as preterm birth, stillbirth, SGA infant, or complication of labor. The vast majority of the patients had mild or inactive disease during conception and throughout the pregnancy.[49] Disease severity and medical therapy were not associated with pregnancy complications or adverse newborn outcomes in this study, implying that women with IBD even in remission are more likely to have adverse pregnancy outcomes than their healthy counterparts.[50]

A meta-analysis by Cornish et al[51] pooled data from 12 studies encompassing 3907 IBD patients (36% CD and 63% UC) found higher incidence of prematurity (1.87-fold), over 2-fold increase in LBW, and 1.5-fold increase in C-section. No increase in incidence of SGA was found in either CD or UC patients. Disease activity could not be accounted for in the pooled data. In another study, maternal IBD was linked to preterm birth in a large Swedish cohort, but LBW was only associated with CD not UC and only after onset of disease, suggesting that disease activity and nutritional status might contribute to adverse neonatal outcomes.[52]

Disease activity was found to be predictor of adverse pregnancy outcomes in several early studies. In a US study by Dominitz et al,[61] active disease at conception or during pregnancy was associated with 3.4-fold increased risk of preterm labor in women with moderate-to-severe disease compared to those with quiescent disease. Active disease at conception was linked to high miscarriage rate[25,26,54] and preterm delivery,[25,26] and disease exacerbation during pregnancy was associated with LBW[55,56] and preterm birth.[56,57] In more recent studies, the role of disease activity and severity has been shown to play a smaller role in adverse birth outcomes beyond the IBD diagnosis itself. In a Danish cohort study, the relative risk of preterm labor was more than 2-fold in women with active CD during pregnancy in relation to those in stable remission with the risk being highest in moderate-high disease activity.[53] On the other hand, they observed no increased risk in LBW, SGA, or congenital anomalies. In the Californian Kaiser population, disease activity was not a predictor of adverse pregnancy outcome, although very few patients had moderate-severe disease.[58]

The largest population-based study to date by Stephansson et al[59] from Scandinavia analyzed pregnancies and births by 2637 primiparous UC women between 1994 and 2006 and reported increased risks of preterm delivery, SGA birth, neonatal death, and C-section but not congenital abnormalities. Women with more severe disease, as measured by history of prior hospital admissions and UC-related surgeries, were more likely to have adverse birth outcomes than those with mild disease. Norgard et al reported 40% increased risk of preterm birth among women with UC in Denmark, the risk being particularly high when the first hospitalization for UC took place during pregnancy; however, no increased risk was found for LBW or SGA.[60] A meta-analysis by Cornish reported that maternal UC is associated with a 3.9-fold increase in congenital anomalies.[51] However, this conclusion was driven by 2 small studies comprising only 170 pregnancies. One of these studies conducted by Dominitz et al[61] used the birth records of Washington state to compare pregnancy outcomes in 107 UC with 1308 patients without IBD and showed that women with UC had a significantly higher rate of congenital malformations (7.9% versus 1.7%). However, the study did not adjust for medical therapy of IBD. No other studies substantiated this finding, including the largest population-based studies (Scandinavian and Northern Californian cohort N = 2937), which showed no increase in incidence of birth defects in babies to UC mothers[58,59] (Table 11-2).

Stephansson et al[62] using the Danish and Swedish Medical Birth Registries to explore gestational risks of CD women (N = 2377) found that the strongest associations with CD were the need for induced preterm delivery and C-section and the risk for SGA infant but no association was found between CD and birth defects. None of the studies examining the incidence of congenital malformation found increased rates among infants born to CD mothers[51,58,61,62] (Table 11-3). The diagnosis of IBD does not appear to have an effect on other common pregnancy-related outcomes such as preeclampsia or eclampsia.

Disease Diagnosis and Activity Assessment During Pregnancy

De novo disease diagnosis and activity assessment can be a challenge during pregnancy. The usefulness of biologic markers is limited due to physiologic changes in pregnancy: hemoglobin and albumin levels are decreased due to hemodilution and the erythrocyte sedimentation rate increased. However, C-reactive protein level remains a reliable indicator of inflammation during gestation. Radiation exposure to the fetus should be minimized, but limited use of abdominal x-rays is justified in appropriate circumstances such as in case of suspected megacolon and bowel obstruction, especially because the potential harm of abdominal radiography to the fetus is minimal.[63] In addition, no single diagnostic radiographic test including abdominal computed tomography (CT) results in radiation exposure to a degree that would disturb the proper development of an embryo or fetus leading to fetal loss or any form of congenital anomaly. Exposure to less than 5 rad has not been reported to increase fetal abnormalities or cause fetal loss. The estimated fetal exposure from the commonly used radiologic procedures ranges between 0.02 rad for chest x-ray to 3.5 rad for abdominal CT.[64]

Table 11-2. Pregnancy-Associated Risks and Birth Outcomes of Women With Ulcerative Colitis Versus Healthy Controls

Authors	Number of Pregnancies Analyzed	Risk of Preterm Birth (OR)	LBW (OR)	SGA Infant (OR)	Congenital Anomalies (OR)	Risk of Cesarean Section (OR)
Stephansson et al[59]	2637	1.77 (1.54 to 2.05)	n/a	1.27 (1.05 to 1.54)	1.05 (0.84 to 1.31)	2.01 (1.84 to 2.19)
Mahadevan et al[58]	300	Pooled risk: 1.48 (0.91 to 2.39)			7% versus 6%	n/a
Cornish et al[51]	1952	N = 1831 1.34 (1.09 to 1.64)	N = 1590 1.66 (0.48 to 0.66)	N = 1546 1.05 (0.51 to 0.16)	N = 170 3.88 (1.41 to 0.67)	N = 204 1.3 (0.86 to 1.96)

LBW = low birth weight; OR = odds ratio; SGA = small for gestational age.

Table 11-3. Pregnancy-Associated Risks and Birth Outcomes of Women With Crohn's Disease Versus Healthy Controls

Authors	Number of Pregnancies Analyzed	Risk of Preterm Birth (OR, 95% CI)	LWB (OR)	SGA Infant (OR)	Congenital Anomalies (OR)	Risk of Cesarean Section (OR)
Stephansson et al[62]	2377	1.76 (1.51 to 2.05)	n/a	1.43 (1.09 to 1.89)	1.01 (0.79 to 1.29)	1.93 (1.76 to 2.12)
Mahadevan et al[58]	154	Pooled risk: 1.4 (0.75 to 2.63)			13% versus 6%	n/a
Cornish et al[51] meta-analysis of 10 studies	1952	N = 1005 1.97 (1.36 to 2.87)	N = 597 2.82 (1.42 to 5.6)	N = 220 5.72 (0.62 to 52.8)	N = 307 2.14 (0.97 to 4.74)	N = 321 1.65 (1.19 to 2.29)

LBW = low birth weight; SGA = small for gestational age; CI = confidence interval; OR = odds ratio.

Nevertheless, ultrasound and magnetic resonance imaging with their novel ancillary techniques are not associated with ionizing radiation and offer a safer alternative to CT in pregnancy. Transabdominal ultrasound can be very helpful particularly with the utilization of color Doppler and contrast-enhanced ultrasound to evaluate bowel wall thickness and surrounding structures including mesenteric inflammatory reaction, extent and localization of involved bowel segments, and detection of extraluminal complications such as fistula or abscesses. Magnetic resonance enterography (MRE) is no longer considered to be just an emerging tool in the evaluation of IBD. It offers disease detection and assessment of the entire gut and the ability to fully evaluate extraluminal disease. MR enteroclysis, when compared to ileocolonoscopy and histology, has a high sensitivity and specificity (96% and 92%, respectively).[65] MRE may well prove itself to be the first-line tool of choice in evaluation of IBD during pregnancy in the future.

There is no evidence that sigmoidoscopy induces labor and may be sufficient to yield the new diagnosis of IBD in the patient presenting with hematochezia, unexplained diarrhea, severe abdominal pain, or severe rectal pain. Likewise, the pregnant IBD patient with worsening symptoms, despite appropriate medical therapy, may also benefit from sigmoidoscopy. Colonoscopy is less often indicated but can be safely performed in the carefully selected pregnant patient. If sedation is required, obstetrical consultation should be obtained prior to endoscopy, and the risks and benefits of endoscopy to both mother and child should be considered. Fetal monitoring is indicated in high-risk or third-trimester patients. Midazolam (Category D) crosses the placenta and few studies reported that it causes transient depression of neonatal respiration and neurobehavioral responsiveness, but it was not associated with cleft lip or palate such as diazepam.[66-68] Fentanyl is a Category C drug and may be used in low dosage for endoscopy during pregnancy. Both midazolam and fentanyl should be used cautiously to provide patient comfort while avoiding oversedation. Propofol (Category B) is relatively safe during pregnancy. Large human studies involving several hundreds of participants failed to report neonatal toxicity from propofol.

Medical Therapy of Inflammatory Bowel Disease During Pregnancy and Lactation

In general, the vast majority of medications used to treat IBD are low risk during pregnancy. The US Food and Drug Administration (FDA) categories provide guidance on medication safety during pregnancy, which is summarized in Table 11-4. The pregnancy risk categories assigned by the FDA for many of these drugs rely on limited studies and animal models and may be of little help for the clinician. There is no current standard FDA classification system to categorize risk for lactation. Table 11-5 summarizes the safety of medications that are commonly used in IBD patients during pregnancy and Table 11-6 during breastfeeding.

Table 11-4. *Food and Drug Administration Categories of Fetal Risk From the Medication Used During Pregnancy*

CATEGORY	DEFINITION
A	Controlled studies in animals and women have shown no risk in the first trimester and overall fetal harm is remote
B	Either animal studies have not demonstrated fetal risk but there are no controlled studies in pregnant women; or animal studies have shown an adverse effect that was not confirmed in controlled studies in women in the first trimester (and there is no evidence of risk in the later trimesters)
C	No controlled studies in pregnant women have been performed and animal studies have revealed adverse effect on the fetus, or reproduction studies in humans and in animals are not available; drug should be used if the potential benefit outweighs the risk
D	There is positive evidence of human fetal risk, but the use of drug is acceptable in severe or life-threatening disease for which safer drugs cannot be used or ineffective
X	Studies in animals or humans have demonstrated fetal abnormalities and the risk clearly outweighs the benefit; the drug is contraindicated

Adapted from Jenss H, Weber P, Hartmann F. 5-aminosalicylic acid and its metabolite in breast milk during lactation. *Am J Gastroenterol.* 1990;85(3):331.

Aminosalicylates

All aminosalicylates are Category B drugs, except for olsalazine, which is a Category C. Mesalamine 400 and 800 mg oral tablets (Asacol and Asacol HD) have been recently assigned to pregnancy Category C by the FDA. Animal studies of mesalamine have failed to reveal evidence of fetal harm. However, dibutyl phthalate (DBP) is an inactive ingredient in the enteric coating of Asacol and Asacol HD tablets, and in animal studies at doses greater than 190 and greater than 80 times the human dose based on body surface area, respectively, maternal DBP was associated with external and skeletal malformations and adverse effects on the male reproductive system. Both sulfasalazine and 5-aminosalicylates (5-ASA) readily cross the placenta, and fetal blood concentrations of sulfasalazine are similar to that of the maternal blood,[69] while 5-ASA concentrations are somewhat lower in the fetal blood at the time of delivery.[70] Although early case reports raised concerns about teratogenicity of sulfasalazine, larger series failed to demonstrate an increased risk of congenital anomalies.

Table 11-5. Safety and Food and Drug Administration Pregnancy Categories of Medications Commonly Used in a Pregnant Inflammatory Bowel Disease Patient

LOW RISK	LIMITED DATA OR CONTROVERSIAL	CONTRAINDICATED (X)
Sulfasalazine (B) Mesalamine (B)* Balsalazine (B) Corticosteroids (C) (prednisone preferred) Budesonide (C) Metronidazole (B) Augmentin (B) Loperamide (B) Infliximab (B) Adalimumab (B) Certolizumab pegol (B) Cholestyramine (B)	Olsalazine (C) Ciprofloxacin (C) Azathioprine and 6-mercaptopurine (D) Cyclosporine and tacrolimus (C) Natalizumab (C) Bisphosphonates (C)	Methotrexate (stop at least 3 months before conception) Thalidomide (stop 1 month before conception) Bismuth subsalicylate (C-D)

*Mesalamine 400 and 800 mg oral tablets (Asacol and Asacol HD) have been assigned to pregnancy Category C by the FDA. Animal studies of mesalamine have failed to reveal evidence of fetal harm. However, dibutyl phthalate (DBP) is an inactive ingredient in the enteric coating of Asacol and Asacol HD tablets, and in animal studies at doses greater than 190 times the human dose, maternal DBP was associated with external and skeletal malformations and adverse effects on the male reproductive system.

Table 11-6. Safety of Inflammatory Bowel Disease Medications During BreastFeeding

COMPATIBLE	LIMITED DATA, POTENTIAL TOXICITY	CONTRAINDICATED
Corticosteroids Sulfasalazine (potential diarrhea) Mesalamine (potential diarrhea) Balsalazine (potential diarrhea) Olsalazine (potential diarrhea) Infliximab Adalimumab Certolizumab pegol Augmentin Ciprofloxacin	Metronidazole Azathioprine/ 6-mercaptopurine Cyclosporine Tacrolimus Loperamide Lomotil Bismuth subsalicylate Natalizumab	Methotrexate Thalidomide

A case-control study of the Hungarian population found no significant teratogenicity associated with the use of sulfasalazine.[71] Moskovitz et al[72] found no increased risk of adverse pregnancy outcome in 170 pregnancies exposed to sulfasalazine or 5-ASAs and concluded that aminosalicylates up to 4 g/day are safe during gestation. In a larger series of 181 pregnancies, Mogadam et al[73] did not report increased incidence of congenital anomalies in women exposed to sulfasalazine. Sulfasalazine appears to be safe in pregnancy as long as aggressive folate supplementation at 2 mg daily dose is taken.[74] Breastfeeding is also considered safe on sulfasalazine therapy. Sulfasalazine, unlike other sulfanomides, does not displace the bilirubin from the albumin binding and does not increase the risk of kernicterus.

Mesalamine exposure during pregnancy is generally considered safe. Numerous case series suggested no increased risk of adverse pregnancy outcomes with oral[75-77] or topical mesalamine.[78] A prospective trial of 165 women matched to nonexposed women showed that mesalamine was not teratogenic at a 2 g daily dose.[79] However, women exposed to mesalamine were more likely to deliver preterm, gain less weight than matched controls, and have LBW babies. Women with active disease and those exposed to multiple IBD medications in addition to mesalamine were more likely to encounter adverse pregnancy outcomes compared to those who were taking mesalamine alone. A Danish cohort study reported no increase in congenital malformations on mesalamine but observed increased frequency of stillbirth and preterm delivery in UC patients exposed to mesalamine.[80] Both of these studies concluded that the increased risk of adverse birth outcomes were due to disease activity rather than medication. None of these studies provided estimates for relative risk adjusted for disease activity or mother's age. The most recent study on this topic by Norgard et al[53] analyzed 179 pregnancies exposed to sulfasalazine/5-ASA, did not indicate increased risk of congenital abnormalities or preterm birth, and found only a very small (0.8%) additional risk for LBW when adjusted for disease activity.

Safety data on larger doses of aminosalicylates in pregnancy are scarce. Although concerns about renal insufficiency in patients taking 5-ASA have been highlighted recently, there was only one case report about interstitial nephritis in an infant exposed to mesalazine in utero.[81] In several studies, mothers were exposed to 3.2 to 4 g/day during the second trimester,[72,79] the period of renal morphogenesis without negative impact on the infant's kidney function. Secondary to paucity of data on high doses, it is best to prescribe the minimum effective dose of mesalazine and/or monitor fetal kidney function during pregnancy.[40]

Breastfeeding on sulfasalazine and 5-ASA is thought to be safe. The concentration of 5-ASA in the breast milk is low, less than 10% of the therapeutic level; thus, the effect of mesalazine on the infant is unlikely to be clinically important.[82,83] However, bloody diarrhea in an infant being breast-fed by a woman taking sulfasalazine has been reported,[84] and watery diarrhea in an infant whose mother was using topical 5-ASA has also been reported.[85] It is recommended that infants who receive breast milk from mothers taking aminosalicylates are monitored for chronic diarrhea or bloody stools.[50]

Corticosteroids

Corticosteroids are classified as Category C drugs. Two large case-control studies reported an increase in the incidence of cleft lip (with or without cleft palate) between 1.7-fold[86] and 6.5-fold[87] with maternal use of corticosteroids in the first trimester. A meta-analysis of 10 studies including the aforementioned case-control studies revealed a 3.4 increased risk in cleft lip (with or without cleft palate) associated with corticosteroid use during pregnancy, although the authors themselves failed to corroborate this finding in a prospective study of 185 pregnancies.[88] Similarly, a prospective controlled study by Gur et al[89] including 311 exposed pregnancies did not demonstrate increased risk of teratogenicity. Overall, corticosteroid exposure in utero, in particular during the first trimester, poses a small but significant risk of cleft lip (with or without cleft palate), which should be communicated to the expecting mother. Prednisone, or its active metabolite prednisolone, should be preferred in pregnancy.[40] Dexamethasone and betamethasone reach higher concentrations than prednisolone in the fetal blood due to differences in placental metabolism and albumin-binding affinities.[90,91] In general, the efficient placental metabolism of corticosteroids appears to protect the fetus from adverse effects, as only sporadic cases of fetal adrenal suppression have been reported in the transplant literature.[92]

Oral budesonide use was reported in 8 women with small bowel CD during pregnancy without adverse outcomes.[93] In addition, a recent systemic evidence review found no increased risk for congenital malformations, preterm birth, or LBW with inhaled budesonide during pregnancy compared with the general population.[94]

Prednisolone is poorly excreted into the breast milk, achieving only 5% to 25% concentrations of that in the serum with increasing doses. At a daily dose of 40 mg prednisolone, the exposure of the infant is minimal (< 5% of the infant's endogenous cortisol production) and unlikely the cause of any adverse effects. At higher doses, the exposure can be minimized if nursing is delayed by 4 hours after the last dose of the medication.[95] Budesonide concentrations are also low in breast milk. It is estimated that the daily infant dose is 0.3% of the daily maternal dose.[96]

Antibiotics

Metronidazole is a pregnancy Category B drug. Numerous studies demonstrated its safety during pregnancy including during the first trimester. A prospective controlled trial followed 228 women exposed to metronidazole in pregnancy, more than 80% of whom had first trimester exposure.[97] No difference was found in the rate of congenital malformations. Metronidazole use was associated with LBW but not premature delivery. In addition, 2 retrospective cohort studies[98,99] and 2 meta-analyses[100,101] concluded that metronidazole was not teratogenic.

Metronidazole is excreted in the breast milk and achieves infant plasma concentrations approximately one-fifth of those observed in the mother's plasma.[102] The American Academy of Pediatrics (AAP) places metronidazole in the category of drugs whose long-term effects are unknown and may be of concern, recommending withholding nursing during therapy for 12 to 24 hours following oral single dose. Some experts suggest that short-course maternal metronidazole therapy during breastfeeding should be well tolerated by the nursing infant.

Fluoroquinolones (ciprofloxacin, levofloxacin, norfloxacin) are Category C drugs. Animal studies showed an increased risk of arthropathy in newborn mice after in utero exposure to quinolones.[103] Based upon animal data, the manufacturer recommends against use in pregnancy and in children. However, a prospective controlled study with 200 women treated with fluoroquinolones during pregnancy failed to demonstrate any adverse effects.[104] Other population-based[105] and retrospective studies also supported the safety of quinolone therapy during pregnancy.

Ciprofloxacin is excreted in human milk in small amounts. The use of quinolones during breastfeeding has not been recommended due to the theoretical potential for arthropathy in the infant. The manufacturer recommends that 48 hours elapse after the last dose before breastfeeding is resumed. However, the AAP considers use of ciprofloxacin compatible with breastfeeding.[106]

Amoxicillin/clavulanic acid is a pregnancy Category B drug. A large, population-based, case-control study and a prospective, controlled study demonstrated no increase in teratogenic risk with its use. It is compatible with breastfeeding.[106]

Antidiarrheals

Loperamide is a pregnancy Category B drug. It has not been shown to be teratogenic in rats. A prospective, controlled study, in which 89 women who were exposed to loperamide in the first trimester were enrolled, showed no increased risk of congenital anomalies, preterm delivery, or spontaneous abortion.[107] However, women who took loperamide throughout their pregnancy were more likely to have babies with smaller birth weight than the controls, and its use late in the pregnancy was associated with bowel obstruction in the newborn. A more recent, large population-based study found a 1.4-fold increased incidence of congenital anomalies in infants with in utero exposure to loperamide during the first trimester,[108] although the lack of specificity among the observed malformations speaks against loperamide teratogenicity in this study. Based upon these data, it is best to avoid long-term use of loperamide in gestation.

Lomotil (diphenoxylate hydrochloride/atropine) is Category C. Human studies are limited, and it is not known whether the drug crosses the placenta. It should be used with caution in pregnant women.[40]

Bismuth subsalicylate is Category C in the first and second trimesters but Category D in the third trimester. Its use in the last trimester has been linked to prolonged gestation and labor, greater blood loss at delivery, and increased perinatal mortality.[109] It should be avoided in pregnancy.

Cholestyramine is a Category B drug. It is not absorbed from the gut, thus it does not have the potential to cross the placenta. Its use is safe during pregnancy and lactation.[40]

Both loperamide and Lomotil are excreted into the breast milk, and their use is not recommended during lactation.[110] Data are limited on bismuth subsalicylate in breastfeeding, so it is best to avoid it.

Azathioprine and 6-Mercaptopurine

Azathioprine (AZA) and 6-mercaptopurine (6-MP) are the most controversial agents with regard to their safety in pregnancy, and they are classified as Category D drugs by the FDA. Animal studies have demonstrated teratogenicity with the use of AZA and 6-MP when administered in higher doses than given in humans.[111] Human studies with regard to congenital anomalies are controversial. AZA can pass through the placenta, but several mechanisms were described that may protect the fetus from AZA exposure. One study showed that the placenta forms a selective barrier to AZA and its metabolites: while AZA and 6-thioguanine passed into the fetal circulation in limited quantities, 6-methylmercaptopurine (MMP) did not at all.[112] No or very limited thiopurine metabolism was detected in a fetus despite the presence of essential enzymes (thiopurine methyltransferase, xanthine oxidase, and hypoxanthinephosporibosyl transferase).[112]

Sporadic congenital malformations,[113] dose-related bone marrow suppression,[114] and transient neonatal immunosuppression[115] were reported in infants of women with rheumatologic conditions taking AZA. In a population-based cohort study, Norgard et al[116] reported significantly elevated risk of congenital abnormalities, preterm birth, and stillbirth associated with maternal use of AZA/6-MP. However, only 11 women (5 women with CD) were exposed to purine analogues in this study, and disease activity or exposure to other potentially teratogenic drugs were not accounted for. The authors surveyed the Danish nationwide databases several years later, this time including 26 women exposed to AZA/6-MP.[117] Concurring with their previous observations, gestational AZA/6-MP exposure was associated with increased prevalence of congenital abnormalities (15.4% compared to 5.7% that of controls) and preterm birth (25% compared to 6.5% that of reference group). One of the limitations of this study is its low statistical power to estimate prevalence of major congenital abnormalities given their rarity (< 1%). In addition, no recurrent pattern or an increased rate of a specific congenital abnormality was observed among birth defects attributed to AZA/6-MP, rendering the causal relationship questionable.

The vast majority of the safety data on AZA comes from the transplant literature. According to the National Transplantation Pregnancy Registry, the incidence of congenital anomalies is 4%, a figure comparable to the 3% reported in the general population. In the IBD literature, Francella et al[118] demonstrated in a large retrospective study that 6-MP taken before, at conception, or during pregnancy did not increase the risk of congenital abnormalities and other adverse pregnancy outcomes. The largest study to date recruited women on AZA/6-MP who called teratogenic information centers in different countries.[119] One hundred eighty-nine women exposed to 50 to 100 mg/day AZA and 230 nonexposed women through delivery were studied. No difference was found in the rate of major congenital abnormalities; however, the AZA group had more cases of prematurity and LBW likely due to active disease that was not adjusted for in this study.

Despite being labeled as Category D drugs, a large body of evidence suggests that AZA and 6-MP are low risk during pregnancy. Discontinuation of maintenance therapy before conception increases the risk of disease flare[118] putting both mother and fetus at risk. Therefore, cessation of AZA/6-MP before planned pregnancy is currently not recommended.[74]

The World Health Organization recommends against breastfeeding while taking AZA/6-MP due to concerns of bone marrow suppression, hepatitis, and pancreatitis in the infant.[50] AZA and its metabolites are excreted into the breast milk, but several studies suggest that the overall exposure of the infant is very low.[120-122] Christensen et al[123] studied 8 lactating women receiving AZA at 75 to 200 mg daily dose. Milk and plasma 6-MP concentrations were obtained 30 and 60 minutes after drug administration and every hour for 5 hours thereafter. All peak levels were within 4 hours of drug intake. The estimated drug exposure was less than 1% of the maternal dose. Based upon the available evidence, breastfeeding appears to be safe while taking AZA/6-MP, especially if nursing is delayed more than 4 hours after the drug is taken.

Methotrexate

Methotrexate (MTX) is Category X, clearly teratogenic, and should be avoided in women considering pregnancy. MTX is an abortifacient, and its use during the critical period of organogenesis (6 to 10 weeks) is associated with craniofacial, digital abnormalities, and often central nervous system defects summarized as fetal MTX syndrome. If conception occurs on treatment, MTX should be stopped and the patient placed on high-dose folic acid. Fertile women on MTX should be counseled on the crucial importance of reliable contraception. Due to prolonged tissue-binding characteristics of MTX, experts recommend the discontinuation of the drug at least 3 to 6 months before attempting conception.[40,50]

The AAP advises against breastfeeding on MTX.[106] MTX is excreted into the breast milk in small quantities, and potential accumulation of the drug in the infant tissues may lead to immunosuppression or other toxicities. Safety of breastfeeding on MTX is unknown.

Cyclosporine

Cyclosporine is Category C. It crosses the placenta in high quantities but is rapidly cleared by the newborn. Although sporadic reports of cataracts and growth delay when given in high doses exist in animal models, cyclosporine has not been associated with any pattern of congenital anomalies.

Data relating to cyclosporine use during pregnancy are mainly derived from the transplant literature. The National Transplantation Pregnancy Registry did not demonstrate an increased risk of teratogenicity with cyclosporine in 2005. A meta-analysis of 15 studies, including 410 pregnancies in transplant recipients, concluded that cyclosporine was not associated with increased frequency of congenital anomalies or other adverse birth outcomes.[124]

To date, case reports are available for a total of 19 IBD patients treated with cyclosporine at 2 to 4 mg/kg dose during pregnancy.[125] The drug was found to be effective in most cases to avoid colectomy, and no congenital defects were observed. Nevertheless, cyclosporine has potentially serious maternal adverse effects including hypertension and seizures, thus its use mandates caution, in particular toward the end of pregnancy. Cyclosporine is not advised for nursing mothers by the AAP because it is excreted into the breast milk in high amounts, and there are concerns about nephrotoxicity and immunosuppression in the fetus.[106]

Tacrolimus

Tacrolimus is a pregnancy Category C drug. The transplant literature has not shown evidence of increased risk for congenital anomalies, but demonstrated a tendency toward preterm delivery and LBW with tacrolimus.[126] The experience with tacrolimus in pregnant IBD patients is very limited. Only one successful pregnancy outcome has been reported in a UC patient who was taking tacrolimus during the entire pregnancy with no side effects to mother or newborn.[127]

Tacrolimus is excreted into the breast milk, and there are no data on its safety in the nursing infant. Therefore, it is currently considered not compatible with breastfeeding by experts.

Thalidomide

Thalidomide is pregnancy Category X drug, and its teratogenic effect has been well documented, including the characteristic bilateral limb reduction defects and abnormalities in multiple inner organs and nervous system, which are collectively called thalidomide embryopathy. Women of childbearing age on thalidomide should be advised to use 2 reliable methods of contraception for 1 month before starting therapy, during therapy, and for 1 month after discontinuation of thalidomide.[50] There are no data on safety while breastfeeding.

Infliximab

All 3 anti-tumor necrosis factor (TNF) antibodies are classified as Category B drugs. Animal reproduction studies were not performed since infliximab only cross reacts with human and chimpanzee TNF-α. They are presumed to be safe in animals. An early case report described poor birth outcome with infliximab in a women with severe active CD.[128] Evidence supporting the safety of infliximab has accumulated from large studies and databases over the past decade. In the IBD population, the largest body of data comes from the TREAT registry and the Infliximab Safety Database. The TREAT registry, a prospective registry of CD patients, reported 36 pregnancies with prior exposure to infliximab without increased risk of congenital anomalies or other adverse pregnancy outcomes. The Infliximab Safety Database, the manufacturer's retrospective adverse event registry, contains data about 96 pregnancies with direct exposure to infliximab. The birth outcomes of these pregnancies were not different than the general population. The first study on intentional use of infliximab for induction and maintenance of remission in 10 pregnant women with CD reported no congenital anomalies.[129] This was the first study to demonstrate that benefits of infliximab in achieving remission of CD during pregnancy outweigh the risk of in utero exposure of the drug.

A recent review of the FDA database on adverse events with anti-TNF antibodies between 1999 and 2005 was reported.[130] The analysis revealed a total of 61 congenital anomalies among 41 children born to mothers treated with anti-TNF antibodies during pregnancy. Of these mothers, 19 received infliximab. Fifty-nine percent of the children had one of more congenital anomalies that are part of the VACTERL spectrum: vertebral abnormalities, anal atresia, cardiac defect, and tracheoeosophageal, renal, and limb abnormalities. These congenital anomalies were observed at a higher rate than historical controls.

The finding of this report contradicts all previous studies, but the study has come under criticism as the data collection in the FDA registry is voluntary, which may introduce selection bias and may not represent the true incidence of congenital anomalies in the population of patients treated with infliximab. Coexisting risks factors such as disease activity were not taken into consideration. The congenital anomalies reported in this study tend to be the most common in the population compromising any causality between drug exposure and specific anomaly incidence; in addition, no patient reported in this study qualifies for the diagnosis of VACTERL syndrome since the diagnosis requires that at least 3 of these VACTERL-associated anomalies present in a single individual.

Infliximab is a chimeric immunoglobulin G (IgG) 1 antibody. IgG is the predominant means of fetal immunity, and it is actively transported across the placenta as early as 13 weeks of pregnancy. The transport occurs in a linear fashion as the pregnancy progresses, with the largest amount transferred in the third trimester. This transport mechanism protects the fetus from infliximab exposure during the period of organogenesis. However, if exposed to infliximab during the third trimester, the newborn has detectable drug levels for several months after delivery.[131] These findings suggest that infliximab should be discontinued after the 30th week of gestation and resumed immediately after delivery.[50] It is currently debated whether, in the case of a disease flare, the expectant mother should be bridged with corticosteroids until the delivery or should she receive a dose of infliximab.[50,124]

Infliximab appears to be compatible with breastfeeding. Kane et al[132] prospectively followed 3 CD patients who were treated with infliximab during pregnancy and postpartum. They received infliximab during pregnancy through the 30th week and resumed the therapy within 14 days of delivery. Infliximab was detected in the mothers' sera but not in the breast milk or in the sera of breast-fed newborns. Another case report confirmed that infliximab was not detected in the breast milk of a woman on infliximab therapy.[131] The mother was treated with 10 mg/kg infliximab with the last dose given 2 weeks before delivery. Accordingly, high infliximab levels were detected in the newborn, suggesting placental transport of the drug. Despite breastfeeding and subsequent retreatment of the mother with infliximab, the infant's infliximab levels slowly declined during the 6 months following delivery. The infant was able to mount an appropriate immune response to vaccinations at 6 months of age.

Adalimumab

Only 3 case reports in the IBD literature documented successful use of adalimumab for therapy in CD during pregnancy without negative pregnancy or birth outcomes.[133-135] One of these cases received adalimumab throughout the entire pregnancy without adverse effects on the mother or baby.[134]

Adalimumab is IgG1 antibody and assumed to cross the placenta in the third trimester in high quantities, similarly to other IgG1 molecules. However, no data exist to confirm this mechanism due to the lack of a commercially available test to measure adalimumab levels. In cases of stable remission, experts recommend to continue adalimumab through week 32 of pregnancy and then give one dose immediately after delivery.[50] On the other hand, if the patient has a flare beyond the 32nd week, it is advisable to continue adalimumab through the remainder of the pregnancy given the low risk-benefit ratio.

Adalimumab, like infliximab, is not thought to be transported into breast milk but objective data are lacking.[50]

Certolizumab

Certolizumab is the newest agent among the anti-TNF agents, and little is known about its safety during gestation and lactation. A single case of a pregnant woman with CD treated with certolizumab during the first and third trimesters delivered a healthy newborn.[136] The molecular structure of certolizumab differs from infliximab and adalimumab: it is a pegylated Fab' fragment of the humanized anti-TNF antibody. It lacks the Fc portion, which is needed for active transport via the placenta. Accordingly, significantly lower drug levels were observed in the fetal blood and breast milk with the Fab' fragment compared to the full antibody.[137] These observations were replicated in two women receiving certolizumab during pregnancy. Although the mothers had high certolizumab levels at the time of delivery, the infants' levels and the cord blood levels were low.[138] Given its minimal transfer across the placenta, some have begun to recommend that certolizumab be continued on schedule throughout the pregnancy.[50]

Natalizumab

An FDA pregnancy Class C agent, the safety of use during pregnancy is not known. In female guinea pigs, natalizumab had no significant effect on a embryo/fetal development, but decreased pregnancy rate was observed when high dose (30 mg/kg) was used.[139] Natalizumab had no adverse effects on the general health, survival, development, or immunologic structure and function of infants born to monkeys treated with the drug during pregnancy.[140]

Human experience with natalizumab is sparse. Recent data presented in abstract form showed that patients with multiple sclerosis and CD exposed to natalizumab during pregnancy had a spontaneous abortion rate comparable to what is expected in the general population.[141] Of the 137 prospectively followed pregnancies, there was no congenital anomaly reported to date.

Natalizumab is a humanized IgG4 antibody. It is suspected that natalizumab crosses the placental preferentially in the third trimester but in smaller quantities than the IgG1 antibodies.[142]

Both animal and human data are lacking with regards to breastfeeding and natalizumab.

Neonatal Outcomes in Women With Inflammatory Bowel Disease Exposed to Immunomodulators and Biologic Therapy

The short- and long-term consequences of in utero exposure to immunosuppressive medications are relatively unknown and had recently become an important area of investigation.

The PIANO Registry[143] is a recently established database that prospectively enrolls pregnant women with IBD from 30 centers in the United States. Data are collected from pregnancy until the first year of the child's life. The aim of the registry is to determine whether the rate of congenital malformations, miscarriages, premature birth, and LBW infants are more prevalent among women with IBD who take AZA/6-MP or anti-TNFs during gestation compared to those with IBD who are not exposed to these medications. As of 2009, 353 women completed the pregnancy with 339 live births.[144] AZA/6-MP exposure was associated with significant delay in developmental milestones at month 9 in the infants. However, there were no differences in the milestones met by the infants at months 4 and 12. No difference in rate of birth defects was observed by drug exposure. In women with IBD, use of AZA/6-MP and anti-TNF did not increase the rate of adverse pregnancy outcomes.

Potential drug-induced immunologic abnormalities in the exposed newborn are an area of concern. In a small case series, infants exposed to infliximab during gestation were able to mount an expected immune response to standard vaccinations.[131,145] Irrespective of in utero immunosuppressant exposure, infants should receive the recommended killed vaccines.[38] Experts suggest that at 7 months of age, infants exposed to anti-TNFs and thiopurines should have serologic confirmation (titers of tetanus toxoid and *Haemophilus influenzae* type B) of their immune response to vaccination. A booster shot can be given in case of undetectable levels.

Live vaccines, such as varicella and measles-mumps-rubella, are usually administered between 12 and 15 months of age when anti-TNF levels should be undetectable.[50] It is recommended that infants should not be exposed to thiopurines via breast milk at least 6 weeks before receiving live vaccines.[38]

There is lack of consensus about the safety of live but highly attenuated rotavirus vaccine given at 2 months of age for infants exposed to immunosuppressive drugs in utero.

Surgery During Pregnancy

Absolute indications for surgery in life-threatening conditions such as toxic megacolon or bowel obstruction are unaltered by pregnancy. Elective surgery should be avoided if possible during pregnancy, or at least delayed from the first to the second trimester to avoid the period of organogenesis and the highest pregnancy loss. However, there is accumulating evidence that nonobstetric abdominal surgeries can be safely performed via laparoscopy in all trimesters.[146] Potential risks of an elective IBD surgery during all trimesters must be weighed against the potential harm active disease poses to both mother and fetus when aggressive medical therapy fails. There is little to no evidence published that any drug used to induce general anesthesia is teratogenic.

Historically, surgical intervention for toxic UC in pregnancy is associated with a high morbidity and mortality for both mother and her fetus. Dozois at al[147] reviewed 37 cases in the literature in where the overall fetal and maternal mortality was 49% and 22%, respectively. However, they reported 5 successfully performed subtotal colectomy cases with Brooke ileostomy for fulminant UC at the Mayo Clinic without adverse outcomes to the mothers or the infants. The authors suggest that a multidisciplinary team that includes a gastroenterologist, high-risk obstetrician, and experienced surgeon is necessary for an optimal outcome. An alternative solution is "blowhole" colostomy and loop ileostomy (Turnbull procedure) for the decompression of toxic megacolon, especially if the procedure is necessary before the 28th week of pregnancy.[148,149]

The indications for bowel surgery in CD are the same in pregnancy as in general: perforation, abscess formation, obstruction, or bleeding not amenable to endoscopic therapy. The maternal and fetal mortality was very high in early case reports. A more recent case series of 6 pregnant patients undergoing surgery for CD complication leading to intraperitoneal sepsis reported good outcomes: all women recovered and 5 had healthy babies, with only one having had a miscarriage due to primary anastomosis dehiscence.[150] Diverting ileostomy is generally preferred during pregnancy with prolongation of ostomy take down after delivery to avoid primary anastomosis-related maternal and fetal complication.[38]

CERVICAL DISEASE AND INFLAMMATORY BOWEL DISEASE

Immunosuppressive therapy is linked to an increased rate of opportunistic infections and malignancies including the female genital tract. Several studies have demonstrated that HIV-induced immunosuppression is associated with higher rates of human papillomavirus (HPV) and increased risk of cervical dysplasia. Similar results were found in patient populations that are exposed to chronic immunosuppressive therapy: women with autoimmune diseases,[151,152] renal transplant recipients, and cancer patients.

Prevalence of cervical disease and abnormal Pap smear as well as screening practices for cervical disease in the IBD population have been the focus of numerous recent studies. The studies analyzing the effect of IBD and immunosuppressive therapy on cervical cytology have resulted in contradictory conclusions. Bhatia et al[153] demonstrated higher prevalence of abnormal Pap smears in 116 women with IBD compared to age-matched controls. They found that 18% of women with IBD had abnormal cervical cytology versus 5% of controls. No association was observed between the use of immunosuppressive therapy and increased risk of abnormal Pap smears. HPV data were only available in a small subgroup of patients precluding the ability to meet any conclusions regarding the role of the virus. In a case-control study of 40 patients, Kane et al[154] also found a higher incidence of abnormal Pap smear in women with IBD compared to healthy, age-, and parity-matched controls, 42.7% versus 7% ($P < 0.001$). In addition, women with IBD were more likely to have "higher-risk" lesions. In their study, exposure to immunosuppressive therapy (steroid, AZA/6-MP, infliximab) for at least 6 months before Pap smears were done was associated with 1.5-fold increased risk. All "higher risk" Pap smears were HPV positive, while only 50% of those were deemed to be the "lower risk" Pap smears. Neither of these studies observed cervical cancer due to the small sample size and potential differences in screening practices between IBD and non-IBD populations. Large case-control studies have shown lack of association between cervical dysplasia and IBD. Hutfless et al,[155] utilizing the Kaiser Permanente system, observed only a trend of elevated cervical cancer risk with the diagnosis of IBD and the use of an immunosuppressant, but the association was not statistically significant. The absolute increase in Pap smear testing was 4% among women with IBD. Lees et al[156] analyzed cervical smear records from more than 350 IBD patients from a single center and 1:4 healthy controls matched by age and geographical location. Women with IBD had no greater risk of cervical dysplasia or neoplasia than the background population except when they smoked. The use of immunosuppressive therapy had no impact on the incidence of abnormal Pap or cervical cancer. The findings of a population-based case-control study from Manitoba did not support a relationship between abnormal cervical pathology and IBD itself.[157] On the other hand, the combination of corticosteroids and immunosuppressants was associated with a 41% increase in absolute risk of abnormal cervical cytology profile. Women with CD but not with UC who were prescribed oral contraceptives on a regular basis also had a higher risk to develop cervical abnormalities. Lyles et al[158] suggested a potential relationship between the duration of AZA therapy and increased risk for cervical dysplasia and cervical cancer. The results of these studies are summarized in Table 11-7.

Table 11-7. Risk of Abnormal Cervical Cytology and Immunosuppression

INDEPENDENT RISK FACTOR	BHATIA ET AL[153] 2006 NYN = 116 ABNORMAL CERVICAL SMEAR	KANE ET AL[154] 2008 MAYO N = 40 ABNORMAL CERVICAL SMEAR	LEES ET AL[156] 2009 SCOTLAND N = 411 ABNORMAL CERVICAL SMEAR	LYLES ET AL[158] 2008 ALABAMA N = 51 ABNORMAL CERVICAL SMEAR	SINGH ET AL[157] 2009 CANADA N = 525 ABNORMAL CERVICAL SMEAR	HUTFLESS ET AL[155] 2008 CALIFORNIA N = 1165 CERVICAL CANCER
IBD alone	Yes 18% versus 5%	Yes 42% versus 7%	No	N/A	No	Only trend
AZA/6-MP	No	Yes 2.5-fold	No	No, but duration of therapy is	No	Yes 3.4-fold
AZA/6-MP plus corticosteroid	No	Yes	No	No	Yes	Yes
Infliximab	No	N/A	No	No	N/A	No

AZA = azathioprine; 6-MP = 6-mercaptopurine

Current guidelines by the American College of Obstetricians and Gynecologists recommend cervical cytologic screening every 2 years for women between the ages 21 and 29 and Pap smears every 3 years in women ages 30 years or older who have had three consecutive negative results. However, women who have HIV or are immunosuppressed require more frequent, at least yearly screening for cervical dysplasia.

Currently, there are no specific recommendations for the interval of cervical cytology screening in women with IBD. Many women with IBD are exposed a to immunosuppressants during their disease course and would benefit from yearly cervical evaluation. A recent cross-sectional study revealed that screening rates are far from optimal. Only 70% of women with IBD receive cervical testing at least once every 3 years in the United States.

Prevention and Treatment Options for Cervical Dysplasia

Currently, two prophylactic HPV vaccines primarily designed for cervical cancer prevention are available. Gardasil (Merck & Co, Inc, Whitehouse Station, NJ) is effective against HPV-16, -18 and -31, three common squamous cell cancer-causing types, associated with >70% of cervical cancers, as well as HPV-6 and -11, both causing genital warts and respiratory papillomatosis. Cervarix (GlaxoSmithKline, Rixensart, Belgium) is effective against HPV-16, -18, -31, -33 and -45, the 5 most common cancer-causing types. HPV vaccines are well tolerated, with serious vaccine-related events occurring in less than 0.1% of patients for both vaccines. The efficacy of Cervarix is proven for 6.4 years and of Gardasil for years. The US Centers for Disease Control and Prevention (CDC) recommends that they be given routinely to females ages 9 to 26, preferably prior to initiation of sexual activity. It is also recommended to those with a history of HPV or an abnormal Pap smear, even though existing data do not provide clear benefit on already developed lesions. Women with IBD, especially those on immunosuppressive therapy, regardless of sexual history, should be considered for HPV vaccination.

In addition to HPV vaccination, there are several nonmedical interventions one can implement to prevent cervical dysplasia and to facilitate treatment of abnormal cytology. Smoking is an established risk factor for cervical dysplasia and neoplasia; thus, smoking cessation should be highly encouraged. OCP use had been linked to increased risk of cervical abnormalities in the IBD population, thus replacement of OCPs with alternative birth control methods should be considered, particularly in women with existing cervical lesions, and alternative methods of birth control should be offered. Consultation on safe sexual practices and on avoidance of promiscuous sexual behavior can be helpful.

Although there is no clear evidence that IBD itself is an independent risk factor for abnormal Pap and cervical neoplasia, there is accumulating evidence that immunomodulator use, especially in combination with steroids, may predispose to development of cervical dysplasia. Data are scarce on anti-TNF agents in this matter, but to date no connection to increased risk of abnormal cervical cytology profile has been reported.

Women with IBD and prior or existing cervical dysplasia present the clinician with a challenging case scenario. Collaboration with the gynecologist is crucial. Lower risk abnormal Pap smears may only require repeat cytology testing, but colposcopy with or without cone biopsy and loop electrosurgical excision procedure may be necessary for higher risk cervical pathology. Since cervical lesions may regress when immunosuppression is withdrawn, changing the IBD therapy to a nonimmunosuppressive drug or even consideration of surgical resection in case of significant cervical pathology is warranted. Occasionally, the cervical dysplasia may dictate the IBD therapy.

☑ Key Points

☑ Overall fertility in IBD is comparable to that of the healthy population. Caveats include women who are status post ileoanal J pouch anastomosis reconstruction or women with disease-related alterations to menstrual cycles and ovulation.

☑ IBD can result in infants that are LBW or SGA, but there is no increased risk for congenital anomalies.

☑ The majority of medications used to treat IBD can be continued throughout pregnancy and should be so as to preserve maternal health.

☑ Breastfeeding should not be discouraged solely because of the presence of IBD. Most medications can be continued throughout the nursing period.

☑ Women with IBD on immunomodulators appear to be at greater risk for abnormal cervical cytology and should be screened appropriately.

REFERENCES

1. Moody GA, Mayberry JF. Perceived sexual dysfunction amongst patients with inflammatory bowel disease. *Digestion.* 1993;54(4):256-260.
2. Timmer A, Kemptner D, Bauer A, Takses A, Ott C, Furst A. Determinants of female sexual function in inflammatory bowel disease: a survey based cross-sectional analysis. *BMC Gastroenterol.* 2008;8:45.
3. Muller KR, Prosser R, Bampton P, Mountifield R, Andrews JM. Female gender and surgery impair relationships, body image, and sexuality in inflammatory bowel disease: patient perceptions. *Inflamm Bowel Dis.* 2010;16(4):657-663.
4. Tiainen J, Matikainen M, Hiltunen KM. Ileal J-pouch—anal anastomosis, sexual dysfunction, and fertility. *Scand J Gastroenterol.* 1999;34(2):185-188.
5. Ording Olsen K, Juul S, Berndtsson I, Oresland T, Laurberg S. Ulcerative colitis: female fecundity before diagnosis, during disease, and after surgery compared with a population sample. *Gastroenterology.* 2002;122(1):15-19.

6. Lepisto A, Sarna S, Tiitinen A, Jarvinen HJ. Female fertility and childbirth after ileal pouch-anal anastomosis for ulcerative colitis. *Br J Surg.* 2007;94(4):478-482.

7. Olsen KO, Juul S, Bulow S, et al. Female fecundity before and after operation for familial adenomatous polyposis. *Br J Surg.* 2003;90(2):227-231.

8. Oresland T, Palmblad S, Ellstrom M, Berndtsson I, Crona N, Hulten L. Gynaecological and sexual function related to anatomical changes in the female pelvis after restorative proctocolectomy. *Int J Colorectal Dis.* 1994;9(2):77-81.

9. Olsen KO, Joelsson M, Laurberg S, Oresland T. Fertility after ileal pouch-anal anastomosis in women with ulcerative colitis. *Br J Surg.* 1999;86(4):493-495.

10. Waljee A, Waljee J, Morris AM, Higgins PD. Threefold increased risk of infertility: a meta-analysis of infertility after ileal pouch anal anastomosis in ulcerative colitis. *Gut.* 2006;55(11):1575-1580.

11. Cornish JA, Tan E, Teare J, et al. The effect of restorative proctocolectomy on sexual function, urinary function, fertility, pregnancy and delivery: a systematic review. *Dis Colon Rectum.* 2007;50(8):1128-1138.

12. Mayberry JF, Weterman IT. European survey of fertility and pregnancy in women with Crohn's disease: a case control study by European collaborative group. *Gut.* 1986;27(7):821-825.

13. Riis L, Vind I, Politi P, et al. Does pregnancy change the disease course? A study in a European cohort of patients with inflammatory bowel disease. *Am J Gastroenterol.* 2006;101(7):1539-1545.

14. Arkuran C, McComb P. Crohn's disease and tubal infertility: the effect of adhesion formation. *Clin Exp Obstet Gynecol.* 2000;27(1):12-13.

15. Hudson M, Flett G, Sinclair TS, Brunt PW, Templeton A, Mowat NA. Fertility and pregnancy in inflammatory bowel disease. *Int J Gynaecol Obstet.* 1997;58(2):229-237.

16. Mountifield R, Bampton P, Prosser R, Muller K, Andrews JM. Fear and fertility in inflammatory bowel disease: a mismatch of perception and reality affects family planning decisions. *Inflamm Bowel Dis.* 2009;15(5):720-725.

17. Marri SR, Ahn C, Buchman AL. Voluntary childlessness is increased in women with inflammatory bowel disease. *Inflamm Bowel Dis.* 2007;13(5):591-599.

18. Janssen NM, Genta MS. The effects of immunosuppressive and anti-inflammatory medications on fertility, pregnancy, and lactation. *Arch Intern Med.* 2000;160(5):610-619.

19. Feagins LA, Kane SV. Sexual and reproductive issues for men with inflammatory bowel disease. *Am J Gastroenterol.* 2009;104(3):768-773.

20. Orholm M, Fonager K, Sorensen HT. Risk of ulcerative colitis and Crohn's disease among offspring of patients with chronic inflammatory bowel disease. *Am J Gastroenterol.* 1999;94(11):3236-3238.

21. Peeters M, Nevens H, Baert F, et al. Familial aggregation in Crohn's disease: increased age-adjusted risk and concordance in clinical characteristics. *Gastroenterology.* 1996;111(3):597-603.

22. Bennett RA, Rubin PH, Present DH. Frequency of inflammatory bowel disease in offspring of couples both presenting with inflammatory bowel disease. *Gastroenterology.* 1991;100(6):1638-1643.

23. Yang H, McElree C, Roth MP, Shanahan F, Targan SR, Rotter JI. Familial empirical risks for inflammatory bowel disease: differences between Jews and non-Jews. *Gut.* 1993;34(4):517-524.

24. Laharie D, Debeugny S, Peeters M, et al. Inflammatory bowel disease in spouses and their offspring. *Gastroenterology.* 2001;120(4):816-819.

25. Nielsen OH, Andreasson B, Bondesen S, Jarnum S. Pregnancy in ulcerative colitis. *Scand J Gastroenterol.* 1983;18(6):735-742.

26. Nielsen OH, Andreasson B, Bondesen S, Jacobsen O, Jarnum S. Pregnancy in Crohn's disease. *Scand J Gastroenterol.* 1984;19(6):724-732.

27. Mogadam M, Korelitz BI, Ahmed SW, Dobbins WO 3rd, Baiocco PJ. The course of inflammatory bowel disease during pregnancy and postpartum. *Am J Gastroenterol.* 1981;75(4):265-269.

28. Korelitz BI. Inflammatory bowel disease and pregnancy. *Gastroenterol Clin North Am.* 1998;27(1):213-224.

29. Agret F, Cosnes J, Hassani Z, et al. Impact of pregnancy on the clinical activity of Crohn's disease. *Aliment Pharmacol Ther.* 2005;21(5):509-513.

30. Moffatt DC, Ilnyckyj A, Bernstein CN. A population-based study of breastfeeding in inflammatory bowel disease: initiation, duration, and effect on disease in the postpartum period. *Am J Gastroenterol.* 2009;104(10):2517-2523.

31. Nwokolo CU, Tan WC, Andrews HA, Allan RN. Surgical resections in parous patients with distal ileal and colonic Crohn's disease. *Gut.* 1994;35(2):220-223.

32. Ravid A, Richard CS, Spencer LM, et al. Pregnancy, delivery, and pouch function after ileal pouch-anal anastomosis for ulcerative colitis. *Dis Colon Rectum.* 2002;45(10):1283-1288.

33. Juhasz ES, Fozard B, Dozois RR, Ilstrup DM, Nelson H. Ileal pouch-anal anastomosis function following childbirth. An extended evaluation. *Dis Colon Rectum.* 1995;38(2):159-165.

34. Ilnyckyji A, Blanchard JF, Rawsthorne P, Bernstein CN. Perianal Crohn's disease and pregnancy: role of the mode of delivery. *Am J Gastroenterol.* 1999;94(11):3274-3278.

35. Brandt LJ, Estabrook SG, Reinus JF. Results of a survey to evaluate whether vaginal delivery and episiotomy lead to perineal involvement in women with Crohn's disease. *Am J Gastroenterol.* 1995;90(11):1918-1922.

36. Rogers RG, Katz VL. Course of Crohn's disease during pregnancy and its effect on pregnancy outcome: a retrospective review. *Am J Perinatol.* 1995;12(4):262-264.

37. Beniada A, Benoist G, Maurel J, Dreyfus M. Inflammatory bowel disease and pregnancy: report of 76 cases and review of the literature. *J Gynecol Obstet Biol Reprod (Paris).* 2005;34(6):581-588.

38. Dubinsky M, Abraham B, Mahadevan U. Management of the pregnant IBD patient. *Inflamm Bowel Dis.* 2008;14(12):1736-1750.

39. Remzi FH, Gorgun E, Bast J, et al. Vaginal delivery after ileal pouch-anal anastomosis: a word of caution. *Dis Colon Rectum.* 2005;48(9):1691-1699.

40. Heetun ZS, Byrnes C, Neary P, O'Morain C. Review article: reproduction in the patient with inflammatory bowel disease. *Aliment Pharmacol Ther.* 2007;26(4):513-533.

41. Castiglione F, Pignata S, Morace F, et al. Effect of pregnancy on the clinical course of a cohort of women with inflammatory bowel disease. *Ital J Gastroenterol.* 1996;28(4):199-204.

42. Kane S, Kisiel J, Shih L, Hanauer S. HLA disparity determines disease activity through pregnancy in women with inflammatory bowel disease. *Am J Gastroenterol.* 2004;99(8):1523-1526.

43. Russell AS, Johnston C, Chew C, Maksymowych WP. Evidence for reduced Th1 function in normal pregnancy: a hypothesis for the remission of rheumatoid arthritis. *J Rheumatol.* 1997;24(6):1045-1050.

44. Rajagopalan S, Long EO. A human histocompatibility leukocyte antigen (HLA)-G-specific receptor expressed on all natural killer cells. *J Exp Med.* 1999;189(7):1093-1100.

45. Kane S, Lemieux N. The role of breastfeeding in postpartum disease activity in women with inflammatory bowel disease. *Am J Gastroenterol.* 2005;100(1):102-105.

46. Bergstrand O, Hellers G. Breastfeeding during infancy in patients who later develop Crohn's disease. *Scand J Gastroenterol.* 1983;18(7):903-906.

47. Whorwell PJ, Holdstock G, Whorwell GM, Wright R. Bottle feeding, early gastroenteritis, and inflammatory bowel disease. *Br Med J.* 1979;1(6160):382.

48. Kornfeld D, Cnattingius S, Ekbom A. Pregnancy outcomes in women with inflammatory bowel disease—a population-based cohort study. *Am J Obstet Gynecol.* 1997;177(4):942-946.

49. Kastrinos F. Maybe a baby? Revisiting the effect of IBD on conception, pregnancy, and newborn outcomes. *Inflamm Bowel Dis.* 2009;15(3):475-477.

50. Mahadevan U. Pregnancy and inflammatory bowel disease. *Med Clin North Am.* 2010;94(1):53-73.

51. Cornish J, Tan E, Teare J, et al. A meta-analysis on the influence of inflammatory bowel disease on pregnancy. *Gut.* 2007;56(6):830-837.

52. Bengtson MB, Solberg IC, Aamodt G, Jahnsen J, Moum B, Vatn MH. Relationships between inflammatory bowel disease and perinatal factors: both maternal and paternal disease are related to preterm birth of offspring. *Inflamm Bowel Dis.* 2010;16(5):847-855.

53. Norgard B, Hundborg HH, Jacobsen BA, Nielsen GL, Fonager K. Disease activity in pregnant women with Crohn's disease and birth outcomes: a regional Danish cohort study. *Am J Gastroenterol.* 2007;102(9):1947-1954.

54. Khosla R, Willoughby CP, Jewell DP. Crohn's disease and pregnancy. *Gut*. 1984;25(1):52-56.

55. Baiocco PJ, Korelitz BI. The influence of inflammatory bowel disease and its treatment on pregnancy and fetal outcome. *J Clin Gastroenterol*. 1984;6(3):211-216.

56. Bush MC, Patel S, Lapinski RH, Stone JL. Perinatal outcomes in inflammatory bowel disease. *J Matern Fetal Neonatal Med*. 2004;15(4):237-241.

57. Fedorkow DM, Persaud D, Nimrod CA. Inflammatory bowel disease: a controlled study of late pregnancy outcome. *Am J Obstet Gynecol*. 1989;160(4):998-1001.

58. Mahadevan U, Sandborn WJ, Li DK, Hakimian S, Kane S, Corley DA. Pregnancy outcomes in women with inflammatory bowel disease: a large community-based study from Northern California. *Gastroenterology*. 2007;133(4):1106-1112.

59. Stephansson O, Larsson H, Pedersen L, et al. Congenital abnormalities and other birth outcomes in children born to women with ulcerative colitis in Denmark and Sweden. *Inflamm Bowel Dis*. 2011;17(3):795-801.

60. Norgard B, Fonager K, Sorensen HT, Olsen J. Birth outcomes of women with ulcerative colitis: a nationwide Danish cohort study. *Am J Gastroenterol*. 2000;95(11):3165-3170.

61. Dominitz JA, Young JC, Boyko EJ. Outcomes of infants born to mothers with inflammatory bowel disease: a population-based cohort study. *Am J Gastroenterol*. 2002;97(3):641-648.

62. Stephansson O, Larsson H, Pedersen L, et al. Crohn's disease is a risk factor for preterm birth. *Clin Gastroenterol Hepatol*. 2010;8(6):509-515.

63. Alstead EM. Inflammatory bowel disease in pregnancy. *Postgrad Med J*. 2002;78(915):23-26.

64. Kilpatrick CC, Monga M. Approach to the acute abdomen in pregnancy. *Obstet Gynecol Clin North Am*. 2007;34(3):389-402, x.

65. Darbari A, Sena L, Argani P, Oliva-Hemker JM, Thompson R, Cuffari C. Gadolinium-enhanced magnetic resonance imaging: a useful radiological tool in diagnosing pediatric IBD. *Inflamm Bowel Dis*. 2004;10(2):67-72.

66. Bland BA, Lawes EG, Duncan PW, Warnell I, Downing JW. Comparison of midazolam and thiopental for rapid sequence anesthetic induction for elective C-section. *Anesth Analg*. 1987;66(11):1165-1168.

67. Crawford ME, Carl P, Bach V, Ravlo O, Mikkelsen BO, Werner M. A randomized comparison between midazolam and thiopental for elective C-section anesthesia. I. Mothers. *Anesth Analg*. 1989;68(3):229-233.

68. Wilson CM, Dundee JW, Moore J, Howard PJ, Collier PS. A comparison of the early pharmacokinetics of midazolam in pregnant and nonpregnant women. *Anaesthesia*. 1987;42(10):1057-1062.

69. Jarnerot G, Into-Malmberg MB, Esbjorner E. Placental transfer of sulphasalazine and sulphapyridine and some of its metabolites. *Scand J Gastroenterol*. 1981;16(5):693-697.

70. Christensen LA, Rasmussen SN, Hansen SH. Disposition of 5-aminosalicylic acid and N-acetyl-5-aminosalicylic acid in fetal and maternal body fluids during treatment with different 5-aminosalicylic acid preparations. *Acta Obstet Gynecol Scand*. 1994;73(5):399-402.

71. Norgard B, Czeizel AE, Rockenbauer M, Olsen J, Sorensen HT. Population-based case control study of the safety of sulfasalazine use during pregnancy. *Aliment Pharmacol Ther*. 2001;15(4):483-486.

72. Moskovitz DN, Bodian C, Chapman ML, et al. The effect on the fetus of medications used to treat pregnant inflammatory bowel-disease patients. *Am J Gastroenterol*. 2004;99(4):656-661.

73. Mogadam M, Dobbins WO 3rd, Korelitz BI, Ahmed SW. Pregnancy in inflammatory bowel disease: effect of sulfasalazine and corticosteroids on fetal outcome. *Gastroenterology*. 1981;80(1):72-76.

74. Mahadevan U, Kane S. American gastroenterological association institute technical review on the use of gastrointestinal medications in pregnancy. *Gastroenterology*. 2006;131(1):283-311.

75. Habal FM, Hui G, Greenberg GR. Oral 5-aminosalicylic acid for inflammatory bowel disease in pregnancy: safety and clinical course. *Gastroenterology*. 1993;105(4):1057-1060.

76. Trallori G, d'Albasio G, Bardazzi G, et al. 5-aminosalicylic acid in pregnancy: clinical report. *Ital J Gastroenterol.* 1994;26(2):75-78.

77. Marteau P, Tennenbaum R, Elefant E, Lemann M, Cosnes J. Foetal outcome in women with inflammatory bowel disease treated during pregnancy with oral mesalazine microgranules. *Aliment Pharmacol Ther.* 1998;12(11):1101-1108.

78. Bell CM, Habal FM. Safety of topical 5-aminosalicylic acid in pregnancy. *Am J Gastroenterol.* 1997;92(12):2201-2202.

79. Diav-Citrin O, Park YH, Veerasuntharam G, et al. The safety of mesalamine in human pregnancy: a prospective controlled cohort study. *Gastroenterology.* 1998;114(1):23-28.

80. Sorensen HT, Pedersen L, Norgard B, Fonager K, Rothman KJ. Does month of birth affect risk of Crohn's disease in childhood and adolescence? *BMJ.* 2001;323(7318):907.

81. Colombel JF, Brabant G, Gubler MC, et al. Renal insufficiency in infant: side-effect of prenatal exposure to mesalazine? *Lancet.* 1994;344(8922):620-621.

82. Silverman DA, Ford J, Shaw I, Probert CS. Is mesalazine really safe for use in breastfeeding mothers? *Gut.* 2005;54(1):170-171.

83. Jenss H, Weber P, Hartmann F. 5-Aminosalicylic acid and its metabolite in breast milk during lactation. *Am J Gastroenterol.* 1990;85(3):331.

84. Branski D, Kerem E, Gross-Kieselstein E, Hurvitz H, Litt R, Abrahamov A. Bloody diarrhea—a possible complication of sulfasalazine transferred through human breast milk. *J Pediatr Gastroenterol Nutr.* 1986;5(2):316-317.

85. Nelis GF. Diarrhoea due to 5-aminosalicylic acid in breast milk. *Lancet.* 1989;1(8634):383.

86. Carmichael SL, Shaw GM, Ma C, Werler MM, Rasmussen SA, Lammer EJ. Maternal corticosteroid use and orofacial clefts. *Am J Obstet Gynecol.* 2007;197(6):585 e581-e587; discussion 683-584, e581-e587.

87. Rodriguez-Pinilla E, Martinez-Frias ML. Corticosteroids during pregnancy and oral clefts: a case-control study. *Teratology.* 1998;58(1):2-5.

88. Park-Wyllie L, Mazzotta P, Pastuszak A, et al. Birth defects after maternal exposure to corticosteroids: prospective cohort study and meta-analysis of epidemiological studies. *Teratology.* 2000;62(6):385-392.

89. Gur C, Diav-Citrin O, Shechtman S, Arnon J, Ornoy A. Pregnancy outcome after first trimester exposure to corticosteroids: a prospective controlled study. *Reprod Toxicol.* 2004; 18(1):93-101.

90. Blanford AT, Murphy BE. In vitro metabolism of prednisolone, dexamethasone, betamethasone, and cortisol by the human placenta. *Am J Obstet Gynecol.* 1977;127(3): 264-267.

91. Dancis J, Jansen V, Levitz M. Placental transfer of steroids: effect of binding to serum albumin and to placenta. *Am J Physiol.* 1980;238(3):E208-E213.

92. McKay DB, Josephson MA. Pregnancy in recipients of solid organs—effects on mother and child. *N Engl J Med.* 2006;354(12):1281-1293.

93. Beaulieu DB, Ananthakrishnan AN, Issa M, et al. Budesonide induction and maintenance therapy for Crohn's disease during pregnancy. *Inflamm Bowel Dis.* 2009;15(1):25-28.

94. Christensson C, Thoren A, Lindberg B. Safety of inhaled budesonide: clinical manifestations of systemic corticosteroid-related adverse effects. *Drug Saf.* 2008;31(11):965-988.

95. Ost L, Wettrell G, Bjorkhem I, Rane A. Prednisolone excretion in human milk. *J Pediatr.* 1985;106(6):1008-1011.

96. Falt A, Bengtsson T, Kennedy BM, et al. Exposure of infants to budesonide through breast milk of asthmatic mothers. *J Allergy Clin Immunol.* 2007;120(4):798-802.

97. Diav-Citrin O, Shechtman S, Gotteiner T, Arnon J, Ornoy A. Pregnancy outcome after gestational exposure to metronidazole: a prospective controlled cohort study. *Teratology.* 2001;63(5):186-192.

98. Piper JM, Mitchel EF, Ray WA. Prenatal use of metronidazole and birth defects: no association. *Obstet Gynecol.* 1993;82(3):348-352.

99. Sorensen HT, Larsen H, Jensen ES, et al. Safety of metronidazole during pregnancy: a cohort study of risk of congenital abnormalities, preterm delivery and low birth weight in 124 women. *J Antimicrob Chemother.* 1999;44(6):854-856.

100. Burtin P, Taddio A, Ariburnu O, Einarson TR, Koren G. Safety of metronidazole in pregnancy: a meta-analysis. *Am J Obstet Gynecol.* 1995;172(2 pt 1):525-529.

101. Caro-Paton T, Carvajal A, Martin de Diego I, Martin-Arias LH, Alvarez Requejo A, Rodriguez Pinilla E. Is metronidazole teratogenic? A meta-analysis. *Br J Clin Pharmacol.* 1997;44(2):179-182.

102. Heisterberg L, Branebjerg PE. Blood and milk concentrations of metronidazole in mothers and infants. *J Perinat Med.* 1983;11(2):114-120.

103. Linseman DA, Hampton LA, Branstetter DG. Quinolone-induced arthropathy in the neonatal mouse. Morphological analysis of articular lesions produced by pipemidic acid and ciprofloxacin. *Fundam Appl Toxicol.* 1995;28(1):59-64.

104. Loebstein R, Addis A, Ho E, et al. Pregnancy outcome following gestational exposure to fluoroquinolones: a multicenter prospective controlled study. *Antimicrob Agents Chemother.* 1998;42(6):1336-1339.

105. Larsen H, Nielsen GL, Schonheyder HC, Olesen C, Sorensen HT. Birth outcome following maternal use of fluoroquinolones. *Int J Antimicrob Agents.* 2001;18(3):259-262.

106. Transfer of drugs and other chemicals into human milk. *Pediatrics.* 2001;108(3):776-789.

107. Einarson A, Mastroiacovo P, Arnon J, et al. Prospective, controlled, multicentre study of loperamide in pregnancy. *Can J Gastroenterol.* 2000;14(3):185-187.

108. Kallen B, Nilsson E, Otterblad Olausson P. Maternal use of loperamide in early pregnancy and delivery outcome. *Acta Paediatr.* 2008;97(5):541-545.

109. Collins E. Maternal and fetal effects of acetaminophen and salicylates in pregnancy. *Obstet Gynecol.* 1981;58(5 suppl):57S-62S.

110. Ferrero S, Ragni N. Inflammatory bowel disease: management issues during pregnancy. *Arch Gynecol Obstet.* 2004;270(2):79-85.

111. Polifka JE, Friedman JM. Teratogen update: azathioprine and 6-mercaptopurine. *Teratology.* 2002;65(5):240-261.

112. de Boer NK, Jarbandhan SV, de Graaf P, Mulder CJ, van Elburg RM, van Bodegraven AA. Azathioprine use during pregnancy: unexpected intrauterine exposure to metabolites. *Am J Gastroenterol.* 2006;101(6):1390-1392.

113. Williamson RA, Karp LE. Azathioprine teratogenicity: review of the literature and case report. *Obstet Gynecol.* 1981;58(2):247-250.

114. Davison JM, Dellagrammatikas H, Parkin JM. Maternal azathioprine therapy and depressed haemopoiesis in the babies of renal allograft patients. *Br J Obstet Gynaecol.* 1985;92(3):233-239.

115. Cederqvist LL, Merkatz IR, Litwin SD. Fetal immunoglobulin synthesis following maternal immunosuppression. *Am J Obstet Gynecol.* 1977;129(6):687-690.

116. Norgard B, Pedersen L, Fonager K, Rasmussen SN, Sorensen HT. Azathioprine, mercaptopurine and birth outcome: a population-based cohort study. *Aliment Pharmacol Ther.* 2003;17(6):827-834.

117. Norgard B, Pedersen L, Christensen LA, Sorensen HT. Therapeutic drug use in women with Crohn's disease and birth outcomes: a Danish nationwide cohort study. *Am J Gastroenterol.* 2007;102(7):1406-1413.

118. Francella A, Dyan A, Bodian C, Rubin P, Chapman M, Present DH. The safety of 6-mercaptopurine for childbearing patients with inflammatory bowel disease: a retrospective cohort study. *Gastroenterology.* 2003;124(1):9-17.

119. Goldstein LH, Dolinsky G, Greenberg R, et al. Pregnancy outcome of women exposed to azathioprine during pregnancy. *Birth Defects Res A Clin Mol Teratol.* 2007;79(10):696-701.

120. Moretti ME, Verjee Z, Ito S, Koren G. Breastfeeding during maternal use of azathioprine. *Ann Pharmacother.* 2006;40(12):2269-2272.

121. Gardiner SJ, Gearry RB, Roberts RL, Zhang M, Barclay ML, Begg EJ. Exposure to thiopurine drugs through breast milk is low based on metabolite concentrations in mother-infant pairs. *Br J Clin Pharmacol.* 2006;62(4):453-456.

122. Sau A, Clarke S, Bass J, Kaiser A, Marinaki A, Nelson-Piercy C. Azathioprine and breastfeeding. is it safe? *Br J Obstet Gynaecol.* 2007;114(4):498-501.

123. Christensen LA, Dahlerup JF, Nielsen MJ, Fallingborg JF, Schmiegelow K. Azathioprine treatment during lactation. *Aliment Pharmacol Ther.* 2008;28(10):1209-1213.

124. Bar Oz B, Hackman R, Einarson T, Koren G. Pregnancy outcome after cyclosporine therapy during pregnancy: a meta-analysis. *Transplantation.* 2001;71(8):1051-1055.

125. Gisbert JP. Safety of immunomodulators and biologics for the treatment of inflammatory bowel disease during pregnancy and breastfeeding. *Inflamm Bowel Dis.* 2010;16(5):881-895.

126. Kainz A, Harabacz I, Cowlrick IS, Gadgil SD, Hagiwara D. Review of the course and outcome of 100 pregnancies in 84 women treated with tacrolimus. *Transplantation.* 2000;70(12):1718-1721.

127. Baumgart DC, Sturm A, Wiedenmann B, Dignass AU. Uneventful pregnancy and neonatal outcome with tacrolimus in refractory ulcerative colitis. *Gut.* 2005;54(12):1822-1823.

128. Srinivasan R. Infliximab treatment and pregnancy outcome in active Crohn's disease. *Am J Gastroenterol.* 2001;96(7):2274-2275.

129. Mahadevan U, Kane S, Sandborn WJ, et al. Intentional infliximab use during pregnancy for induction or maintenance of remission in Crohn's disease. *Aliment Pharmacol Ther.* 2005;21(6):733-738.

130. Carter JD, Ladhani A, Ricca LR, Valeriano J, Vasey FB. A safety assessment of tumor necrosis factor antagonists during pregnancy: a review of the Food and Drug Administration database. *J Rheumatol.* 2009;36(3):635-641.

131. Vasiliauskas EA, Church JA, Silverman N, Barry M, Targan SR, Dubinsky MC. Case report: evidence for transplacental transfer of maternally administered infliximab to the newborn. *Clin Gastroenterol Hepatol.* 2006;4(10):1255-1258.

132. Kane S, Ford J, Cohen R, Wagner C. Absence of infliximab in infants and breast milk from nursing mothers receiving therapy for Crohn's disease before and after delivery. *J Clin Gastroenterol.* 2009;43(7):613-616.

133. Coburn LA, Wise PE, Schwartz DA. The successful use of adalimumab to treat active Crohn's disease of an ileoanal pouch during pregnancy. *Dig Dis Sci.* 2006;51(11):2045-2047.

134. Vesga L, Terdiman JP, Mahadevan U. Adalimumab use in pregnancy. *Gut.* 2005;54(6):890.

135. Mishkin DS, Van Deinse W, Becker JM, Farraye FA. Successful use of adalimumab (Humira) for Crohn's disease in pregnancy. *Inflamm Bowel Dis.* 2006;12(8):827-828.

136. Oussalah A, Bigard MA, Peyrin-Biroulet L. Certolizumab use in pregnancy. *Gut.* 2009;58(4):608.

137. Nesbitt A, Stephens S, Foulkes R. Placental transfer and accumulation in milk of the anti-TNF antibody TN3 in rats: immunoglobulin G1 versus PEGylated Fab'. *Am J Gastroenterol.* 2006;101:1119.

138. Mahadevan U, Abreu M. Certolizumab use in pregnancy: low levels detected in cord blood. *Gastroenterology.* 2009;136(5):960.

139. Wehner NG, Skov M, Shopp G, Rocca MS, Clarke J. Effects of natalizumab, an alpha4 integrin inhibitor, on fertility in male and female guinea pigs. *Birth Defects Res B Dev Reprod Toxicol.* 2009;86(2):108-116.

140. Wehner NG, Shopp G, Oneda S, Clarke J. Embryo/fetal development in cynomolgus monkeys exposed to natalizumab, an alpha4 integrin inhibitor. *Birth Defects Res B Dev Reprod Toxicol.* 2009;86(2):117-130.

141. Mahadevan U, Nazareth M, Christiano L. Natalizumab use during pregancy. *Am J Gastroenterol.* 2008;103(4 suppl 1):A1150.

142. Kane SV, Acquah LA. Placental transport of immunoglobulins: a clinical review for gastroenterologists who prescribe therapeutic monoclonal antibodies to women during conception and pregnancy. *Am J Gastroenterol.* 2009;104(1):228-233.

143. Mahadevan U, Martin CF, Sandler RS, Kane SV. A Multi-Center National Prospective Study of pregnancy and neonatal outcomes in women with inflammatory bowel disease exposed to immunomodulators and biologic therapy. *Gastroenterology.* 2009;136(5 suppl 1):A88.

144. Mahadevan U, Martin CF, Sandler RS, et al. One year newborn outcomes among offspring of women with inflammatory bowel disease: The PIANO Registry. *Gastroenterology.* 2010;138(5 suppl 1):S106.

145. Mahadevan U, Kane SV, Church JA. The effect of maternal peripartum infliximab use on neonatal immune response. *Gastroenterology.* 2009;136(5 suppl 1):A69.

146. Chohan L, Kilpatrick CC. Laparoscopy in pregnancy: a literature review. *Clin Obstet Gynecol.* 2009;52(4):557-569.

147. Dozois EJ, Wolff BG, Tremaine WJ, et al. Maternal and fetal outcome after colectomy for fulminant ulcerative colitis during pregnancy: case series and literature review. *Dis Colon Rectum.* 2006;49(1):64-73.

148. Ooi BS, Remzi FH, Fazio VW. Turnbull-Blowhole colostomy for toxic ulcerative colitis in pregnancy: report of two cases. *Dis Colon Rectum.* 2003;46(1):111-115.

149. Haq AI, Sahai A, Hallwoth S, Rampton DS, Dorudi S. Synchronous colectomy and caesarean section for fulminant ulcerative colitis: case report and review of the literature. *Int J Colorectal Dis.* Jul 2006;21(5):465-469.

150. Hill J, Clark A, Scott NA. Surgical treatment of acute manifestations of Crohn's disease during pregnancy. *J R Soc Med.* 1997;90(2):64-66.

151. Bateman H, Yazici Y, Leff L, Peterson M, Paget SA. Increased cervical dysplasia in intravenous cyclophosphamide-treated patients with SLE: a preliminary study. *Lupus.* 2000;9(7):542-544.

152. Bernatsky S, Ramsey-Goldman R, Gordon C, et al. Factors associated with abnormal Pap results in systemic lupus erythematosus. *Rheumatology (Oxford).* 2004;43(11):1386-1389.

153. Bhatia J, Bratcher J, Korelitz B, et al. Abnormalities of uterine cervix in women with inflammatory bowel disease. *World J Gastroenterol.* 2006;12(38):6167-6171.

154. Kane S, Khatibi B, Reddy D. Higher incidence of abnormal Pap smears in women with inflammatory bowel disease. *Am J Gastroenterol.* 2008;103(3):631-636.

155. Hutfless S, Fireman B, Kane S, Herrinton LJ. Screening differences and risk of cervical cancer in inflammatory bowel disease. *Aliment Pharmacol Ther.* 2008;28(5):598-605.

156. Lees CW, Critchley J, Chee N, et al. Lack of association between cervical dysplasia and IBD: a large case-control study. *Inflamm Bowel Dis.* 2009;15(11):1621-1629.

157. Singh H, Demers AA, Nugent Z, Mahmud SM, Kliewer EV, Bernstein CN. Risk of cervical abnormalities in women with inflammatory bowel disease: a population-based nested case-control study. *Gastroenterology.* 2009;136(2):451-458.

158. Lyles TE, Oster RA, Gutierrez A. Prevalance of abnormal PAP smears in patients with inflammatory bowel disease on immune modulator therapy. *Gastrotenterology.* 2008;134 (4 suppl 1):A143.

Suggested Readings

Cornish J, Tan E, Teare J, et al. A meta-analysis on the influence of inflammatory bowel disease on pregnancy. *Gut.* 2007;56(6):830-837.

Dubinsky M, Abraham B, Mahadevan U. Management of the pregnant IBD patient. *Inflamm Bowel Dis.* 2008;14(12):1736-1750.

Heetun ZS, Byrnes C, Neary P, O'Morain C. Review article: reproduction in the patient with inflammatory bowel disease. *Aliment Pharmacol Ther.* 2007;26(4):513-533.

Mahadevan U. Pregnancy and inflammatory bowel disease. *Med Clin North Am.* 2010;94(1): 53-73.

Mahadevan U, Kane S. American gastroenterological association institute technical review on the use of gastrointestinal medications in pregnancy. *Gastroenterology.* 2006;131(1):283-311.

Nutritional Complications of IBD

*Sulieman Abdal Raheem MD; Omer J. Deen MD; and
Donald F. Kirby MD, FACP, FACN, FACG, AGAF, CNSC, CPNS*

Nutrition is an important part of daily life. However, for many patients with inflammatory bowel disease (IBD) eating can be a particular challenge because the associated disease affects the gastrointestinal tract. This may lead to a variety of nutritional problems that influence the intake, absorption, and utilization of both macro- and micronutrients. Furthermore, the resulting nutritional deficiencies may alter normal development and growth, significantly decreasing the patient's quality of life. This chapter will cover the nutritional aspects of what clinicians need to know and should consider when caring for patients with IBD.

EPIDEMIOLOGY

Patients with IBD are at risk for a variety of nutritional deficiencies, particularly micronutrients. These deficiencies are more common among patients with Crohn's disease (CD) because of small bowel involvement. For example, 9.5% of pediatric CD patients present with growth retardation at diagnosis and 32% are severely malnourished.[1] The resulting growth failure from undernutrition is significant; 40% to 50% of CD children suffer from temporary growth failure and another 10% to 20% from prolonged failure.[2] In adults, this undernutrition leads to a 65% to 75% body mass loss in CD patients and a corresponding 18% to 62% loss in ulcerative colitis (UC) patients.[3,4]

Regueiro MD, Swoger JM, eds.
Clinical Challenges and Complications of IBD (pp 231-240).
© 2013 Taylor & Francis Group.

Table 12-1. Factors Affecting Nutritional Status in IBD Patients

MECHANISM	CAUSE	EFFECT
Decreased enteral intake	• Nausea and vomiting • Abdominal pain • Diarrhea • Mucosal aphthous ulcers • Loss of appetite and taste changes • Restricted diets • Small bowel strictures	• Fear of eating • Decreased caloric intake • Abdominal pain
Decreased absorptive surface	• Active disease • Bowel resection • Fistula	• Maldigestion • Malabsorption
Intestinal loss of nutrients	• Protein wasting enteropathy • Diarrhea • Acute and chronic blood loss • Steatorrhea • Bacterial overgrowth	• Protein deficiency • Anemia • Electrolyte loss • Vitamins A, D, E, K and divalent cation loss
Hypermetabolism	• Resting energy expenditure changes	• Increased caloric needs
Medications	• Drug-nutrients interaction • Side effects	• Loss of appetite • Malabsorption

PATHOPHYSIOLOGY

The pathophysiology of the nutritional deficiencies associated with IBD is multifactorial (Table 12-1) and may include any or a combination of the following:

◊   Decreased food intake
◊   Decreased intestinal absorptive surface
◊   Intestinal loss of nutrients
◊   Hypermetabolism (i.e., increased energy requirements)
◊   Medication-nutrient interactions

A fear of eating and decreased appetite leading to reduced food intake are often seen in IBD patients. Patients may suffer from painful oral lesions, severe abdominal pain, or painful diarrhea that can all lead to a negative association with eating and, therefore, reduce oral intake. Reduced intake of food may also be a result of the altered taste and loss of appetite resulting from the release of inflammatory markers, such as tumor necrosis factor (TNF), interleukin-1 (IL1), and interleukin-6 (IL6).[5-7] Furthermore, rat models have demonstrated that colitis may result in increased serotonin levels inducing anorexia, an additional source of reduced food intake in IBD patients.[8]

Many nutritional deficiencies may result from a decrease in absorptive surface as portions of the intestine are lost to either active disease or surgical resection. Proper identification of the extent of any active disease, either endoscopically or radiologically, along with surgical records delineating any prior loss of intestinal length, may elucidate which specific nutrient deficiencies a patient is vulnerable to. For example, loss of the last 100 cm of the terminal ileum, whether due to active disease or surgical resection, may lead to a deficiency of bile acids and fat malabsorption, resulting in steatorrhea. Additionally, since vitamin B_{12} has special receptors in the terminal ileum, its loss can result in vitamin B_{12} deficiency. IBD patients may also suffer from dramatic protein losses due to inflamed ulcerated sections of the intestinal mucosa.[9] Profuse chronic diarrhea, intestinal bleeding, and an intestinal microflora imbalance may also contribute to significant intestinal nutrient losses.

Energy metabolism is altered in IBD, increasing caloric needs.[10] If these increased caloric requirements go unmet, further nutrient deficiencies and weight loss can result. Histological and laboratory analysis of 24 children with CD, 19 malnourished females with anorexia nervosa, and 22 healthy subjects elucidated a possible mechanism for the increased resting energy expenditure seen in IBD.[11] The IBD patients suffered significant losses in lean body mass. Thus, at a cellular level there was a considerable decrease in intracellular water relative to extracellular water. In healthy individuals, resting energy expenditure is directly correlated to body cell mass measured by intracellular water. However, in CD there is a failure to downregulate the resting energy expenditure in response to weight loss. The cytokines previously mentioned (TNF, IL1, and IL6) may play a role in this failure, propagating nutrient and weight loss.

There are also medication-nutrient interactions that may lead to nutrient deficiency and/or weight loss. For example, sulfasalazine inhibits folate absorption, as its sulfa moiety binds to folate and methotrexate inhibits folic acid activation.[12] Both of these interactions leads to folic acid deficiency and anemia. Awareness of these drug interactions indicates a potential need for folate supplementation to reduce dysplasia and colorectal cancer risk. Additionally, medications such as metronidazole can cause taste alterations that may decrease patients' oral intake as well. Other medications, such as infliximab, can adversely affect protein metabolism, while systemic steroids can alter protein and mineral metabolism.[13,14]

Clinical Features

The clinical features of nutrient deficiencies vary depending on the specific nutrient in deficit (Table 12-2).[15-18] As previously mentioned, undernutrition in IBD leads to significant weight loss and in children, growth retardation or failure. Specific micronutrient deficiencies may be observed in the following:

◊ Water-soluble vitamins
◊ Fat-soluble vitamins
◊ Antioxidant vitamins
◊ Minerals and trace elements

Table 12-2. Nutritional Deficiencies Reported in Adults With IBD

NUTRIENT DEFICIENCY	PERCENT (%)
Vitamin B_{12}	18.4 to 60[15-16]
Vitamin B_6	29[16]
Folic acid	19 to 54[15-16]
Vitamin A	11 to 26[15]
Vitamin D	17.6 to 75[15-16]
Vitamin C	84[17]
Vitamin E	16[18]
Iron	39.2 to 81[15-16]
Magnesium	14 to 33[15]
Potassium	6 to 20[15]
Copper	84[17]
Selenium	82[17]
Zinc	15.2 to 65[16,17]
Calcium	13 to 23[15]
Carotene	23.4[16]

Common water-soluble vitamin deficiencies include folic acid, vitamins B_6, B_{12}, and/or niacin. Deficiencies in the first 3 vitamins can lead to anemia, while a deficiency in the latter leads to pellagra that can be characterized by dermatitis, worsening diarrhea, dementia, and in severe cases, death. Both sulfasalazine and methotrexate, common medications utilized to treat IBD, interfere with folic acid absorption and activation, leading to a deficit. For this reason, folic acid should be supplemented when these medications are used. A disease distribution that includes the proximal small bowel where folic acid is primarily absorbed may also lead to folic acid deficiency, and thus anemia. Niacin deficiency is generally rare in IBD; however, it has been reported to be present in as high as 77% of CD patients in remission.[17]

Fat-soluble vitamin deficiencies may occur as a result of terminal ileal disease/resection, poor intake, and/or cholestyramine use. Any of these contributing factors can lead to bile acid deficiency and, therefore, fat malabsorption, potentially worsening deficits in vitamins A, D, E, and/or K. In patients with CD, plasma retinol levels may drop below 0.8 mmol/L in vitamin A deficiency, resulting in night blindness.[19] Also, in a study of 82 CD patients, 65% demonstrated a low serum 25-hydroxyvitamin D concentration and 25% demonstrated levels below 10 ng/ml.[20] Such vitamin D deficiencies put patients at high risk for metabolic bone disease.

In a study of 37 nonsmoking CD patients, plasma antioxidant vitamins such as ascorbic acid, carotene, lycopene, and cryptoxanthin were significantly lower than in their non CD counterparts.[21] The increased production of reactive oxygen species from activated neutrophils in CD may reduce plasma concentrations of antioxidant vitamins, resulting in increased oxidative stress.

In IBD, mineral deficiencies are common, including iron, zinc, calcium, phosphate, selenium, copper, and magnesium. Iron deficiency may result from vitamin B_{12} or folic acid deficiencies, drug interaction (i.e. sulfasalazine), or bleeding. In fact, 35% to 90% of adults with IBD exhibit iron deficiency, making it the primary cause of anemia in this population.[22] Proper management with iron supplementation is necessary. A fixed dose of IV ferric carboxymaltose regimen resolves iron deficiency more effectively than IV Iron Sucrose that, in turn, is more effective than oral iron supplementation.[23,24] Ostomies, fistulae, and profuse diarrhea in patients with IBD may also lead to increased loss of zinc that can result in dry scaly eczematous plaques in the facial and anogenital regions. Oral or parenteral zinc supplementation is necessary in these patients. It is also important to include zinc replacement for patients on long term parenteral nutrition to avoid deficiency. Bone disease due to calcium deficiency is seen in 13% of patients with CD.[25] For this reason, vitamin D and calcium intake should be reviewed and supplemented as required.

In patients with IBD, chronic diarrhea leading to the malabsorption of phosphate and/or refeeding syndrome may lead to a deficit in phosphate.[26] In patients with CD who have had small bowel resection or significant stool losses, selenium deficiency may be present and can potentially lead to erythrocyte macrocytosis, muscle dysfunction, cardiomyopathy, and/or encephalitis.[27,28] IBD patients with decreased oral intake, malabsorption, and/or increased intestinal losses of magnesium may suffer from neuromuscular symptoms or osteopenia. Although the least common mineral deficiency, copper deficiency in IBD may also result from increased intestinal losses, diarrhea, and/or prolonged zinc supplementation. Deficiency of copper can manifest as both neuromuscular as well as hematologic symptoms.[29] Furthermore, copper deficiency leads to a microcytic hypochromic anemia, as is seen with iron deficiency anemia. If copper deficiency is not recognized, these patients can be mistakenly treated with excess iron that competes with copper for absorption, leading to worsening copper deficiency.[30]

In general, prolonged parenteral nutrition without adequate vitamin/mineral replacement may result in grave nutrient deficiencies. Regardless of the etiology of the nutrient deficiencies present in the treatment of IBD, care should be taken to carefully assess nutritional status and supplement as necessary. This has been particularly challenging in the last few years as a result of several vitamin and mineral shortages.

DIAGNOSIS

Prudent nutritional assessment is of the utmost importance in the management of IBD. In a study of 155 hospital in-patients receiving treatment for gastrointestinal or other internal disease, the severity of malnutrition in inpatients directly predicted the occurrence of complications during their stay.[31] Specifically in patients with IBD, it has been demonstrated that poor nutritional status may be directly correlated to the development of osteoporosis and anxiety/depressive disorders.[32,33] Thus, nutrition plays an important role in IBD management with regards to both the treatment and prevention of complications.

However, nutritional status cannot be determined by any single indicator; proper assessment relies on medical, surgical, and nutritional histories, physical exam, and laboratory evaluation. A thorough nutritional status assessment may include the following:

- ◊ Body composition evaluation:
  - • Anthropometric measurements—Height, weight, body mass index (BMI), and triceps skinfold measurement
  - • Bioelectric Impedance Analysis—To measure percentage fat and percentage fat free mass
  - • Air Plethysmography (BodPod)—Another method to measure percent fat and lean body mass
- ◊ Subjective global assessment (SGA)—A qualitative assessment of nutrition status, categorizing patients as either well nourished (Group A), moderately nourished (Group B), or severely malnourished (Group C).[34] Numerous studies have demonstrated the SGA's reliability in predicting prognosis for a wide spectrum of diseases.[35,36]
- ◊ Dietary intake assessment—Evaluate macro- and micronutrient intake as well as caloric intake.
- ◊ Physical activity assessment—Categorize patients activity levels as either low, intermediate, or high.[37]
- ◊ Laboratory testing—Laboratory evaluation plays an important role in evaluating nutritional status and guidelines for its implementation vary by a patient's disease activity and location, nutritional status, and method of nutrition (i.e., parenteral versus enteral nutrition).

Overall, current surveys demonstrate a shift from undernutrition and, thereby, low BMIs to malnutrition in patients with IBD as treatment options have changed (i.e., increased utilization of immunosuppression drugs).[18] Therefore, a nutritional assessment beyond simple anthropometrics is suggested to avoid oversight in treating patients.

Management

In general, macro- or micronutrient deficiencies must be corrected to improve treatment outcome and reduce the occurrence of negative sequelae for patients with IBD. Specifically, the supplementation technique to correct a micronutrient deficiency depends on the vitamins and/or mineral in deficit. Furthermore, when oral ingestion to maintain adequate nutrition is not possible due to patient preference, oral disease, or lesions, severe anorexia and nausea, high aspiration risk, or any other limiting factors, then enteral or parenteral nutrition may be indicated.

According to a meta-analysis of 29 trials completed by 2008, which included 2552 patients, enteral nutrition is strongly preferred over parenteral for the nutritional management of patients with IBD.[38] Secondly, enteral nutrition is less expensive and requires less training to administer and helps to avoid negative complications.[39] It has also been suggested by animal studies that enteral nutrition is superior to parenteral nutrition because it may prevent intestinal mucosal atrophy and prevent bacterial translocation. However, these assertions have not been fully validated by human studies.[40] Enteral nutrition may utilize either a nasogastric or a postpyloric feeding tube. A postpyloric feeding tube is useful when the stomach needs to be bypassed due to gastroparesis, intractable nausea and vomiting, or a severe risk of aspiration. In children, it is especially important to make every effort to maintain appropriate growth and development. In some cases, in addition to daytime oral intake, nocturnal tube feeding by way of a nasogastric tube may be utilized to help provide additional nutrition.[41]

Despite the seemingly superior performance of enteral nutrition in managing IBD, under certain circumstances parenteral nutrition may be indicated. One such circumstance is in patients with IBD who have enterocutaneous fistulas. These patients may be particularly challenging to feed enterally. If feeding causes an increase in output, or if a tube cannot be placed past the enterocutaneous fistulas, then parenteral nutrition may be indicated. In general, parenteral nutrition is indicated for hospitalized patients with small bowel obstruction/ileus or intestinal failure, if a feeding tube cannot be placed, or in perioperative cases where prolonged nil per os (NPO) status is required. In the past, it was suggested that bowel rest may provide benefit in the management of IBD. However, in 1998, Greenberg et al concluded that "bowel rest was not a major factor in achieving a remission during nutritional support" in IBD.[42] When administering parenteral nutrition, it is crucial to keep potential iatrogenic deficiencies in micronutrients in mind and include these in formulations.

In some cases of IBD, surgical resection or severity of the disease decrease the functional length of the small intestine, leading to malabsorption and short bowel syndrome. When the functional length remaining does not allow for intestinal rehabilitation, parenteral nutrition may be indicated. Intestinal rehabilitation strives to decrease transit time and increase absorption, and may include the use of diphenoxylate/atropine, loperamide, codeine, tincture of opium, a bulk-forming diet, and oral rehydration solutions.[43] Many patients with short bowel syndrome receiving parenteral nutrition may eventually be transitioned judiciously to enteral or oral nutrition. However, patients with less than 100 cm of remaining jejunum will most likely remain on parenteral nutrition indefinitely.[44] Home parenteral nutrition with close monitoring may be a means for improved quality of life for patients with short bowel syndrome. At some institutions of excellence, patients can be maintained on home parenteral nutrition indefinitely with minimal complications. Frequent office visits may be necessary in this setting to monitor routine lab work inclusive of trace elements and vitamins with subsequent adjustment of the parenteral nutrition formula. Additionally, oral rehydration solutions and appropriate diets can be reviewed and modified as needed for optimal nutrition.

☑ Key Points

☑ Patients with IBD are at high risk for many macro- and micronutrient deficiencies and, thus, require prudent nutritional assessment.

☑ These nutritional deficiencies may be due to decreased ingestion, decreased intestinal absorption surface, intestinal loss of nutrients, hypermetabolism, and/or medication-nutrient interactions.

☑ Proper nutritional assessment may include use of the SGA.

☑ Management of malnutrition in IBD may include enteral or parenteral nutrition. Enteral nutrition is preferred over parenteral nutrition.

☑ All attempts should be made to first rehabilitate the remaining small intestine in cases of short bowel syndrome. When such attempts are unable to provide adequate nutrition, enteral or parenteral nutrition may be administered.

☑ In extreme cases, patients may require lifelong use of parenteral nutrition or consideration of intestinal transplantation.

REFERENCES

1. Vasseur F, Gower Rousseau C, Vernier-Massouille G, et al. Nutritional status and growth in pediatric Crohn's disease: a population-based study. *Am J Gastroenterol.* 2010;105(8):1893-1900.
2. Cezard JP, Touati G, Alberti C, Hugot JP, Brinon C, Czernichow, P. Growth in paediatric Crohn's disease. *Horm Res.* 2002;58(Suppl 1):11-15.
3. Fleming CR. Nutrition in patients with Crohn's disease: another piece of the puzzle. JPEN *J Parenter Enteral Nutr.* 1995;19(2):93-94.
4. Geerling BJ, Badart-Smook A, Stockbrugger RW, Brummer RJ. Comprehensive nutritional status in patients with long-standing Crohn disease currently in remission. *Am J Clin Nutr.* 1998;67(5):919-926.
5. Murch SH. Local and systemic effects of macrophage cytokines in intestinal inflammation. *Nutrition.* 1998;14(10):780-783.
6. DeLegge MH. Nutrition and dietary interventions in adults with inflammatory bowel disease. In Rutgeerts P, Lipman TO, Grover S, Waltham, MA, UpToDate (Eds.). 2012.

7. Rigaud D, Angel LA, Cerf M, et al. Mechanisms of decreased food intake during weight loss in adults Crohn's disease patients without obvious malabsorption. *Am J Clin Nutr.* 1994;60 (5):775-781.

8. Ballinger A, El-Haj T, Perrett D, et al. The role of medial hypothalamic serotonin in the suppression of feeding in a rat model of colitis. *Gastroenterology.* 2000;118(3):544-553.

9. Miura S, Yoshioka M, Tanaka S, et al. Faecal clearance of alpha 1-antitrypsin reflects disease activity and correlates with rapid turnover proteins in chronic inflammatory bowel disease. *J Gastroenterol Hepatol.* 1991;6(1):49-52.

10. Zoli G, Katelaris PH, Garrow J, Gasbarrini G, Farthing MJ. Increased energy expenditure in growing adolescents with Crohn's disease. *Dig Dis Sci.* 1996;41(9):1754-1759.

11. Azcue M, Rashid M, Griffiths A, Pencharz P. Energy expenditure and body composition in children with Crohn's disease: effect of enteral nutrition and treatment with prednisolone. *Gut.* 1997;41(2):203–208.

12. Selhub J, Dhar GJ, Rosenberg IH. Inhibition of folate enzymes by sulfasalazine. *J Clin Invest.* 1978;61(1):221–224.

13. Steiner SJ, Pfefforkorn MD, Fitzgerald JF, Denne SC. Protein and energy metabolism response to the initial dose of infliximab in children with Crohn's disease. *Inflamm Bowel Dis.* 2007;13(6):737-744.

14. Gokhale R, Favus MJ, Karrison T, Sutton MM, Rich B, Kirschner BS. Bone mineral density assessment in children with inflammatory bowel disease. *Gastroenterology.* 1998;114(5):902-911.

15. Perkal, MF, Seashore, JH. Nutrition and inflammatory bowel disease. *Gastroenterol Clin North Am.* 1989;18(3):567-578.

16. Vagianos K, Bector S, McConnell J, Bernstein CN. Nutrition assessment of patients with inflammatory bowel disease. *JPEN J Parenter Enteral Nutr.* 2007;31(4):311-319.

17. Filippi J, Al-Jaouni R, Wiroth JB, Hebuterne X, Schneider, SM. Nutritional deficiencies in patients with Crohn's disease in remission. *Inflamm Bowel Dis.* 2006;12(3):185-191.

18. Sousa Guerreiro C, Cravo M, Costa AR, et al. A comprehensive approach to evaluate nutritional status in Crohn's patients in the era of biologic therapy: a case control study. *Am J Gastroenterol.* 2007;102(11):2551-2556.

19. Main AN, Mills PR, Russell RI, et al. Vitamin A deficiency in Crohn's disease. *Gut.* 1983;24(12):1169-1175.

20. Driscoll RH Jr, Meredith SC, Sitrin M, Rosenberg IH. Vitamin D deficiency and bone disease in patients with Crohn's disease. *Gastroenterology.* 1982;83(6):1252-1258.

21. Wendland BE, Aghdassi E, Tam C, et al. Lipid peroxidation and plasma antioxidant micronutrients in Crohn disease. *Am J Clin Nutr.* 2001;74(2):259-264.

22. Gisbert JP, Gomollón F. Common misconceptions in the diagnosis and management of anemia in inflammatory bowel disease. *Am J Gastroenterol.* 2008;103(5):1299-1307.

23. Lindgren S, Wikman O, Befrits R, et al. Intravenous iron sucrose is superior to oral iron sulphate for correcting anaemia and restoring iron stores in IBD patients: a randomized, controlled, evaluator-blind, multicentre study. *Scand J Gastroenterol.* 2009;44(7):838-845.

24. Evstatiev R, Marteau P, Iqbal T. FERGIcor, a randomized controlled trial on ferric carboxymaltose for iron deficiency anemia in inflammatory bowel disease. *Gastroenterology.* 2011;141(3):846-853.

25. Hechtman L. Crohn's Disease. *In: Clinical Naturopathic Medicine.* New South Wales, Australia. Elsevier Australia. 2012;192.

26. Mehanna HM, Moledina J, Travis J. Refeeding syndrome: what it is, and how to prevent and treat it. *BMJ.* 2008;336(7659):1495-1498.

27. Rannem T, Ladefoged K, Hylander E, Hegnhoj J, Staun M. Selenium depletion in patients with gastrointestinal diseases: are there any predictive factors? *Scand J Gastroenterol.* 1998;33(10):1057-1061.

28. Fleming CR, McCall JT, O'Brien JF, Forsman RW, Ilstrup DM, Petz J. Selenium status in patients receiving home parenteral nutrition. *JPEN J Parenter Enteral Nutr.* 1984;8(3):258-262.

29. Kumar N, Gross JB Jr, Ahlskog JE. Copper deficiency myelopathy produces a clinical picture like subacute combined degeneration. *Neurology*. 2004;63(1):33-39.

30. Barclay SM, Aggett PJ, Lloyd DJ, Duffty P. Reduced erythrocyte superoxide dismutase activity in low birth weight infants given iron supplements. *Pediatr Res*. 1991;29(3):297-301.

31. Naber TH, Schermer T, de Bree A, et al. Prevalence of malnutrition in nonsurgical hospitalized patients and its association with disease complications. *Am J Clin Nutr*. 1997;66(5):1232-1239.

32. Boot AM, Bouquet J, Krenning EP, de Muinck Keizer-Schrama. Bone mineral density and nutritional status in children with chronic inflammatory bowel disease. *Gut*. 1998;42(2):188-194.

33. Addolorato G, Capristo E, Stefanini GF, Gasbarrini G. Inflammatory bowel disease: A study of the association between anxiety and depression, physical morbidity, and nutritional status. *Scand J Gastroenterol*. 1997;32(10):1013-1021.

34. Detsky AS, McLaughlin JR, Baker JP, et al. What is the subjective global assessment of nutritional status? *JPEN J Parenter Enteral Nutr*. 1987;11(1):8-13.

35. Sacks GS, Dearman K, Replogle WH, Cora VL, Meeks M, Canada T. Use of subjective global assessment to identify nutrition-associated complication and death in geriatric long-term care facility residents. *J Am Coll Nutr*. 2000;19(5):570-577.

36. Enia G, Sicuso C, Alati G, Zoccali C. Subjective global assessment of nutrition in dialysis patients. *Nephrol Dial Transplant*. 1993;8(10):1094-1098.

37. Arroll B, Jackson R, Beaglehole R. Validation of a three month physical activity recall questionnaire with a seven day food intake and physical activity diary. *Epidemiology*. 1991;2(4):296-299.

38. Mazaki T, Ebisawa K. Enteral versus parenteral nutrition after gastrointestinal surgery: a systematic review and meta-analysis of randomized controlled trials in the English literature. *J Gastrointest Surg*. 2008;12(4):739-755.

39. Gonzalez-Huix F, Fernandez-Banares F, Esteve-Comas M, et al. Enteral versus parenteral nutrition as adjunct therapy in acute ulcerative colitis. *Am J Gastroenterol*. 1993;88(2):227-232.

40. Jeejeebhoy KN. Total parenteral nutrition: potion or poison. *Am J Clin Nutr*. 2001;74(2):160-163.

41. Aiges H, Markowitz J, Rosa J, Daum F. Home nocturnal supplemental nasogastric feedings in growth-retarded adolescents with Crohn's disease. *Gastroenterology*. 1989;97(4):905-910.

42. Greenberg GR, Fleming CR, Jeejeebhoy KN, Rosenberg IH, Sales D, Tremaine WJ. Controlled trial of bowel rest and nutritional support in the management of Crohn's disease. *Gut*. 1988;29(10):1309-1315.

43. Shatnawei A, Parekh NR, Rhoda KM, et al. Intestinal failure management at the Cleveland Clinic. *Arch Surg*. 2010;145(6):521-527.

44. Lennard-Jones JE. Indications and need for long-term parenteral nutrition: implications for intestinal transplantation. *Transplant Proc*. 1990; 22(6):2427-2429.

Suggested Readings

Evans JP, Steinhart AH, Cohen Z, McLeod RS. Home total parenteral nutrition: an alternative to early surgery for complicated inflammatory bowel disease. *J Gastrointest Surg*. 2003;7(4):562-566.

Geerling BJ, Stockbrügger RW, Brummer RJ. Nutrition and inflammatory bowel disease: an update. *Scand J Gastroenterol Suppl*. 1999;230:95-105.

Husain A, Korzenik JR. Nutritional issues and therapy in inflammatory bowel disease. *Semin Gastrointest Dis*. 1998;9(1):21-30.

Kirby DF. Improving outcomes with parenteral nutrition. *Gastroenterol Hepatol* (N.Y.). 2012;8(1):39-41.

Chapter 13

Vaccination and Immunization Issues for Patients With IBD

Gil Y. Melmed, MD, MS

The mainstay of medical therapy for patients with inflammatory bowel disease (IBD) increasingly involves the use of immunosuppression, including corticosteroids, immunomodulators, and biologic therapies. The most common adverse events associated with immunosuppressive therapies are infections, including vaccine-preventable diseases.[1,2] Patients with IBD are at an increased risk for infection, not only due to immunosuppressive therapies, but also due to malnutrition, hospitalization, and surgery. Many infections are preventable with prophylactic immunizations. Furthermore, some infections can be serious, or even fatal, in the at-risk patient, including pneumococcal pneumonia,[3] disseminated varicella,[4] fulminant liver failure due to viral hepatitis,[5] and human papillomavirus (HPV)-associated cervical cancer. Unfortunately, multiple studies have demonstrated that vaccines are underutilized in the IBD patient population. In general, standard pediatric and adult immunization guidelines should be followed in IBD patients, but live-virus vaccines should be avoided in those who are immunosuppressed (Figures 13-1 and 13-2). Special considerations for the immunization of immunosuppressed IBD patients may include travel medicine, vaccination of household contacts, and living in a college dormitory environment. Among immunosuppressed patients with IBD, vaccine antibody response may be somewhat blunted, particularly among patients on multiple immunosuppressive therapies. However, most patients still develop protective antibody titers following vaccination.

Regueiro MD, Swoger JM, eds.
Clinical Challenges and Complications of IBD (pp 241-252).
© 2013 Taylor & Francis Group.

Recommended Adult Immunization Schedule—United States - 2012

Note: These recommendations must be read with the footnotes that follow containing number of doses, intervals between doses, and other important information.

Recommended adult immunization schedule, by vaccine and age group[1]

VACCINE ▼ / AGE GROUP ▶	19-21 years	22-26 years	27-49 years	50-59 years	60-64 years	≥ 65 years
Influenza [2,*]	1 dose annually					
Tetanus, diphtheria, pertussis (Td/Tdap) [3,*]	Substitute 1-time dose of Tdap for Td booster; then boost with Td every 10 yrs					Td/Tdap[3]
Varicella [4,*]	2 Doses					
Human papillomavirus (HPV) Female [5,*]	3 doses					
Human papillomavirus (HPV) Male [5,*]	3 doses					
Zoster [6]					1 dose	
Measles, mumps, rubella (MMR) [7,*]	1 or 2 doses			1 dose		
Pneumococcal (polysaccharide) [8,9]	1 or 2 doses					1 dose
Meningococcal [10,*]	1 or more doses					
Hepatitis A [11,*]	2 doses					
Hepatitis B [12,*]	3 doses					

*Covered by the Vaccine Injury Compensation Program

Legend: For all persons in this category who meet the age requirements and who lack documentation of vaccination or have no evidence of previous infection — Recommended if some other risk factor is present (e.g., on the basis of medical, occupational, lifestyle, or other indications) — Tdap recommended for ≥65 if contact with <12 month old child. Either Td or Tdap can be used if no infant contact — No recommendation

Report all clinically significant postvaccination reactions to the Vaccine Adverse Event Reporting System (VAERS). Reporting forms and instructions on filing a VAERS report are available at www.vaers.hhs.gov or by telephone, 800-822-7967.

Information on how to file a Vaccine Injury Compensation Program claim is available at www.hrsa.gov/vaccinecompensation or by telephone, 800-338-2382. To file a claim for vaccine injury, contact the U.S. Court of Federal Claims, 717 Madison Place, N.W., Washington, D.C. 20005, telephone, 202-357-6400.

Additional information about the vaccines in this schedule, extent of available data, and contraindications for vaccination is also available at www.cdc.gov/vaccines or from the CDC-INFO Contact Center at 800-CDC-INFO (800-232-4636) in English and Spanish, 8:00 a.m. - 8:00 p.m. Eastern Time, Monday - Friday, excluding holidays.

Use of trade names and commercial sources is for identification only and does not imply endorsement by the U.S. Department of Health and Human Services.

Figure 13-1. Current vaccination guidelines for adults. For further details and footnotes regarding CDC recommendations for specific vaccines, please visit www.cdc.gov/vaccines/pubs/acip-list.htm.

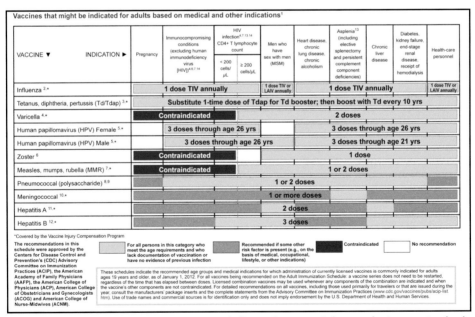

Figure 13-2. Current vaccination guidelines for special populations—including immunocompromised individuals and health care workers. For further details and footnotes regarding CDC recommendations for specific vaccines, please visit www.cdc.gov/vaccines/pubs/acip-list.htm.

General Considerations

Guiding Principles

Several guiding principles should be considered when contemplating vaccination of patients with IBD, especially for those on immunosuppressive therapies.[6-8] The diagnosis of IBD is rare before the age of 5, so most childhood vaccines (including the live-virus measles-mumps-rubella [MMR] vaccine) will have likely been administered prior to a diagnosis of IBD. IBD itself is not thought to impact the immune response to vaccination, and patients not on immunosuppressive therapy should undergo all routine childhood and adult vaccinations.[7,9] Additionally, all recommended non-live vaccines can be safely administered to patients on immunosuppressive therapy. However, individuals receiving immunosuppressant medications represent a population requiring additional considerations (see Figure 13-2). Specific concerns include a general avoidance of live-virus vaccines and consideration for checking postvaccination immune titers if possible. For these patients, an approach that considers not just the patient but the environment as well is critical. Physicians must consider the overall risks and benefits of vaccination, particularly in settings of a high exposure potential to infectious pathogens to which the host is naive. Special considerations in the IBD populations also include travel, the immunization of household contacts, and the immunization of neonates exposed in utero to immunosuppressive therapies taken by a mother with IBD.

In general, all IBD patients should receive standard recommended immunizations as outlined by the Advisory Committee on Immunization Practices of the Centers for Disease Control and Prevention.[6] Ideally, patients either newly diagnosed with IBD or at their initial IBD consultation should be queried regarding vaccination status, travel history, and risk factors for various infections.[7,9] Where possible, all indicated vaccines should be administered to patients prior to starting immunosuppressive therapy in order to maximize the chance of mounting an adequate immune response and to allow for the administration of live vaccines, if indicated.[9,10] However, in cases where patients require a more immediate initiation of immunosuppressive therapy, live-virus immunizations may need to be postponed.

Knowledge and Practice Gaps

Despite specific immunization guidelines for IBD patients published in 2004, vaccines are underutilized in IBD patients.[11] This may be due to a lack of awareness of appropriate indications for vaccination on the part of both patients and physicians. For example, in a survey of 169 patients at a tertiary IBD referral center in 2006, only 28% had received an influenza vaccination within the previous year, despite nearly 90% having been exposed to long-term immunosuppressive therapy.[11] Less than 10% had ever received a pneumococcal vaccine, and 11% could not recall a history of prior chickenpox infection or varicella vaccination. When asked why they had not received a flu shot within the previous year, over half the respondents indicated that

Table 13-1. Live-Virus Vaccines

Varicella
Yellow fever
Anthrax
Bacille calmette-guérin
Measles-mumps-rubella
Smallpox (Vaccinia)
Adenovirus
Live cholera
Typhoid (oral)
Influenza (intranasal)
Zoster

they were not aware that it was recommended. Notably, over 80% of these patients had seen their primary care provider at least once within the prior 12 months.

General Safety of Vaccines in Inflammatory Bowel Disease

Studies in immunosuppressed populations, including those with IBD, rheumatoid arthritis, and a history of organ transplant, demonstrate that vaccinations are safe and well tolerated. Most patients with IBD respond to common vaccines including influenza,[12,13] pneumococcal,[14] and tetanus.[15] However, patients on multiple concomitant immunosuppressive agents may have diminished serologic responses.[14] Vaccinations with non-live vaccines are considered safe. Prospective studies in children and adults with IBD have included subjects who safely received influenza, pneumococcal, and hepatitis A virus (HAV) vaccinations, although there are case reports of ulcerative colitis disease flare after vaccination with influenza.[16] Multiple epidemiologic studies have assessed the risk of IBD following MMR or measles vaccination, and have not found any association between vaccination and the development of Crohn's disease or ulcerative colitis.[17,18]

Live-virus Vaccines

In general, live-virus vaccines should not be given to patients on immunosuppressive medications. Common live-virus vaccines include intranasal influenza, bacille Calmette-Guérin, varicella, zoster, yellow fever, and MMR (Table 13-1). In general it is advised that live vaccines be given prior to the initiation of immunosuppressive therapy or 2 to 3 months after immunosuppressive therapy is discontinued. To avoid the risk of systemic infection from live-virus vaccination, it would be conservative to wait 6 weeks prior to restarting immunosuppressive therapy. However, there are very limited data assessing this approach, which is likely to vary based on vaccine-specific viral shedding and medication-specific half-life.

SPECIFIC VACCINE RECOMMENDATIONS

Influenza

In the United States, 30,000 people die annually from seasonal influenza, and patients on immunosuppressive medications remain at risk for seasonal and H1N1 influenza. Annual influenza vaccination with the injectable vaccine is recommended for all patients with IBD. The inactivated trivalent influenza vaccine which, in 2010, includes H1N1 is safe in immunosuppressed recipients. Conversely, the live attenuated intranasal vaccine is generally contraindicated in individuals receiving immunosuppressive therapy. Influenza vaccination is effective in inducing immune responses in children with IBD but may be less effective among those on anti-tumor necrosis factor (TNF) therapies. The majority of those with IBD develop protective antibody titers following influenza vaccination, regardless of immunosuppressive medication use. However, 2 studies performed in children with IBD suggest that responses to at least 1 of the 3 antigens may be blunted in those on immunosuppressive therapies at the time of vaccination.[12,13]

Pneumococcus

Indications for vaccination against pneumococcal disease largely overlap with indications for influenza vaccination. Pneumococcal vaccination with the conjugated pneumococcal vaccine (Prevnar) is recommended for all children <5 years of age, while the pneumococcal polysaccharide vaccine (Pneumovax 23) is recommended for adults considered at risk, including those with chronic diseases such as IBD, especially if on immunosuppressive medications. Common risks, even among nonimmunosuppressed individuals with IBD, include concomitant asthma and other respiratory conditions. Vaccinations against influenza and pneumococcal are safe, and simultaneous administration is recommended in order to maximize opportunities for vaccination.

The pneumococcal polysaccharide vaccine is safe and effective in patients receiving immunosuppression, although response rates may vary depending on the type and number of concomitant immunosuppressive therapies. In patients with rheumatoid arthritis, the proportion of those achieving response to PPV23 was actually higher among those treated with anti-TNF medications (infliximab or etanercept) alone, as compared with either methotrexate alone or in combination with anti-TNF therapy.[19] In this study, monotherapy with methotrexate showed the poorest response and vaccination was less effective than combination therapy with an anti-TNF agent and methotrexate. In a randomized controlled trial, Kaine et al showed that subjects with rheumatoid arthritis treated with adalimumab had similar vaccine response rates to those receiving placebo, suggesting that monotherapy with anti-TNF agents does not impair vaccine response rates.[20] Others have shown that those treated with combination anti-TNF and methotrexate therapy had lower response rates than those treated with methotrexate alone.[21] It is unclear whether information obtained from the rheumatoid arthritis population can be extrapolated to patients with IBD, who are treated with similar drug classes but may have additional factors (eg, younger age, malnutrition) that may influence vaccine response.

In patients with IBD, one study assessed response rates to pneumococcal polysaccharide vaccination in 21 adults with IBD on combination anti-TNF and immunomodulator therapy, 25 nonimmunosuppressed IBD patients, and 19 healthy controls.[14] Immunosuppressed subjects had significantly impaired postvaccination titers, while those with IBD who were not immunosuppressed had response rates similar to healthy controls. This study suggests that in patients with IBD, the combined use of anti-TNF agents and immunomodulators may in fact dampen response to the pneumococcal polysaccharide vaccine.

Given that those treated with combination immunosuppressive therapy may not mount an adequate vaccine response, and that the likelihood for immunosuppression is unpredictable, it is reasonable to consider vaccination against pneumococcal disease in all patients with IBD early in the course of the disease. However, for those patients already on immunosuppression, vaccination is safe, and most patients do have at least a partial response to the vaccine.

Hepatitis A Virus

Vaccination against hepatitis A utilizes a non-live vaccine and can be administered alone or can be coadministered with the hepatitis B virus (HBV) vaccine. Although historically HAV was recommended primarily for travel to endemic areas, it is now recommended for children and at-risk adults. People with compromised immunity are not specifically considered at risk, but the vaccine is well tolerated, non-live, and affords protection against a potentially life-threatening infection. Experts suggest vaccination for all naive patients with IBD.[22] A study of 66 children in Poland with IBD and 68 healthy controls demonstrated that vaccination with HAV was similar in both groups after 2 doses and was safe and well tolerated.[23]

Hepatitis B Virus

Treatment with anti-TNF agents has been associated with fulminant and fatal liver failure in patients with reactivated latent HBV infection.[5,24] Assessment for HBV is therefore recommended prior to initiation of anti-TNF therapy, although there is variability in how assessment should be performed. Some advocate HBV screening and vaccination only among those with risk factors, including intravenous drug use, travel to endemic regions, high-risk sexual behavior, hemodialysis patients, and health care providers (Table 13-2). Others recommend screening all patients with HBV serology and vaccination of all seronegative patients.[9] The 3-dose hepatitis B vaccination series is safe

Table 13-2. Risk Factors for Hepatitis B Virus Infection
Intravenous drug use
Travel to endemic regions
High-risk sexual behaviors
Prisoners
Hemodialysis
Health care providers
Household contacts of chronic HBV carriers
Sharing personal items with HBV carrier (razor, toothbrush, nail clippers)
Vertical transmission—mother to infant
Blood transfusion prior to 1987

in immunosuppressed patients and well tolerated. A Spanish retrospective assessment of 129 patients with IBD suggested impaired antibody responses to the HBV vaccine.[25]

Diphtheria, Tetanus, and Pertussis Vaccines

Vaccination against tetanus and diphtheria toxoids (Td) is recommended for children, and for adults, as a Td or Tdap (Td plus pertussis vaccination) booster shot every 10 years. Td and Tdap are noninfectious, safe, and can be given to all IBD patients as part of routine immunization.[6] In 2010, a pertussis epidemic was reported in California and all adults were advised to undergo booster vaccination to protect susceptible infants who are naive to the infection and the vaccine.[26]

Meningococcus

Meningococcal vaccination is recommended for 2- to 55-year-olds with risk factors for meningococcal infection, such as travelers to endemic areas and those with splenic dysfunction or who have had a splenectomy.[27] The vaccine is also recommended for children aged 11 to 18 years old and for adults with risk factors, such as college freshmen, military recruits, or travelers to endemic areas. This vaccine, previously a polysaccharide vaccine, is now available as a conjugate vaccine, which is considered to be more immunogenic.[28] It is thought to be safe in immunocompromised patients.[22]

Human Papillomavirus

The HPV vaccine includes the 4 HPV serotypes most strongly associated with progression to cervical dysplasia and cancer. A 3-dose series is recommended for males and females ages 9 to 26 years and is considered safe in immunosuppressed patients, although studies are lacking. Women with IBD may have a higher risk for HPV and abnormal Pap smears, especially those receiving immunosuppressive medications.[29-31] However, not all studies support an increased risk.[32] Although the vaccine is licensed for individuals up to the age of 26, it may be reasonable to consider vaccination in women of any age who are immunosuppressed and thus considered at increased risk.

Varicella (Chickenpox) and Zoster (Shingles)

The varicella vaccine is a live-virus vaccine recommended as a 2-dose series in children, beginning at 12 months age, and in all healthy persons aged >13 years without evidence of immunity. During the initial health care visit of a patient with IBD, varicella immune status should be assessed by inquiring about previous varicella infection or immunization and checking varicella titers if there is doubt regarding prior exposure.[7] Patients not on immunosuppressive therapy, who are naive to varicella, should receive the vaccine. This live-virus vaccine remains contraindicated in immunosuppressed patients. However, careful assessment of the risks of vaccination in a naive patient recently discontinued from immunosuppressive therapy needs to be carefully weighed against the benefits of vaccination, especially when the potential for environmental exposure is high.

The zoster vaccine, also a live-virus vaccine, is indicated for all persons aged >60 years, including those with a history of zoster or varicella. Herpes zoster is associated with immunosuppression among patients with IBD,[33] and its risk increases with the use of 2 or 3 immunosuppressants.[31] The zoster vaccine is a live-virus vaccine that should generally be avoided among immunosuppressed individuals. Experts suggest that the zoster vaccine is considered safe in patients receiving "low-dose" immunosuppressive therapy (≤20 mg/day prednisone, 3 mg/kg azathioprine, 1.5 mg/kg 6-mercaptopurine), although no data support this recommendation.[34] However, for those requiring anti-TNF therapy, the vaccine should be administered prior to initiation of therapy or deferred for a period of time after therapy is discontinued.

Measles, Mumps, and Rubella

Current guidelines advise a 2-dose MMR immunization series in children aged >1 year. In naive adults born after 1957, a single-dose MMR vaccination is generally indicated, and a second MMR dose can be given to adults >50 years of age if risk factors are present.[6] This vaccine contains live attenuated viruses and is generally contraindicated in immunocompromised IBD patients. Household contacts of immunosuppressed individuals with IBD should receive MMR vaccination.

Yellow Fever and Travel Medicine

Travelers to endemic countries often require proof of yellow fever vaccination, usually within the previous 10 years. Vaccination with this live-virus vaccine poses rare theoretical risk of severe neurologic impairment, or death, in immunocompromised individuals. Therefore, some experts advise against travel to endemic areas for yellow fever if vaccination is required.[35] However, travelers who choose to visit endemic areas without vaccination may require a medical letter of exemption and should be advised to wear protective clothing and use mosquito nets and repellent to reduce the risks of mosquito vector transmission. Decisions regarding yellow fever and other travel-related vaccinations among immunosuppressed individuals should be made in consultation with a travel medicine specialist.

Household Contacts

The vaccination of household contacts of immunosuppressed individuals with IBD is generally recommended and considered safe, although certain live-virus vaccines require special consideration. Vaccinations considered contraindicated for household contacts of immunosuppressed individuals include the live oral polio vaccine and the smallpox vaccine. The live influenza intranasal vaccination can shed live vaccine-strain virus for several days following vaccination of the healthy recipient and can thus theoretically increase the risk of infection in an immunosuppressed household contact. Therefore, the inactivated (injected) influenza vaccine is recommended for household contacts of immunosuppressed individuals.[36] The varicella vaccine is generally considered safe, and no special precautions are recommended for household contacts, unless the vaccine recipient develops a rash, in which case direct contact should be avoided until resolution of the rash.[37] Rotavirus vaccination is considered safe for household contacts of individuals with IBD, although rigorous hand-washing precautions are advised following changing the diaper of a rotavirus recipient for 1 week following vaccination.[38]

Health Care Providers

Health care providers are considered at risk for certain vaccine-preventable illnesses due to frequent contact with potentially infectious patients, as well as their role in serving as a vector for infection transmission to susceptible patients. In particular, recommendations for vaccination against influenza, pneumococcus, varicella, MMR, Td, and hepatitis B specifically single out health care providers as a target group for immunization, based on both an increased risk of transmission and on general adult vaccination guidelines.[39]

CONCLUSION

Ideally, vaccinations should be considered at the time of initial IBD diagnosis or consultation. A complete vaccination history should be obtained as early as possible, and appropriate recommendations made. In adults, immunizations with influenza (in season) and pneumococcal vaccines are almost always appropriate, regardless of immunosuppression status (see Figure 13-2). Assessment for HBV and varicella should be performed, particularly prior to the initiation of immunosuppressive therapy. If possible, varicella-naive patients who are not receiving immunosuppressive therapy should be vaccinated, given the significant morbidity associated with varicella in adults, as well as in immunocompromised populations. HPV vaccination should be considered in women and men, particularly those on immunosuppressive therapy. Special situations involving travel should be determined together with a travel medicine specialist, particularly if patients are travelling to endemic areas for yellow fever. Finally, health care providers who manage patients with IBD and prescribe immunosuppressive medications should recognize their role in educating patients and colleagues about vaccination recommendations.

Note: Recommendations for vaccinations and immunizations vary by country and region. Unless otherwise specified, recommendations described in this chapter are based on guidelines provided by the Centers for Disease Control and Prevention (www.cdc.gov/vaccines).

☑ Key Points

☑ Infections are the most common adverse events associated with immunosuppression in IBD, and many infections are preventable with routine immunizations.

☑ All adults with IBD should receive annual influenza vaccination and a one-time pneumococcal vaccine, regardless of immunosuppressed status.

☑ Immune responses to many vaccines are blunted among those on immunosuppressive therapies, so ideally vaccinations should be considered prior to starting such therapy.

☑ In general, live-virus vaccines should be avoided in patients who are immunosuppressed (with the possible exception of the zoster [shingles] vaccine in specific situations).

☑ Special considerations are warranted for travel to endemic areas requiring proof of vaccination against yellow fever, a live-virus vaccine.

☑ Household contacts of immunosuppressed individuals can safely receive most live-virus vaccines, with a few exceptions including the live intranasal flu-mist.

REFERENCES

1. Viget N, Vernier-Massouille G, Salmon-Ceron D, Yazdanpanah Y, Colombel JF. Opportunistic infections in patients with inflammatory bowel disease: prevention and diagnosis. *Gut.* 2008;57:549-558.
2. Toruner M, Loftus EV Jr, Harmsen WS, et al. Risk factors for opportunistic infections in patients with inflammatory bowel disease. *Gastroenterology.* 2008;134:929-936.

3. Ritz MA, Jost R. Severe pneumococcal pneumonia following treatment with infliximab for Crohn's disease. *Inflamm Bowel Dis*. 2001;7:327.

4. Leung VS, Nguyen MT, Bush TM. Disseminated primary varicella after initiation of infliximab for Crohn's disease. *Am J Gastroenterol*. 2004;99:2503-2504.

5. Esteve M, Saro C, Gonzalez-Huix F, Suarez F, Forne M, Viver JM. Chronic hepatitis B reactivation following infliximab therapy in Crohn's disease patients: need for primary prophylaxis. *Gut*. 2004;53:1363-1365.

6. Kroger AT, Atkinson WL, Marcuse EK, Pickering LK. General recommendations on immunization: recommendations of the Advisory Committee on Immunization Practices (ACIP). *MMWR Recomm Rep*. 2006;55:1-48.

7. Sands BE, Cuffari C, Katz J, et al. Guidelines for immunizations in patients with inflammatory bowel disease. *Inflamm Bowel Dis*. 2004;10:677-692.

8. National Advisory Committee on Immunization. *Canadian Immunization Guide*. 6th ed. Ottawa, Canada: Public Health Agency of Canada; 2006.

9. Rahier JF, Ben-Horin S, Chowers Y, et al. European evidence-based consensus on the prevention, diagnosis and management of opportunistic infections in inflammatory bowel disease. *J Crohns Colitis*. 2009;3:47-91.

10. Melmed GY. Vaccination strategies for patients with inflammatory bowel disease on immunomodulators and biologics. *Inflamm Bowel Dis*. 2009;15:1410-1416.

11. Melmed GY, Ippoliti AF, Papadakis KA, et al. Patients with inflammatory bowel disease are at risk for vaccine-preventable illnesses. *Am J Gastroenterol*. 2006;101:1834-1840.

12. Mamula P, Markowitz JE, Piccoli DA, Klimov A, Cohen L, Baldassano RN. Immune response to influenza vaccine in pediatric patients with inflammatory bowel disease. *Clin Gastroenterol Hepatol*. 2007;5:851-856.

13. Lu Y, Jacobson DL, Ashworth LA, et al. Immune response to influenza vaccine in children with inflammatory bowel disease. *Am J Gastroenterol*. 2009;104:444-453.

14. Melmed GY, Agarwal N, Frenck RW, et al. Immunosuppression impairs response to pneumococcal polysaccharide vaccination in patients with inflammatory bowel disease. *Am J Gastroenterol*. 2010;105:148-154.

15. Nielsen HJ, Mortensen T, Holten-Andersen M, Brunner N, Sorensen S, Rask-Madsen J. Increased levels of specific leukocyte- and platelet-derived substances during normal anti-tetanus antibody synthesis in patients with inactive Crohn's disease. *Scand J Gastroenterol*. 2001;36:265-269.

16. Fields SW, Baiocco PJ, Korelitz BI. Influenza vaccinations: should they really be encouraged for IBD patients being treated with immunosuppressives? *Inflamm Bowel Dis*. 2009;15:649-651.

17. Seagroatt V, Goldacre MJ. Crohn's disease, ulcerative colitis, and measles vaccine in an English population, 1979-1998. *J Epidemiol Community Health*. 2003;57:883-887.

18. Davis RL, Kramarz P, Bohlke K, et al. Measles-mumps-rubella and other measles-containing vaccines do not increase the risk for inflammatory bowel disease: a case-control study from the Vaccine Safety Datalink project. *Arch Pediatr Adolesc Med*. 2001;155:354-359.

19. Kapetanovic MC, Saxne T, Sjoholm A, Truedsson L, Jonsson G, Geborek P. Influence of methotrexate, TNF blockers and prednisolone on antibody responses to pneumococcal polysaccharide vaccine in patients with rheumatoid arthritis. *Rheumatology*. 2006;45:106-111.

20. Kaine JL, Kivitz AJ, Birbara C, Luo AY. Immune responses following administration of influenza and pneumococcal vaccines to patients with rheumatoid arthritis receiving adalimumab. *J Rheumatol*. 2007;34:272-279.

21. Elkayam O, Caspi D, Reitblatt T, Charboneau D, Rubins JB. The effect of tumor necrosis factor blockade on the response to pneumococcal vaccination in patients with rheumatoid arthritis and ankylosing spondylitis. *Semin Arthritis Rheum*. 2004;33:283-288.

22. Kotton CN. Vaccines and inflammatory bowel disease. *Dig Dis*. 2010;28:525-535.

23. Radzikowski A, Banaszkiewicz A, Lazowska-Przeorek I, et al. Immunogenecity of hepatitis A vaccine in pediatric patients with inflammatory bowel disease. *Inflamm Bowel Dis* 2011;17:1117-1124.

24. Shale MJ, Seow CH, Coffin CS, Kaplan GG, Panaccione R, Ghosh S. Review article: chronic viral infection in the anti-tumour necrosis factor therapy era in inflammatory bowel disease. *Aliment Pharmacol Ther.* 2010;31:20-34.

25. Vida Perez L, Gomez Camacho F, Garcia Sanchez V, et al. Adequate rate of response to hepatitis B virus vaccination in patients with inflammatory bowel disease. *Med Clin.* 2009;132:331-335.

26. California Department of Public Health. http://www.cdph.ca.gov. Accessed October 2010.

27. Bilukha OO, Rosenstein N. Prevention and control of meningococcal disease. Recommendations of the Advisory Committee on Immunization Practices (ACIP). *MMWR Recomm Rep.* 2005;54:1-21.

28. Advisory Committee on Immunization Practices. Licensure of a meningococcal conjugate vaccine (Menveo) and guidance for use—Advisory Committee on Immunization Practices (ACIP), 2010. *MMWR Morb Mortal Wkly Rep.* 2010;59:273.

29. Kane S, Khatibi B, Reddy D. Higher incidence of abnormal Pap smears in women with inflammatory bowel disease. *Am J Gastroenterol.* 2008;103:631-636.

30. Bhatia J, Bratcher J, Korelitz B, et al. Abnormalities of uterine cervix in women with inflammatory bowel disease. *World J Gastroenterol.* 2006;12:6167-6171.

31. Marehbian J, Arrighi HM, Hass S, Tian H, Sandborn WJ. Adverse events associated with common therapy regimens for moderate-to-severe Crohn's disease. *Am J Gastroenterol.* 2009;104:2524-2533.

32. Lees CW, Critchley J, Chee N, et al. Lack of association between cervical dysplasia and IBD: a large case-control study. *Inflamm Bowel Dis.* 2009;15:1621-1629.

33. Gupta G, Lautenbach E, Lewis JD. Incidence and risk factors for herpes zoster among patients with inflammatory bowel disease. *Clin Gastroenterol Hepatol.* 2006;4:1483-1490.

34. Harpaz R, Ortega-Sanchez IR, Seward JF. Prevention of herpes zoster: recommendations of the Advisory Committee on Immunization Practices (ACIP). *MMWR Recomm Rep.* 2008;57:1-30.

35. Cetron MS, Marfin AA, Julian KG, et al. Yellow fever vaccine. Recommendations of the Advisory Committee on Immunization Practices (ACIP), 2002. *MMWR Recomm Rep.* 2002;51:1-11.

36. Kamboj M, Sepkowitz KA. Risk of transmission associated with live attenuated vaccines given to healthy persons caring for or residing with an immunocompromised patient. *Infect Control Hosp Epidemiol.* 2007;28:702-707.

37. Prevention of varicella. Update recommendations of the Advisory Committee on Immunization Practices (ACIP). *MMWR Recomm Rep.* 1999;48:1-5.

38. Cortese MM, Parashar UD. Prevention of rotavirus gastroenteritis among infants and children: recommendations of the Advisory Committee on Immunization Practices (ACIP). *MMWR Recomm Rep* 2009;58:1-25.

39. Immunization of health-care workers: recommendations of the Advisory Committee on Immunization Practices (ACIP) and the Hospital Infection Control Practices Advisory Committee (HICPAC). *MMWR Recomm Rep.* 1997;46:1-42.

SUGGESTED READINGS

Melmed GY. Vaccination strategies for patients with inflammatory bowel disease on immuno-modulators and biologics. *Inflamm Bowel Dis.* 2009;15:1410-1416.

Melmed GY, Ippoliti AF, Papadakis KA, et al. Patients with inflammatory bowel disease are at risk for vaccine-preventable illnesses. *Am J Gastroenterol.* 2006;101:1834-1840.

Moscandrew M, Mahadevan U, Kane S. General health maintenance in IBD. *Inflamm Bowel Dis.* 2009;15:1399-1409.

Rahier JF, Ben-Horin S, Chowers Y, et al. European evidence-based consensus on the prevention, diagnosis and management of opportunistic infections in inflammatory bowel disease. *J Crohn Colitis.* 2009;3:47-91.

Sands BE, Cuffari C, Katz J, et al. Guidelines for immunizations in patients with inflammatory bowel disease. *Inflamm Bowel Dis.* 2004;10:677-692.

Chapter 14

Psychiatric Complications of IBD

David Benhayon, MD, PhD and Eva Szigethy, MD, PhD

Approximately 1.4 million Americans struggle with inflammatory bowel disease (IBD),[1] and 25% of cases are diagnosed during childhood.[2] The peak age of incidence is adolescence and young adulthood, although patients frequently develop IBD later in life as well.[3] Certain ethnicities, particularly Whites and Ashkenazi Jews, have higher rates of IBD; however, IBD is seen in numerous different ethnic groups, and rates of diagnosis as a whole are rising.[4,5] It is unknown whether this increase in diagnosis is secondary to better detection methods or to an actual increase in numbers of affected patients.

Both Crohn's disease (CD) and ulcerative colitis (UC) are thought to be multifactorial in etiology, with genetic and environmental factors contributing to the pathogenesis of the illnesses. Additionally, psychological stress has been increasingly linked to disease course and outcomes.[6] However, psychological symptoms and psychosocial stressors in IBD are often undetected and undertreated. A multitude of factors have contributed to this underrecognition: (1) gastroenterologists often lack the time or resources in busy clinics to detect psychopathology, (2) a shortage of mental health professionals to refer such medically complex cases, and (3) an assumption by the field that psychological symptoms (eg, depression), which occur during disease flare-ups, do not require attention beyond medical treatments for IBD. This chapter is aimed at providing an educational overview for medical specialists working with the IBD population, so that psychological factors can be addressed and suffering can be decreased. A biopsychosocial model will be used to provide a framework in which to understand psychiatric-medical comorbidity in IBD. This model incorporates biologic (genetics, physical factors, and psychiatric illness-related factors), psychological (coping styles), and environmental factors (external stressors, social supports) to formulate etiologies for illness. This chapter focuses on psychopathology that may be present in patients with IBD, ranging from mild stress, adjustment, and coping difficulties to full-blown psychiatric diagnoses, most often depressive and anxiety disorders

Regueiro MD, Swoger JM, eds.
Clinical Challenges and Complications of IBD (pp 253-284).
© 2013 Taylor & Francis Group.

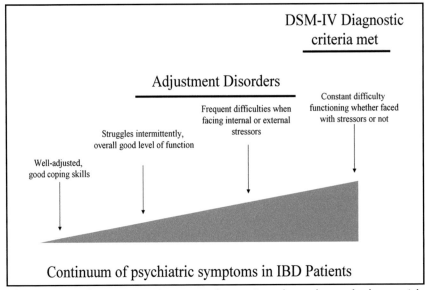

Figure 14-1. The varying degrees of severity of psychopathology with which IBD patients struggle. A significant number of patients cope well with the difficulties induced by IBD (the left end of the continuum), but a number struggle with stressors, either intermittently or chronically. When patients are unable to function in the face of these stressors, they often meet criteria for DSM-IV psychiatric diagnoses. The presence or absence of protective factors, either biologic or social, can moderate the severity of illness.

(Figure 14-1 and Tables 14-1 through 14-3). In addition, information is provided regarding screening, treatment, and prevention options for psychological stress in patients dealing with chronic illnesses such as CD and UC.

STRESS AND IBD

The literature to date supports a bidirectional relationship between stress and IBD. Stress may be defined as a threat or a perceived threat to an individual's homeostasis that overwhelms the brain's capacity to deal with the event effectively. In patients with IBD, such threats include physical manifestations of the disease (eg, inflammation-related gastrointestinal symptoms), environmental events (eg, trauma, life stress), stress-induced changes in the microbiome, or psychological states (eg, anxiety or depression). In the short term, such stressors may be adaptive for survival, by activating allostasis to re-establish physiologic homeostasis within the organism. Chronic stress, however, has been shown to be detrimental in IBD, with documented negative physiologic, neurologic, immune, and psychological consequences.[6]

There are many different ways in which to categorize stressors, one of which includes dividing stressors into internal and external types (Figure 14-2). Although arbitrary, this designation is preferable to characterizing stressors as medical or psychiatric, as the medical and psychiatric factors contributing to

Table 14-1. DSM-IV Diagnostic Criteria for Psychiatric Disorders Commonly Seen in Inflammatory Bowel Disease

MAJOR DEPRESSIVE EPISODE

A. Five or more of the following symptoms have been present during the same 2-week period and represent a change from previous functioning; at least 1 of the symptoms is either (1) depressed mood or (2) loss of interest or pleasure.

  1. Depressed mood most of the day, nearly every day. In children and adolescents, this may be irritable mood.

  2. Markedly diminished interest or pleasure in all activities most of the day, nearly every day.

  3. Significant weight loss when not dieting, weight gain, or change in appetite nearly every day.

  4. Insomnia or hypersomnia nearly every day.

  5. Psychomotor retardation or agitation nearly every day, observable by others.

  6. Fatigue or loss of energy nearly every day.

  7. Feelings of worthlessness or excessive or inappropriate guilt nearly every day.

  8. Diminished ability to think or concentrate, or indecisiveness, nearly every day.

  9. Recurrent thoughts of death, recurrent suicidal ideation without a specific plan, or a suicide attempt or a specific plan for committing suicide.

B. The symptoms cause clinically significant distress or impairment in social, occupational, or other areas of functioning.

C. The symptoms are not due to the direct physiologic effects of a substance (medications or drugs of abuse) or a general medical condition.

Adapted from American Psychiatric Association. Task Force on D-I. *Diagnostic and Statistical Manual of Mental Disorders: DSM-IV-TR*. Washington, DC: American Psychiatric Association; 2000.

IBD are closely intertwined. Whereas it is generally accepted that the innate biologic factors that worsen IBD are able to worsen psychological illness, there are data to suggest that problems with depression, anxiety, coping, or sleep worsen the course of IBD, thus creating a positive feedback loop.

Internal stressors include IBD activity, as well as innate physical and psychological factors, including their genetic underpinnings, that predispose one to developing psychopathology. An inflammatory response to illness may result in permanent changes to the autonomic (ANS) and enteric

Table 14-2. Generalized Anxiety Disorder

A.	Excessive anxiety and worry, occurring more days than not for at least 6 months, about a number of events or activities.
B.	The person finds it difficult to control the worry.
C.	The anxiety and worry are associated with 3 or more of the following symptoms for the last 6 months (on more days than not). Only one item is required in children.
	1. Restlessness or feeling keyed up or on edge
	2. Being easily fatigued
	3. Difficulty concentrating or mind going blank
	4. Irritability
	5. Muscle tension
	6. Sleep disturbance (difficulty falling asleep or staying asleep, or restless, unsatisfying sleep)
D.	The anxiety, worry, or physical symptoms cause clinically significant distress or impairment in social, occupational, or other important areas of functioning.
E.	The disturbance is not due to the direct physiologic effects of a substance (a drug of abuse or medication) or a general medical condition and does not occur exclusively during another psychiatric disorder.

Table 14-3. Pain Disorder

A.	Pain in one or more anatomical sites is the predominant focus of the clinical presentation and is of sufficient severity to warrant clinical attention.
B.	The pain causes significant distress or impairment in social, occupational, or other important areas of functioning.
C.	Psychological factors are judged to have an important role in the onset, severity, exacerbation, or maintenance of the pain.
D.	The symptom of deficit is not intentionally produced or feigned.
E.	The pain is not better accounted for by a mood, anxiety, or psychotic disorder.

Pain disorders are categorized into those that are associated with psychological factors, those associated with a general medical condition, and those associated with both psychological factors and a general medical condition.

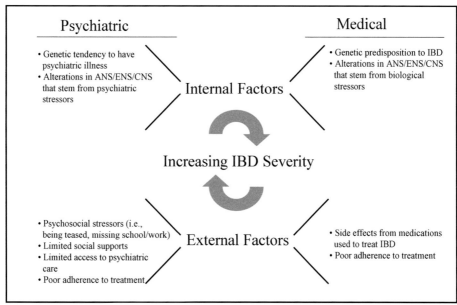

Figure 14-2. A representation of the positive feedback loop that exists between internal and external stressors. The buildup of stressors exacerbates IBD severity. The figure separates stressors into psychiatric as well as medical categories, but also separates them into internal and external stressors. Although these are arbitrary designations, this diagram illustrates the interactions between psychiatric, biologic, genetic, and social factors and emphasizes the notion that any of these factors may worsen the other, thereby worsening IBD. ANS = autonomic nervous system; CNS = central nervous system; ENS = enteric nervous system

nervous systems (ENS), thereby worsening gut function and abdominal pain. Concurrently, these inflammatory changes may induce or worsen psychiatric illness. Psychoneuroimmunology is in the early stages of attempting to elucidate the specifics of these cytokine-mediated effects on brain and body function.

External stressors include difficulties in the environment, early life adversity, social difficulties (including lack of adequate support systems), and ongoing life stressors. Such external stressors have also been associated with IBD-related inflammation and disease course.[7-9] Additionally, stress-induced maladaptive coping strategies or behaviors (eg, medication nonadherence) can adversely impact IBD-related outcomes and are categorized as external stressors, even though self-induced.

Internal Stress and IBD

Specific support for the relationship between internal stress and IBD comes from both animal models and human studies. Dysregulation in pathways linking the ANS, hypothalamic-pituitary-adrenal (HPA) axis, and the ENS in the gastrointestinal system[10] have been associated with IBD-related pathology.[6] The ENS is a component of the ANS, uniquely able to function independently of the central nervous system (CNS). However, it is exquisitely sensitive to the inflammatory changes common to IBD.[11] At the level of the ENS, inflammation-related changes in gut permeability may lead to diarrhea, while damage to nerve endings leads to visceral hyperalgesia and pseudo-obstruction. Research has shown that the underlying neurobiology involves hypertrophy and hyperplasia of neuronal cell fibers and cell bodies, axonal damage, and hyperplasia of glial cells in CD, and to a lesser extent in UC.[11,12] In addition to these hyperplastic changes, studies have shown that necrosis and neurodegeneration occur in the gastrointestinal tract in response to IBD.[13] It appears that inflammation in the gastrointestinal tract may cause a hyper-excitability of neurons, one that remains even after the inflammation resolves[11] and that may lead to permanent alterations in visceral sensitivity to distention stimuli (eg, rectal balloons).

In addition to inflammation, electrolyte imbalances secondary to diarrhea, anemia due to blood loss, and nutritional abnormalities due to malabsorption (eg, vitamin B_{12}) can stress patients with IBD and impact the nervous system-HPA-gastrointestinal axis. Changes in neurotransmitters localized in the ENS, including serotonin and catecholamines, have been implicated in IBD-related dysfunction in gastrointestinal motility and nociception.[14-17] In fact, the gastro-intestinal tract contains more serotonin than the brain, and this neurotrans-mitter has been implicated in many gastrointestinal processes.[18]

External Stress and Inflammatory Bowel Disease

There is growing evidence to support the role of psychological stress in the exacerbation of inflammation in animal models of colitis[19] and worsening IBD activity and relapse.[20-23] Proposed etiologies for this relationship include ANS dysfunction leading to inhibition of the vagal anti-inflammatory pathway, damage to the ENS due to chronic inflammation, and activation of cytokine cascades in the brain mimicking the increased levels of circulating proinflam-matory cytokines that are present in the gut.[24] Although UC appears to operate more through a Th2 pathway, and CD is more predominantly mediated by Th1 and the newly discovered Th17 pathways, cytokines released by each pathway have clear effects on the CNS. External psychological stress can also cause degranulation of mast cells locally in the gut, and this response is increased in patients with IBD, even when disease is in remission.[7]

In humans, many studies support the notion that adverse life events and perceived stress play a role in exacerbation of existing IBD activity and disease course,[25,26] although there is less support for such stress playing a causative role in IBD. This is controversial, however, and there are studies that do not support this relationship,[23,27,28] likely due to differences in how stress was measured and over what period of time. There also may be differences in how UC and CD respond to stress. Finally, there is some evidence in both rodent models of colitis and humans with IBD that early life stress and trauma may predispose to the development of IBD.[29,30]

In humans, psychological stress can take the form of anxiety and depression. The presence of depression in patients with IBD has also been shown to negatively impact IBD activity in most,[31-33] but not all studies.[34] In one study of patients with CD, depressed patients were less likely to respond to infliximab.[35] Finally, persistent abdominal pain in the absence of active IBD is another form of stress that has been associated with decreased quality of life in patients with IBD.[36]

EPIDEMIOLOGY OF PSYCHIATRIC ILLNESS IN IBD

The preponderance of data supports a correlation between increased psychiatric illness and IBD, both CD and UC. Furthermore, this correlation appears to be higher than that observed in other chronic illnesses, leading many to speculate that there is something intrinsic to IBD that lends itself to development of psychiatric symptoms. Of all mental illnesses, depressive disorders have been best characterized in IBD patients. Although the most severe symptoms result in the diagnosis of major depressive disorder (see Table 14-1), many patients are more mildly affected. Rates of depressive illness in IBD patients are variable, for reasons listed in the previous section, but studies seem to indicate a clear correlation between depressive disorders and IBD.

Although it is perhaps not surprising that patients with a chronic illness might have higher rates of psychiatric illness than healthy controls, multiple studies have compared IBD sufferers to patients with other chronic illnesses. The prevalence rates for depression in patients with IBD vary depending upon the study, but they are usually estimated at 25% to 35%,[6] approximately twice the lifetime prevalence in healthy individuals. Other studies have reported lifetime prevalence of psychiatric disorders as high as 65% in patients with IBD.[37] Epidemiologic studies have been performed in children and adolescents, and pediatric IBD patients seem to have more psychiatric illness than children with cystic fibrosis[38] or diabetes mellitus.[39]

Several studies have also shown a correlation between anxiety and IBD, although this does not seem to be as robust as the link between IBD and depression.[40,41] Although many patients do not meet criteria for generalized anxiety disorder, subsyndromal symptoms of anxiety may still be present and debilitating. In adolescents with IBD, anxiety symptoms have been shown to precede the diagnosis of IBD, while depression is most commonly diagnosed post-IBD, suggestive of different causal relationships between these psychological states and IBD.[42]

Although depressive disorders and anxiety disorders are the most commonly observed psychiatric illnesses in IBD sufferers,[43] other psychiatric comorbidities have been reported. Anxiety is extremely common, and it can manifest in several forms, including ruminative worrying, muscle tension, insomnia, or panic attacks. Suicidal ideation, narcotic dependence, and panic disorders have all been associated with IBD in adult populations.[44-47] In adolescents with IBD, eating disorders such as bulimia nervosa have also been reported after IBD onset, although causal associations remain to be determined.[48] Finally, comorbid functional pain disorders such as irritable bowel syndrome (IBS) can lead to iatrogenic opiate use, which in vulnerable patients can develop into narcotic dependence.[49] In hospitalized IBD patients, risk factors for narcotic use included having a psychiatric diagnosis, smoking, comorbid IBS, and previous IBD-related surgery.

CAVEATS IN DIAGNOSING PSYCHIATRIC DISORDERS IN INFLAMMATORY BOWEL DISEASE

Although numerous studies have been performed, certain caveats accompany many of the analyses of the epidemiology of psychiatric syndromes, limiting their generalizability. There are fewer objective criteria for diagnosing psychiatric illness (eg, blood tests, brain imaging), so these studies are dependent on more subjective patient-reported measures or clinician-reported measures. Many of these rating scales require the clinician to undergo costly and time-consuming training. There is a wide range of symptom severity, and the cutoffs for psychiatric illness differ by study. Often, there is no information about comparing severity scales with the criterion standard for psychiatric diagnosis, a structured psychiatric interview based on *Diagnostic and Statistical Manual of Mental Disorders* (DSM-IV) nosology.[50] In addition, some of the studies focus on IBD patients in remission, whereas others are performed in medically compromised patients, which can make comparisons between studies difficult. Certain studies include CD and UC together, but it is well known that, mechanistically, these are 2 separate illnesses. Finally, differences in IBD duration, course, or medical treatment regimens are often not accounted for. Therefore, it seems reasonable to suspect there may be multiple different mechanisms that lead to common psychiatric symptoms in each distinct IBD subtype.

According to DSM-IV criteria for major depression (see Table 14-1), symptoms may be designated as neurovegetative (changes in mood, sleep, appetite, concentration, energy, anhedonia) or neurocognitive (guilt, low self-esteem, suicidal ideation). The neurovegetative symptoms are consistent with cytokine-induced serum sickness,[51,52] but this may not be the complete etiologic explanation. For example, infliximab (anti-tumor necrosis factor [TNF]-α) infusion improved quality of life and depression in adults with CD but did not improve fatigue, suggesting that the molecular mechanisms driving psychiatric illness are extremely complex.[53]

Not every patient with mood or anxiety symptoms will meet criteria for a DSM-IV diagnosis, as there is a continuum of severity of psychiatric symptoms (see Figure 14-1). A significant percentage of patients with mild as well as severe symptoms will never actively seek psychiatric care, and this should be kept in mind when evaluating any patient with IBD. These symptoms impact quality of life, and the health care provider should probe for psychiatric illness.

ETIOLOGY AND PATHOPHYSIOLOGY OF PSYCHIATRIC CONDITIONS

It is likely that there are several different pathways that may lead to phenotypically similar depressive or anxiety disorders. Proinflammatory cytokines interleukin-1 (IL-1), IL-6, TNF-α in the periphery can signal across the blood-brain barrier to induce "serum sickness" in animals (fatigue, anhedonia, sleep disturbance, psychomotor retardation) and depression in humans.[54] The immune response that is the cornerstone of IBD is known to have effects on the CNS. Although it has not been shown specifically in IBD, it seems logical to suspect that high levels of cytokines induced in the gut mediate the psychiatric disturbances seen in IBD. Although IL-1, IL-6, and TNF-α are proinflammatory, there are anti-inflammatory cytokines as well (IL-4, IL-10), and the mechanisms by which serum sickness is induced are unclear. Although a few cytokines that may be transported across the blood-brain barrier have been mentioned here, this is by no means an exhaustive list.[55]

Dysautonomia is prominent in IBD and has been linked both to a decreased quality of life and an increase in health care utilization.[56] The parasympathetic nervous system is altered in chronic illness and modulates the immune response. Research has shown that sympathetic function is increased,[57] and parasympathetic nervous system function is decreased in patients with UC,[58] although they are unchanged compared to controls in patients with CD. These researchers also found that increased "personality-related anxiety" was correlated with worsening UC activity as well as decreased quality of life.[57] In addition, depression has been linked to autonomic dysfunction and systemic inflammation in other illnesses.[59,60]

Visceral pain is also associated with anxiety and depression in pediatric IBD and may represent another pathway to psychopathology.[61] Pain signals in the gut are transmitted centrally along spinal cord tracts where they synapse at numerous regions of the brain, including the hypothalamus, where they integrate emotional and visceral information.[62,63] A pediatric study has suggested that CD may induce lasting changes in the visceral nerves of the gut.[64] This visceral hypersensitivity persists even when CD is in remission, and it has been linked to functional abdominal pain as well as anxiety. A recent study in adults suggests that persistent pain in IBD patients in remission may be due to persistent microscopic inflammation detected only by fecal calprotectin, a highly sensitive marker of polymorphonuclear cell inflammation.[65] Changes in autonomic dysfunction and related persistent pain also may be due to chronic inflammation-related damage to peripheral nerves from nitric oxide or other free radicals.

In addition to pathways to psychopathology related to IBD, it is likely that a subset of patients have anxiety and depression as independent comorbidities due to the same underlying genetic or environmental factors (eg, trauma) that are seen in non-IBD cohorts. Future studies will need to identify different endophenotypes of various psychiatric disorders. Preliminary evidence has described changes in cortical brain metabolism in humans with IBD. In depressed adolescents with IBD, decreased activity on functional magnetic resonance imaging was observed in the anterior cingulate cortex and dorsolateral prefrontal cortex, regions of the brain associated with emotional regulation.[42]

MEDICATION-RELATED PSYCHOPATHOLOGY

Medications are a prominent part of treatment of IBD, and several are known or hypothesized to have effects on mental health. The major categories of medications used in IBD are aminosalicylates, antibiotics, corticosteroids, immunomodulators, and biologic agents. Many of these medications have limited psychiatric effects. On the other hand, corticosteroids are well known to have major effects on an array of psychiatric symptoms, including depression, anxiety, and psychosis. These data have been reviewed elsewhere,[66] but it appears that as many as 60% of patients on low-dose, long-term prednisone have developed symptoms of anxiety or depression.[67] In IBD, steroids have been found to be correlated with depressive disorders in children and adolescents as well as cognitive symptoms such as attention and memory.[68,69]

In terms of other classes of IBD-related medications, there are no data to date indicating a relationship between psychiatric symptoms and aminosalicylates or most antibiotics. There are 2 case reports of acute psychosis related to ciprofloxacin administration.[70,71]

The class of biologics used in IBD primarily consists of adalimumab, infliximab, certolizumab, and natalizumab. There is no significant evidence in the literature to suggest that this class of medications worsens depression or anxiety disorders. Indeed, one could hypothesize that these medications may be beneficial for psychiatric illness, as these medications inhibit the cytokine-mediated signaling pathways that are thought to be partially responsible for changes in mental status. This has been postulated, although the data to support this hypothesis are limited thus far.[72] Notably, the antidepressant bupropion (Wellbutrin) has been shown to have anti-TNF-α effects,[73,74] although the clinical relevance of this finding is unclear.

The relationship between immunomodulators and psychiatric illness is variable and complicated in certain instances, particularly with regard to tacrolimus or FK-506 (Prograf). As this drug modulates the HPA axis, which is known to have an effect on anxiety and depression, it is not surprising that this medication would have an impact on mental health. Tacrolimus acts specifically by binding to a chaperone for the glucocorticoid receptor, *FKBP5*.[75] Pharmacogenetic analysis has noted polymorphisms in this gene (*FKBP5*), and Brent et al found an increased risk of suicidality associated with certain polymorphisms.[76] This is thought to be due to increasing the subsensitivity of the glucocorticoid receptor, thereby underscoring the importance of the HPA axis on mental health.

On the other hand, 6-mercaptopurine and methotrexate seem to have minimal effect on psychiatric function. Anxiety and obsessive-compulsive disorder have been reported to occur as a result of azathioprine in a single case report,[77] but otherwise, it appears to be relatively free of psychiatric adverse effects.

SLEEP AND IBD

One issue that is often neglected in patients with IBD is that of sleep. Sleep is a prime example of the interface between the realms of medicine and psychiatry, and it is clear that both medical and psychiatric problems impact sleep. It is also fairly well accepted that sleep disturbances may exacerbate either psychiatric or medical illnesses. Studies suggest that alterations in sleep are present in inactive IBD,[78,79] and anecdotal reports suggest that sleep disruption is a prominent concern in patients with active IBD, whether secondary to nocturnal abdominal pain, diarrhea, or direct effects on sleep quality or cytoarchitecture. Regardless of the etiology, sleep disturbances are important to consider when addressing the mental health of IBD sufferers, given the adverse effects of poor sleep on both medical and psychiatric processes.

The relationship between sleep and immune function is quite complex, but it is clear that chronic sleep loss dysregulates immune function.[80] One current paradigm is that CD is largely mediated by T-helper (Th1) cellular immune system and Th17 cell types, whereas UC is more a consequence of T-helper (Th2) humoral immune system.[81,82] Each of these different T-cell lines secretes a different set of cytokines, which, in turn, exert differing effects on patient sleep patterns.

PAIN AND IBD

Even in the absence of IBD, patients with psychiatric illness are often more sensitive to pain, and functional abdominal pain is one of the most frustrating issues related to IBD, both for caregivers and patients. Up to 82% of adults[83] and 37% of children and adolescents with inactive IBD have persistent abdominal pain.[84] Long and Drossman recently suggested a biopsychosocial model linking a genetic predisposition both to sensitivity to life stressors via the HPA axis and to infection by altered bacterial flora, which induces abdominal pain.[36] This visceral pain signal can be further amplified by psychological distress or poor coping via CNS dysregulation. As mentioned previously, chronic abdominal pain has also been linked to narcotic use, which can worsen pain over time due to decreased gastric motility, nausea, and gastroparesis.[49]

HEALTH-RELATED QUALITY OF LIFE

Health-related quality of life has been the subject of study in many chronic illnesses, including IBD. Depression and anxiety have been correlated with lower quality of life in IBD. In 2002, Guthrie et al found that, in both UC and CD, the presence of a psychiatric condition was correlated with a lower health-related quality of life, independent of the severity of medical disease.[85] Several psychosocial factors have been identified as being risk factors for decreased quality of life. Being single, young, or having limited social support were all significant risk factors for perceiving a more severe impact of UC.[86] Other risk factors for perception of decreased quality of life in IBD include female gender,[87,88] African American race,[89] and belonging to a lower socioeconomic group.[90] In terms of personality styles, neuroticism has been found to correlate most closely with low health-related quality of life in IBD.[91] Interestingly, steroid dosage, anxiety, and depression were correlated with a decrease in health-related quality of life in patients with CD.[31]

COGNITIVE COPING STYLES

Certain patients have more effective coping mechanisms than others, and those who cope more effectively tend to function much better with a chronic illness such as IBD. The reasons for these differences in coping styles is the subject of much research, and it is difficult to predict which patients will be more resilient and adjust more easily to their diagnosis. Coping styles are critical in IBD, and it has been suggested that a depressive coping style is maladaptive. It has been more closely correlated with lower quality of life than any other factor, medical or psychosocial.[92] Maladaptive coping styles are marked by a tendency to blame oneself, avoidant behavior, and a lack of self-control. Perceptions of illness experience have also been shown to have impact on coping with IBD.[93] Kinash et al found that patients with IBD using emotion-focused coping strategies reported poorer quality of life than those using more problem-focused strategies.[94] Adult patients report numerous areas that are major concerns directly related to IBD, and these should be addressed by caregivers. The most common concerns reported by adults in an outpatient setting are the effects of medications, the possibility of having an ostomy bag, and the uncertain nature of IBD.[92] Most patients perceive a stigma that is associated with IBD, and this is associated with lower quality of life, more psychological distress, decreased self-esteem, and poorer adherence to treatment.[95]

Similarly, perceptions of illness have been studied in children and adolescents with IBD, and several disease-related themes emerged. These included seeing themselves as vulnerable and different from their healthy peers. Loss of control over their lives was frequently reported.[96] Another study found a feeling of damaged self as well as limited self-competence.[84] Shame and embarrassment about using public restrooms has been noted.[96] Although grief regarding IBD diagnosis has not been well characterized, it is another cognition that is pervasive among patients. Concerns about having an ostomy were noted in a study of 20 adolescents. Teens mentioned fears of humiliation that their diagnosis would be discovered by peers, guilt that they were monopolizing their family's time, and a loss of independence.[97]

Interestingly, the adolescents drew strength from family and social supports, and they appeared to adapt and develop appropriate coping skills over time. This is an important finding, suggesting that illness-related themes in adolescents are more easily repaired compared to the relatively fixed cognitions and behavioral repertoires of adults.

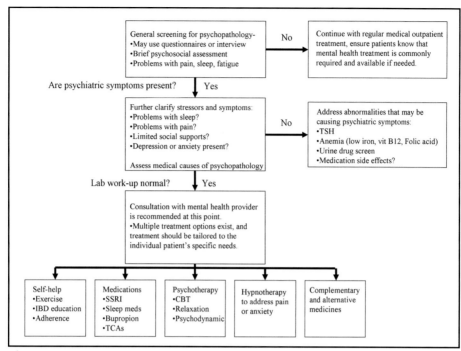

Figure 14-3. This algorithm is an example of how we would recommend assessing an IBD patient seen in the outpatient clinic. Work-up of patients includes psychiatric assessment, correction of laboratory abnormalities, consideration of potential medication side effects, and referral to a mental health provider if needed. Several options for treatment exist, and these options should be guided by patient preference, whenever possible. TSH = thyroid stimulating hormone; SSRI = selective serotonin reuptake inhibitor; TCA = tricyclic antidepressant; CBT = cognitive behavioral therapy

DIAGNOSTIC EVALUATION

Although there are objective clinical data that can measure the physical manifestations of IBD, this is not always the case for the psychiatric comorbidities of the illness. The goal of all mental health practitioners is to make psychiatric diagnosis less subjective and more standardized, and this has led to the institution of validated measures that assess multiple different mental health parameters (Figure 14-3). There are measures of depression, anxiety, quality of life, sleep, pain, and compliance with treatment. Although most of these questionnaires are patient reported, the majority have been validated statistically and are thought to be reliable measures of psychiatric symptoms. Many of these measures are quite simple and brief, and they may be given to patients in the waiting room,[69] thereby providing clinically relevant information to the physician in a very brief period of time.

As with any patient suffering from a mental illness, we recommend a thorough psychiatric evaluation, including laboratory markers. In addition to the diagnostic interview, basic laboratory work that is indicated includes a urine drug screen, thyroid stimulating hormone (TSH) to rule out thyroid abnormalities that may mimic depression or anxiety, a complete blood count with differential, and vitamin B_{12} and folic acid levels, particularly if there is concern about malabsorption or poor dietary habits. Anemia may be the result of a number of factors (poor diet, poor absorption, resection of bowel, blood loss). Iron deficiency has been suggested to have numerous psychiatric effects in IBD, including increased fatigue, poor cognitive function, and decreased quality of life.[98] A fasting lipid panel and glucose are also recommended, particularly if a patient is likely to be started on psychotropic medications. Although many of these values will be obtained during the regular care of a patient with IBD, these laboratory values are frequently affected by certain psychotropic medications; therefore, baseline levels are recommended.

Quality of life should be considered when evaluating any patient with IBD,[99] particularly when there are concerns about psychiatric comorbidities. The short and full-length[100] Inflammatory Bowel Disease Questionnaires (IBDQ) are commonly administered to assess quality of life in IBD patients. This is paralleled in the pediatric IBD population with the IMPACT-III quality of life assessment tool.[101] Evaluation of the patient's social support network as well as life stressors is critical, as this has been shown to be beneficial to his or her quality of life, as well as to his or her psychological distress.[102]

As depressive and anxiety disorders are often comorbid with IBD, it is worthwhile to regularly screen all patients for these illnesses. Although this may be determined with an unstructured interview, a number of validated screening tools may efficiently be employed. In adults, screens such as the Hamilton Depression or Anxiety Rating Scales, Beck Depression Inventory, Beck Anxiety Inventory, or McGill Pain Index may all provide useful information regarding psychiatric symptoms. In children, the Childhood Depression Inventory, Screen for Child Anxiety Related Emotional Disorders, or Pediatric Symptom Checklist are scales that can provide symptom information. Some of these are parent reported, and some of these scales are patient reported, but all may be useful, depending upon the situation. As with all clinical probes, it is important to make sure that questionnaires utilized require author permission or a fee or whether they are available in the public domain. The use of such objective measures allows for better screening for psychopathology, tracking of outcomes, and provides important data for insurance coverage for psychological assessments and treatment in this patient group. Interestingly, assessment of comorbid psychiatric symptoms in physical illness is a major focus of the National Institutes of Health, and they have recently implemented the Patient-Reported Outcomes Measurement Information System (PROMIS). PROMIS is a free resource that contains brief (4 to 8 items), well-validated screening tools that may be used to probe an array of symptoms, including depression, anxiety, sleep, fatigue, and pain.

If depression or other severe psychiatric disorders are suggested by either the clinical interaction or the scales obtained, the clinician should ask about suicidality. This should be done when alone with the patient, and the question should be asked in a nonjudgmental fashion. If the patient does endorse thoughts of self-harm, subsequent questions should focus on his or her plan, access to guns, and steps the patient may have already taken (writing a suicide note, making plans for family or pets, purchasing a weapon, etc). Depending upon the severity and intensity of the patient's thoughts, immediate referral to trained mental health providers or even involuntary hospitalization may be required.

Sleep concerns are often debilitating to patients with IBD, and there are a number of brief measures that can be used to assess sleep disorders. These include the Pittsburgh Sleep Quality Index (PSQI) and the Epworth Sleepiness Scale (ESS).[103,104] The PSQI identifies several domains that are often disturbed in patients with IBD.[42] These include difficulty falling asleep, pain, and the need for nighttime trips to the bathroom. The ESS is a measure of daytime sleepiness, which is not to be confused with fatigue, another common symptom reported by IBD sufferers. Sleep diaries are an effective way for patients to track sleep duration, awakenings, and sleep quality.

Finally, a thorough evaluation should also include an evaluation for substance abuse, especially opiates, cannabis, and alcohol. There are several brief screens available in the public domain on the National Institute on Drug Abuse Web site (www.nida.nih.gov/nidamed).

MANAGEMENT/TREATMENT

Most gastroenterologists who specialize in IBD are well aware that mental illnesses commonly occur in these patients. Even if the etiology is unclear, there is generally agreement that there is an unmet need for mental health care in this population. An optimal setting with which to care for IBD patients would include access to mental health practitioners, including psychiatrists, psychotherapists, and social workers who are skilled in dealing with the unique problems faced by this population.

Fortunately, there are a number of treatment options available, including several different types of psychotherapy, psychotropic medications, and support networks. Education about IBD has been shown to be important to patients, and this may be a useful adjunct to treatment.

SCHOOL INTERVENTIONS

For young people with IBD, school is a significant issue, and patients are often penalized due to their need to miss frequent amounts of class time. These children are often embarrassed by their illness, and they may be hypersensitive to criticism by teachers or peers. We recommend a 504 Plan to ensure that the school systems provide proper accommodations for patients with IBD. A 504 Plan is a federally mandated intervention that forces public schools to make individualized education plans for children who miss school due to illness or disability.[105] Frequent suggestions made in these plans include bathroom passes as needed and extra time to catch up on school work when time is missed due to physician appointments or hospitalizations. Teachers and school administrators often require education about the nature of IBD, and serving as a liaison between families and schools is often extremely useful in alleviating the anxiety and stress levels of pediatric patients.

EDUCATION REGARDING ILLNESS/SELF-MANAGEMENT/ ADHERENCE TO TREATMENT

Additionally, education about their disease is often beneficial for patients suffering from IBD. This is particularly critical for patients who are newly diagnosed, as they will need to make significant adjustment to a new chronic illness. Studies have shown that patients diagnosed with IBD often feel that they are not given enough information regarding the nature of their illness, and this has been shown to translate to the perception of poorer health.[106] A Canadian study showed that patients who received an educational intervention intended to teach them about IBD had greater satisfaction with their medical care.[107] This study also suggested that increased levels of education result in lower health care utilization costs, which has been replicated elsewhere.[108]

Adherence to medical treatment is a major barrier in IBD, one that is associated with enormous health care costs. Jackson et al recently published a systematic review of factors that contribute to poor adherence with oral medications.[109] They found that reported rates of nonadherence to treatment ranged between 7% and 72%, but the bulk of studies reported nonadherence rates in the range of 30% to 45%. They noted that psychiatric stressors were not always measured, but they were clearly associated with nonadherence to treatment in the studies in which they were assessed. The factors specifically associated with worsened adherence to treatment included depression,[110,111] anxiety,[110] and chronically perceived stress.[112] Conversely, a positive doctor-patient relationship was found to be protective against nonadherence to IBD therapy.[112]

SUPPORT GROUPS

Social support from other patients with IBD is thought to normalize the experience of having a chronic illness. Several studies have illustrated that both children and adults with IBD benefit from involvement in social networks that include other patients. Improved social support has been shown to improve quality of life in adults[113] as well as to enhance coping skills in children.[114] Another study followed female adolescents with IBD and their mothers as they participated in monthly support groups. Both the adolescent patients and their mothers found this intervention useful, and the patients' emotional and social functioning improved as measured by the IMPACT-III.[115]

PSYCHOTHERAPY

Cognitive-Behavioral Therapy

Psychotherapy can be a very useful tool for many patients suffering from chronic illnesses, and it comes in many different forms. Cognitive-behavioral therapy (CBT) has been the best-studied therapeutic modality and has shown a great deal of promise in patients with chronic illnesses, including IBD. The premise of CBT involves teaching the patients to recognize their negative and distorted thought processes. They subsequently learn to challenge these maladaptive thoughts and beliefs. By continually recognizing and challenging these negative thoughts, patients will modify their autonomic negative thoughts, which are prevalent in depressive and anxiety disorders.

One of the benefits of CBT is that it may be tailored to fit the needs of the individual. In the case of patients with IBD, illness-related problems may be targeted. For instance, many IBD sufferers note extreme anxiety about leaving home or being in social situations for fear that they will need to access a bathroom. Or, they may become extremely depressed, feeling as though they have a loss of control in their lives due to illness. This may cause them to become disinterested in medication compliance, feeling as though it makes little difference whether they regularly take their medications or not. These are all maladaptive thought processes that can result in worsening mental health and quality of life. CBT encourages IBD patients to challenge these negative ideas, examining the evidence for and against them. CBT can be extremely beneficial, although it requires a fairly large time investment on the part of the patient, as well as several sessions with a skilled therapist.

The efficacy of CBT in IBD has been studied on numerous occasions, primarily in adults. Several groups have incorporated CBT, relaxation techniques, coping strategies, and psychoeducation into studies of patients with IBD. Milne et al found that stress management groups were effective in decreasing disease activity (as measured by the Crohn's Disease Activity Index [CDAI]) and stress levels.[116] This is in contrast to the work of Mussell et al, which did not show any change in CDAI in patients with IBD who underwent CBT.[117] This group did find gender differences in response to psychotherapy, with females showing an improvement in depressive coping styles that was not seen in males. In 2004, a cohort of adult CD patients was assigned to receive either stress management or treatment as usual.[118] This study determined that stress management improved abdominal pain, constipation, and fatigue, but they did not assess disease activity, mood symptoms, or quality of life. These improvements persisted 1 year post-treatment. A Spanish group showed improvement in depressive and anxious symptoms in adult IBD patients who received group intervention consisting of CBT teaching along with social and coping skills training.[119] A more recent retrospective study compared the disease course of adult IBD patients who underwent CBT with IBD patients receiving treatment as usual.[120] This study found that CBT improved psychological functioning and was correlated with fewer relapses of IBD in the following year.

The work of Szigethy and colleagues has clearly illustrated that depressed adolescents with IBD respond to CBT, with significant improvements in depression and feeling more control over their illness.[68,121] Additionally, the benefits of CBT in patients with chronic illness persist at 1 year postpsychotherapy.[122] In depressed adolescents with IBD, CBT was modified to include incorporation of an illness narrative (eg, patient's illness experience, sense of control over IBD, and coping strategies utilized) as part of the CBT behavioral and cognitive skills being taught. Not only did the resultant 8- to 12-week intervention lead to improvement in depression and global functioning compared to treatment as usual, these results persisted up to 1 year.[123] These results are promising but need to be replicated in larger samples and compared to other active treatment for depression.

Psychodynamic Psychotherapy for Inflammatory Bowel Disease

Psychodynamic psychotherapy focuses upon examining interpersonal relations and attempts to repair insecure attachment styles. This school of therapy is based in psychoanalysis, and there are a few groups that have looked at the impact of this type of therapy on IBD patients. The results of these studies are not particularly impressive, although some benefits have been noted. A study from 1964 in UC patients suggested that psychodynamic psychotherapy for as long as 2 years had some improvement in symptoms, but these were nonvalidated measures that were not statistically driven.[124] A German group examined the effect of psychodynamic psychotherapy on CD patients over a 1-year period. They found no difference in depressive symptoms, disease activity, or quality of life in these patients,[125,126] but the therapy did decrease the number of hospital-days over the following year.[127] Finally, a Canadian group analyzed the impact of a group intervention that used supportive-expressive psychotherapy to treat IBD patients.[128] Although there was an improvement in coping styles, there was no improvement in depressive or anxious symptoms, and disease symptoms were also unchanged. These studies are more thoroughly reviewed elsewhere.[6]

Exercise

Exercise is well known to be associated with improved quality of life and better physical and mental health in the general population. However, it is less clear how this applies to patients with IBD. One group looked at the benefits of a low-impact exercise program on patients with inactive CD.[129] They found improvements in psychological and physical health, and the activity was not associated with relapse of illness. Since that time, low-impact activity has been linked with improvements in IBDQ scores, disease activity, and stress levels.[130] A 2008 review examined the link between physical activity and IBD.[131] The authors concluded that exercise has no effect on delaying or hastening onset of IBD; however, exercise may ameliorate some of the extraintestinal manifestations of IBD. Specific areas where improvement may occur include ankylosing spondylitis, osteoporosis, mental stress, and even enhancing the immune system. Although the data are fairly limited, it seems safe to suggest that IBD patients who are able and motivated will benefit from a regular exercise regimen, particularly in terms of stress management.

Hypnosis

Another form of therapy that has shown a great deal of promise in IBD is hypnosis. This technique may be extremely useful in targeting abdominal pain, as well as anxiety, both of which can be quite debilitating in IBD. Szigethy et al reviewed the usage of hypnosis in both adults and children with IBD, and the data are overwhelmingly positive.[84] Most of the data have come from studies of patients with IBS, but several groups are providing impressive data in support of its usage in children[132] and adults.[133,134] Regardless of whether hypnotherapy is used to treat IBD or IBS, certain common findings have emerged. The dose of treatment is important to efficacy, and sessions must be tailored to support the needs of the individual. Perhaps most impressively, the benefits of hypnosis are sustained as much as 6 years post-treatment.

Adults with active UC were treated with gut-directed hypnotherapy, and a single 50-minute session decreased several inflammatory markers, including the release of substance P, histamine, and IL-13 from rectal mucosa. Rectal blood flow was also decreased, as was serum IL-6 concentration.[135] Another group found a significant increase in quality of life scores in females with inactive IBD who underwent hypnotherapy.[136] Changes in autonomic or inflammatory variables were not correlated with hypnotizability or changes in psychological stressors.

Another study looked at patients with severe IBD and found an excellent response to gut-focused hypnotherapy.[137] Fifteen patients with IBD received 12 sessions of hypnosis and were followed for 5 years. Although there was a range of responses in the cohort that was tested, 80% of patients were found to have good or excellent quality of life at 5 years, and their corticosteroid requirement was significantly decreased. Only 2 of 15 patients in the sample required surgery during the 5-year interval.

Complementary and Alternative Medicines

Hilsden et al have published numerous papers showing that complementary and alternative medicine (CAM) usage is quite common in IBD patients in North America and Europe.[138-142] In their definition, CAM includes homeopathy, acupuncture, herbal and dietary supplements, meditation, and prayer. They report that the percentage of patients that currently use CAM ranges from 11% to 34%. When looking at lifetime prevalence, the values increase to 21% to 60% of all IBD patients.[142] The most common reason given by patients for using CAM is that it provides a greater feeling of control over their IBD. As stated elsewhere, this feeling of empowerment and control over illness can be extremely beneficial for mental health.

One technique that has been studied in IBD patients is acupuncture. A recent review points out several small randomized controlled trials that suggest acupuncture decreases disease activity in CD and UC.[143] The comparison groups received sham-acupuncture, implying that the placebo effect is insufficient to explain the improvement. Regardless of how much credence one lends to CAM, it is important to recognize that patients will frequently use it; thus, it is important to be well versed in these topics.

Psychotropic Medications

Medications are often used to treat psychiatric symptoms that are not adequately responsive to psychotherapy. There are a number of reasons why psychiatric symptoms might not remit with psychotherapy alone. These include disinterest on the part of the patient, lack of enough resources to give the patient a full trial of therapy, and on occasion, a patient may be so impaired by mental illness that he or she may be unable to participate in psychotherapy. In these cases, selective serotonin reuptake inhibitors (SSRIs) are used as first-line treatment. These medications are often very effective in targeting symptoms of depression and anxiety. As pain in the gut is modulated through serotonin receptors, SSRIs often have the additional benefit of downregulating pain pathways. Caution is encouraged when considering addition of a psychotropic medication, as there are numerous drug-drug interactions that must be considered, particularly in medically complex patients that are often on a large number of medications. Ciprofloxacin is a strong inhibitor of several cytochrome P450 enzymes in the liver, and many psychotropic medications are substrates of these enzymes. Conversely, many antidepressant medications are strong inhibitors of other cytochrome P450 isoforms, emphasizing the need to be cautious when selecting medications.

Citalopram (Celexa) is very well tolerated, and this is a first-line choice when treating IBD-related psychopathology, particularly in children. There are some data indicating that citalopram is useful in children with IBS or functional abdominal pain,[144,145] although a more recent study contradicts this finding.[146] Overall, citalopram may be a useful medication for both children and adults, and it seems to be accompanied by relatively few side effects. As with most SSRIs, the majority of side effects that occur are usually transient. These include diarrhea or constipation, insomnia, headache, or hidrosis. Despite the tendency to cause insomnia briefly, citalopram is a mild antihistamine, and it may result in some sedation in the long term, thus requiring that it be given at night. The most troubling long-term side effect is decreased libido in both genders.

Paroxetine (Paxil) has some data supporting its usage in IBD as well, although these studies are quite limited.[147] Although the results were positive in the largest trial of patients with IBD,[148] this study was open label, including only 8 patients. However in a double-blinded study of patients receiving interferon-α for malignant melanoma, paroxetine was shown to be protective against development of depressive symptoms.[149] Since interferon-α is present and part of the immune response in IBD, paroxetine may be a useful medication for IBD as well.

Sertraline (Zoloft) is an SSRI that has not been reported upon in patients with IBD. It is commonly used to target depression and anxiety, although the data for its usage in chronic illness are not impressive. A large, randomized-controlled double-blinded trial in patients with heart failure showed no improvement in either depression or heart failure with sertraline.[150] A case report describes the successful usage of sertraline to treat an adolescent boy with psychosis and depression induced by long-term steroid usage.[151]

Although SSRIs have become the mainstay of psychiatric treatment, there are other antidepressant medications that may be particularly effective in certain situations. Bupropion (Wellbutrin) is a medication that functions through a number of different neurotransmitters, and it is often efficacious as an adjunct for depressive disorders. There are reports that it has TNF-α inhibitory activity,[73,74] making it an intriguing candidate for use in IBD. Kast et al have been firm proponents of bupropion in IBD, showing an improved course of IBD,[152] as well as an increase in bone density in patients with CD.[153] Although it is not particularly effective in treating anxiety disorders, it is usually well tolerated. Mirtazapine (Remeron) also seems to be well tolerated. Although it can be somnogenic and increase appetite, these side effects may be beneficial in patients with chronic gastrointestinal problems and sleep alterations. However, it has been noted that mirtazapine increases circulating levels of TNF-α, thus it has been suggested to be a second-line treatment in patients with IBD.[152]

Medications such as mood stabilizers and antipsychotics are utilized relatively infrequently in the IBD population. Mood stabilizers have been effective for abdominal pain secondary to abdominal migraines, while antipsychotics have been used for steroid-induced psychosis or mania, as well as disease-related delirium. Side effects of both mood stabilizers and antipsychotics include increased appetite, weight gain, and sedation. Whereas in the general population this is not often a desired outcome, in patients suffering from IBD, these may be beneficial. Consultation with a psychiatrist is indicated if these medications are being considered, particularly since many of these medications do not have approval from the Food and Drug Administration for use in medically ill populations and require careful monitoring for serious side effects, including suicidality and agitation.

Sleep Treatments

Since sleep is so frequently disrupted in IBD sufferers, we strongly encourage asking directly about patient sleep problems. There are numerous etiologies for sleep disturbance in this population. Problems with sleep may be a result of need for nighttime bowel movements, medications, pain, or autonomic dysfunction. Sleep-disordered breathing is always a consideration as well, particularly in an overweight individual. On the other hand, there is an expanding literature to suggest a bidirectional relationship between circadian rhythms and the immune system.[154] If sleep is an issue, both medical and behavioral options for treatment exist. In all patients, sleep habits should be reviewed in detail, and there are often behavioral changes that alone may be effective in improving sleep. When the diagnosis is unclear, referral to a sleep specialist for further assessment is indicated.

In all situations, behavioral changes are recommended prior to using medications. For instance, patients are encouraged to avoid daytime napping or vigorous exercise before bedtime and limit caffeine intake, particularly late in the day. Patients should be encouraged to avoid using their bed for activities other than sex and sleep. These alterations are often extremely effective; however, patients often struggle due to the difficulty of making broad lifestyle changes.

CBT has been shown to have outstanding efficacy in treating sleep disorders in several different populations and studies. In particular, CBT for insomnia has been demonstrated to have a great deal of utility in patients with medical and psychiatric comorbidities.[155]

In terms of medications used for sleep in IBD patients, the options are essentially the same as those in healthy individuals. The choice depends upon the type of sleep problem, the severity of symptoms, and the comfort of the prescriber with each type of medication. We would encourage providers who are uncomfortable treating sleep problems with medications to refer to a specialist in sleep disorders. Unfortunately, there is very little information about the use of these medications in treating patients with IBD. Trazodone (Desyrel) is a weak antidepressant that also has significant antihistaminic effects, making it similar to medications such as diphenhydramine (Benadryl), which can be useful in induction of sleep. Although these medications are usually well tolerated, they can have side effects including oversedation and weight gain. A second option is the nonbenzodiazepine medications such as zolpidem (Ambien) or eszopiclone (Lunesta). These medications may be quite useful, although opinions vary regarding their addictive potential.

When circadian rhythms become disrupted, melatonin may be a useful adjunctive treatment to try to normalize sleep onset. This medication is available over the counter; however, there is little information about melatonin usage in IBD patients. What evidence does exist is fairly mixed,[156] although animal studies suggest that melatonin may have some anti-inflammatory properties in the gut.[157-159] Melatonin is an interesting medication in that it possesses both inflammatory as well as anti-inflammatory properties.[160] There are other medications that may be useful in certain situations, particularly when comorbid psychiatric illness is present. Mirtazapine (Remeron) is a very sedating antidepressant, and it is often beneficial in treating depressive disorders mixed with insomnia. Other options in more complicated situations include the atypical antipsychotics, tricyclic antidepressants (TCAs), and monoamine oxidase inhibitors. All of these are somnogenic medications that have their uses in the management of psychiatric disorders in patients with IBD, but they are beyond the scope of this chapter. For daytime fatigue, modafinil (Provigil) or stimulant medications can be helpful for some patients, but patients need to be monitored for appetite suppression.

Restless legs syndrome (RLS) is another sleep disorder that may be comorbid with depression and anxiety. The diagnosis of RLS is made clinically,[161] and patients with this disorder have significant sleep disruption. A recent association was reported between CD and RLS, and it is thought that this occurs as a result of iron deficiency secondary to blood loss and malabsorption of iron.[162] As RLS is a condition that disrupts sleep and has been associated with mood disorders[163] and CD, it is important to screen for it in adult and pediatric patients. First-line treatment of RLS usually includes iron replacement therapy and dopamine agonists.[164] Other options for therapy include gabapentin (Neurontin) and pregabalin (Lyrica), medications that are often useful for managing neuropathic pain.

Pain Management

Functional abdominal pain is an extremely challenging problem for virtually all gastroenterologists, both in the pediatric and adult settings. Narcotics are not recommended due to their slowing of gastrointestinal transit time as well as their addictive potential; thus, alternative means of pain management are necessary. Most of the options for treating pain have been discussed previously and could be considered variants of the management techniques discussed previously. These include CBT to teach distraction strategies, cognitive reframing of pain, hypnotherapy, and relaxation techniques.

CBT has been used successfully in numerous studies of patients with abdominal pain. Although it has not been well studied in patients with IBD, a large amount of data have been obtained in patients with IBS. In 2006, a study showed that CBT taught by nurses was effective at managing symptoms of IBD, and these improvements persisted after 12 months.[165] Unfortunately, this intervention is not cost effective due to the number of staff required.[166] Recently, a self-administered CBT was tested in patients with IBS, and this intervention was found to be quite effective in decreasing symptoms of IBS.[167] Studies by Sanders et al in pediatric patients with recurrent abdominal pain have shown CBT to be quite effective in managing pain, with benefits persisting 12 months post-treatment.[168,169]

Regarding pharmacologic treatment of functional abdominal pain, lowdose SSRIs and TCAs have most support in adults with IBS.[144,170,171] Of the TCAs, desipramine has the most empirical evidence for efficacy and is least associated with sedation and constipation. Of the SSRI medications, citalopram, fluoxetine, and sertraline have the most support for efficacy. In a recent review of psychological therapies and antidepressants for IBS, CBT and antidepressants showed the greatest efficacy.[172]

CONCLUSION

Either IBD or psychiatric illness may be debilitating, and in combination, the level of impairment may be even more severe. Each of these illnesses results in very high medical utilization and financial expenditure, and IBD and psychiatric illness are frequently comorbid with one another. It has been clearly illustrated that IBD is an illness in which medical complications exacerbate psychiatric comorbidities. However, accumulating data are showing that psychiatric comorbidities worsen the medical complications of IBD in a significant number of patients. Therefore, we would argue that effective treatment of IBD requires addressing both the physical and psychiatric issues concurrently. It is important to screen for and aggressively treat comorbid mental illness as part of comprehensive medical care of IBD. The causes for individual differences in psychiatric comorbidities are unclear and are the subject of genetic research, just as they are in IBD. Individualized psychiatric treatments integrated within a medical treatment regimen reduce stigma, improve adherence to treatment, and ultimately decrease patient suffering.

☑ Key Points

- ☑ IBD is clearly associated with increased rates of psychiatric illness in certain subgroups of patients, and psychiatric illness impacts quality of life in patients suffering from this chronic medical illness.

- ☑ Psychiatric factors and medical issues seem to exacerbate one another in a bidirectional fashion in patients suffering with IBD.

- ☑ Patients with IBD should be screened for psychiatric symptoms using simple tools when presenting to clinic visits. Problems with mood, anxiety, and sleep are easily assessed using basic instruments or clinical interview.

- ☑ Psychiatric treatment has been shown to be very effective in improving quality of life and psychiatric symptoms in patients with IBD and comorbid psychiatric illness.

- ☑ In many patients with IBD, the optimal treatment situation requires the gastroenterologist to have access to a mental health professional who is well-versed in working with patients with chronic illnesses.

REFERENCES

1. Abraham C, Cho JH. Inflammatory bowel disease. *N Engl J Med.* 2009;361(21):2066-2078.
2. Szigethy E, McLafferty L, Goyal A. Inflammatory bowel disease. *Child Adolesc Psychiatr Clin North Am.* 2010;19(2):301-318, ix.
3. Hanauer SB. Inflammatory bowel disease: epidemiology, pathogenesis, and therapeutic opportunities. *Inflamm Bowel Dis.* 2006;12(suppl 1):S3-S9.
4. Malaty HM, Fan X, Opekun AR, Thibodeaux C, Ferry GD. Rising incidence of inflammatory bowel disease among children: a 12-year study. *J Pediatr Gastroenterol Nutr.* 2010;50(1): 27-31.

5. Ahuja V, Tandon RK. Inflammatory bowel disease in the Asia-Pacific area: a comparison with developed countries and regional differences. *J Dig Dis.* 2010;11(3):134-147.

6. Goodhand J, Wahed M, Rampton D. Management of stress in inflammatory bowel disease: a therapeutic option? *Expert Rev Gastroenterol Hepatol.* 2009;3(6):661-679.

7. Farhadi A, Keshavarzian A, Van de Kar L, et al. Heightened responses to stressors in patients with inflammatory bowel disease. *Am J Gastroenterol.* 2005;100(8):1796-1804.

8. Maunder RG, Greenberg GR, Nolan RP, Lancee WJ, Steinhart AH, Hunter JJ. Autonomic response to standardized stress predicts subsequent disease activity in ulcerative colitis. *Eur J Gastroenterol Hepatol.* 2006;18(4):413-420.

9. Mawdsley JE, Macey MG, Feakins RM, Langmead L, Rampton DS. The effect of acute psychologic stress on systemic and rectal mucosal measures of inflammation in ulcerative colitis. *Gastroenterology.* 2006;131(2):410-419.

10. Glaser R, Kiecolt-Glaser JK. Stress-induced immune dysfunction: implications for health. *Nat Rev Immunol.* 2005;5(3):243-251.

11. Lakhan SE, Kirchgessner A. Neuroinflammation in inflammatory bowel disease. *J Neuroinflammation.* 2010;7:37.

12. Geboes K, Collins S. Structural abnormalities of the nervous system in Crohn's disease and ulcerative colitis. *Neurogastroenterol Motil.* 1998;10(3):189-202.

13. Vasina V, Barbara G, Talamonti L, et al. Enteric neuroplasticity evoked by inflammation. *Auton Neurosci.* 2006;126-127:264-272.

14. Forrest CM, Gould SR, Darlington LG, Stone TW. Levels of purine, kynurenine and lipid peroxidation products in patients with inflammatory bowel disease. *Adv Exp Med Biol.* 2003;527:395-400.

15. Coates MD, Johnson AC, Greenwood-Van Meerveld B, Mawe GM. Effects of serotonin transporter inhibition on gastrointestinal motility and colonic sensitivity in the mouse. *Neurogastroenterol Motil.* 2006;18(6):464-471.

16. Wolf AM, Wolf D, Rumpold H, et al. Overexpression of indoleamine 2,3-dioxygenase in human inflammatory bowel disease. *Clin Immunol.* 2004;113(1):47-55.

17. Gershon MD, Tack J. The serotonin signaling system: from basic understanding to drug development for functional GI disorders. *Gastroenterology.* 2007;132(1):397-414.

18. Targan SR, Karp LC. Defects in mucosal immunity leading to ulcerative colitis. *Immunol Rev.* 2005;206:296-305.

19. Qiu BS, Vallance BA, Blennerhassett PA, Collins SM. The role of CD4+ lymphocytes in the susceptibility of mice to stress-induced reactivation of experimental colitis. *Nat Med.* 1999;5(10):1178-1182.

20. Bernstein CN, Walker JR, Graff LA. On studying the connection between stress and IBD. *Am J Gastroenterol.* 2006;101(4):782-785.

21. Maunder RG, Levenstein S. The role of stress in the development and clinical course of inflammatory bowel disease: epidemiological evidence. *Curr Mol Med.* 2008;8(4):247-252.

22. North CS, Alpers DH. A review of studies of psychiatric factors in Crohn's disease: etiologic implications. *Ann Clin Psychiatry.* 1994;6(2):117-124.

23. North CS, Alpers DH, Helzer JE, Spitznagel EL, Clouse RE. Do life events or depression exacerbate inflammatory bowel disease? A prospective study. *Ann Intern Med.* 1991;114(5):381-386.

24. Ghia JE, Blennerhassett P, Deng Y, Verdu EF, Khan WI, Collins SM. Reactivation of inflammatory bowel disease in a mouse model of depression. *Gastroenterology.* 2009;136(7):2280-2288, e2281-e2284.

25. Duffy L, Zielezny M, Marshall J, et al. Relevance of major stress events as an indicator of disease activity prevalence in inflammatory bowel disease. *Behav Med.* 1991;17(3):101-110.

26. Levenstein S, Prantera C, Varvo V, et al. Stress and exacerbation in ulcerative colitis: a prospective study of patients enrolled in remission. *Am J Gastroenterol.* 2000;95(5):1213-1220.

27. Riley S, Mani V, Goodman M, Lucas S. Why do patients with ulcerative colitis relapse? *Gut.* 1990;31(2):179-183.

28. Vidal A, Gómez-Gil E, Sans M, et al. Life events and inflammatory bowel disease relapse: a prospective study of patients enrolled in remission. *Am J Gastroenterol.* 2006;101(4):775-781.

29. Agostini A, Rizzello F, Ravegnani G, et al. Parental bonding and inflammatory bowel disease. *Psychosomatics.* 2010;51(1):14-21.

30. Gue M, Bonbonne C, Fioramonti J, et al. Stress-induced enhancement of colitis in rats: CRF and arginine vasopressin are not involved. *Am J Physiol.* 1997;272(1 pt 1):G84-G91.

31. Bitton A, Dobkin P, Edwardes M, et al. Predicting relapse in Crohn's disease: a biopsycho-social model. *Gut.* 2008;57(10):1386-1392.

32. Mardini H, Kip K, Wilson J. Crohn's disease: a two-year prospective study of the association between psychological distress and disease activity. *Dig Dis Sci.* 2004;49(3):492-497.

33. Mittermaier C, Dejaco C, Waldhoer T, et al. Impact of depressive mood on relapse in patients with inflammatory bowel disease: a prospective 18-month follow-up study. *Psychosom Med.* 2004;66(1):79-84.

34. Mikocka-Walus A, Turnbull D, Andrews JM, Moulding N, Wilson I, Holtmann G. Psychogastroenterology: a call for psychological input in Australian gastroenterology clinics. *Intern Med J.* 2009;39(2):127-130.

35. Persoons P, Vermeire S, Demyttenaere K, et al. The impact of major depressive disorder on the short- and long-term outcome of Crohn's disease treatment with infliximab. *Aliment Pharmacol Ther.* 2005;22(2):101-110.

36. Long MD, Drossman DA. Inflammatory bowel disease, irritable bowel syndrome, or what?: a challenge to the functional-organic dichotomy. *Am J Gastroenterol.* 2010;105(8):1796-1798.

37. Walker EA, Gelfand MD, Gelfand AN, Creed F, Katon WJ. The relationship of current psychiatric disorder to functional disability and distress in patients with inflammatory bowel disease. *Gen Hosp Psychiatry.* 1996;18(4):220-229.

38. Burke P, Meyer V, Kocoshis S, et al. Depression and anxiety in pediatric inflammatory bowel disease and cystic fibrosis. *J Am Acad Child Adolesc Psychiatry.* 1989;28(6):948-951.

39. Engstrom I. Mental health and psychological functioning in children and adolescents with inflammatory bowel disease: a comparison with children having other chronic illnesses and with healthy children. *J Child Psychol Psychiatry.* 1992;33(3):563-582.

40. Kurina LM, Goldacre MJ, Yeates D, Gill LE. Depression and anxiety in people with inflammatory bowel disease. *J Epidemiol Community Health.* 2001;55(10):716-720.

41. Lerebours E, Gower-Rousseau C, Merle V, et al. Stressful life events as a risk factor for inflammatory bowel disease onset: a population-based case-control study. *Am J Gastroenterol.* 2007;102(1):122-131.

42. Benhayon D, Binion DG, Regueiro M, et al. Characterization of sleep in a pediatric population with inflammatory bowel disease and depression. *Gastroenterology.* 2011;140(5, suppl 1): S-506-S-507.

43. Arfaoui D, Elloumi H, Debbebi W, Bel Hadj Ali N, Ajmi S. Psychological disorder associated to inflammatory bowel disease. *Tunis Med.* 2007;85(3):189-191.

44. Addolorato G, Capristo E, Stefanini G, Gasbarrini G. Inflammatory bowel disease: a study of the association between anxiety and depression, physical morbidity, and nutritional status. *Scand J Gastroenterol.* 1997;32(10):1013-1021.

45. Tarter R, Switala J, Carra J, Edwards K, Van Thiel D. Inflammatory bowel disease: psychiatric status of patients before and after disease onset. *Int J Psychiatry Med.* 1987;17(2):173-181.

46. Kaplan M, Korelitz B. Narcotic dependence in inflammatory bowel disease. *J Clin Gastroenterol.* 1988;10(3):275-278.

47. Fuller-Thomson E, Sulman J. Depression and inflammatory bowel disease: findings from two nationally representative Canadian surveys. *Inflamm Bowel Dis.* 2006;12(8):697-707.

48. Szigethy E. Therapy for the brain and gut. *J Psychiatr Pract.* 2005;11(1):51-53.

49. Long MD, Barnes EL, Herfarth HH, Drossman DA. Narcotic use for inflammatory bowel disease and risk factors during hospitalization. *Inflamm Bowel Dis.* 2012;18(5):869-876.

50. American Psychiatric Association. Task Force on D-I. *Diagnostic and Statistical Manual of Mental Disorders: DSM-IV-TR.* Washington, DC: American Psychiatric Association; 2000.

51. Maier SF, Watkins LR. Cytokines for psychologists: implications of bidirectional immune-to-brain communication for understanding behavior, mood, and cognition. *Psychol Rev.* 1998;105(1):83-107.

52. Yirmiya R, Pollak Y, Morag M, et al. Illness, cytokines, and depression. *Ann N Y Acad Sci.* 2000;917:478-487.

53. Minderhoud IM, Samsom M, Oldenburg B. Crohn's disease, fatigue, and infliximab: is there a role for cytokines in the pathogenesis of fatigue? *World J Gastroenterol.* 2007;13(14):2089-2093.

54. Aubert A, Vega C, Dantzer R, Goodall G. Pyrogens specifically disrupt the acquisition of a task involving cognitive processing in the rat. *Brain Behav Immun.* 1995;9(2):129-148.

55. Banks WA. The blood-brain barrier in psychoneuroimmunology. *Neurol Clin.* 2006;24(3):413-419.

56. Ananthakrishnan AN, Issa M, Barboi A, et al. Impact of autonomic dysfunction on inflammatory bowel disease. *J Clin Gastroenterol.* 2010;44(4):272-279.

57. Ganguli S, Kamath M, Redmond K, et al. A comparison of autonomic function in patients with inflammatory bowel disease and in healthy controls. *Neurogastroenterol Motil.* 2007;19(12):961-967.

58. Sharma P, Makharia G, Ahuja V, Dwivedi S, Deepak K. Autonomic dysfunctions in patients with inflammatory bowel disease in clinical remission. *Dig Dis Sci.* 2009;54(4):853-861.

59. Kamphuis MH, Geerlings MI, Dekker JM, et al. Autonomic dysfunction: a link between depression and cardiovascular mortality? The FINE Study. *Eur J Cardiovasc Prev Rehabil.* 2007;14(6):796-802.

60. Pizzi C, Manzoli L, Mancini S, Costa GM. Analysis of potential predictors of depression among coronary heart disease risk factors including heart rate variability, markers of inflammation, and endothelial function. *Eur Heart J.* 2008;29(9):1110-1117.

61. Srinath AI, Goyal A, Keljo DJ, Binion DG, Szigethy E. Predictors of abdominal pain in depressed pediatric Crohn's disease patients. *Gastroenterology.* 2011;140(5):S91.

62. Drossman DA. Functional abdominal pain syndrome. *Clin Gastroenterol Hepatol.* 2004;2(5):353-365.

63. Jones MP, Dilley JB, Drossman D, Crowell MD. Brain-gut connections in functional GI disorders: anatomic and physiologic relationships. *Neurogastroenterol Motil.* 2006;18(2):91-103.

64. Faure C, Giguere L. Functional gastrointestinal disorders and visceral hypersensitivity in children and adolescents suffering from Crohn's disease. *Inflamm Bowel Dis.* 2008;14(11):1569-1574.

65. Keohane J, O'Mahony C, O'Mahony L, O'Mahony S, Quigley EM, Shanahan F. Irritable bowel syndrome-type symptoms in patients with inflammatory bowel disease: association or reflection of occult inflammation? *Am J Gastroenterol.* 2010;105(8):1788-1794; quiz 1795.

66. Graff LA, Walker JR, Bernstein CN. Depression and anxiety in inflammatory bowel disease: a review of comorbidity and management. *Inflamm Bowel Dis.* 2009;15(7):1105-1118.

67. Bolanos SH, Khan DA, Hanczyc M, Bauer MS, Dhanani N, Brown ES. Assessment of mood states in patients receiving long-term corticosteroid therapy and in controls with patient-rated and clinician-rated scales. *Ann Allergy Asthma Immunol.* 2004;92(5):500-505.

68. Szigethy E, Craig AE, Iobst EA, et al. Profile of depression in adolescents with inflammatory bowel disease: implications for treatment. *Inflamm Bowel Dis.* 2009;15(1):69-74.

69. Szigethy E, Levy-Warren A, Whitton S, et al. Depressive symptoms and inflammatory bowel disease in children and adolescents: a cross-sectional study. *J Pediatr Gastroenterol Nutr.* 2004;39(4):395-403.

70. Norra C, Skobel E, Breuer C, Haase G, Hanrath P, Hoff P. Ciprofloxacin-induced acute psychosis in a patient with multidrug-resistant tuberculosis. *Eur Psychiatry.* 2003;18(5):262-263.

71. Reeves RR. Ciprofloxacin-induced psychosis. *Ann Pharmacother.* 1992;26(7-8):930-931.

72. Soczynska JK, Kennedy SH, Goldstein BI, Lachowski A, Woldeyohannes HO, McIntyre RS. The effect of tumor necrosis factor antagonists on mood and mental health-associated quality of life: novel hypothesis-driven treatments for bipolar depression? *Neurotoxicology.* 2009;30(4):497-521.

73. Kast RE. Evidence of a mechanism by which etanercept increased TNF-alpha in multiple myeloma: new insights into the biology of TNF-alpha giving new treatment opportunities—the role of bupropion. *Leuk Res.* 2005;29(12):1459-1463.

74. Kast RE, Altschuler EL. Anti-apoptosis function of TNF-alpha in chronic lymphocytic leukemia: lessons from Crohn's disease and the therapeutic potential of bupropion to lower TNF-alpha. *Arch Immunol Ther Exp (Warsz).* 2005;53(2):143-147.

75. Binder EB, Salyakina D, Lichtner P, et al. Polymorphisms in FKBP5 are associated with increased recurrence of depressive episodes and rapid response to antidepressant treatment. *Nat Genet.* 2004;36(12):1319-1325.

76. Brent D, Melhem N, Ferrell R, et al. Association of FKBP5 polymorphisms with suicidal events in the Treatment of Resistant Depression in Adolescents (TORDIA) study. *Am J Psychiatry.* 2010;167(2):190-197.

77. van der Hoeven J, Duyx J, de Langen JJ, van Royen A. Probable psychiatric side effects of azathioprine. *Psychosom Med.* 2005;67(3):508.

78. Keefer L, Stepanski EJ, Ranjbaran Z, Benson LM, Keshavarzian A. An initial report of sleep disturbance in inactive inflammatory bowel disease. *J Clin Sleep Med.* 2006;2(4):409-416.

79. Ranjbaran Z, Keefer L, Farhadi A, Stepanski E, Sedghi S, Keshavarzian A. Impact of sleep disturbances in inflammatory bowel disease. *J Gastroenterol Hepatol.* 2007;22(11):1748-1753.

80. Krueger JM, Rector DM, Churchill L. Sleep and cytokines. *Sleep Med Clin.* 2007;2(2):161-169.

81. Abraham C, Cho J. Interleukin-23/Th17 pathways and inflammatory bowel disease. *Inflamm Bowel Dis.* 2009;15(7):1090-1100.

82. Xavier RJ, Podolsky DK. Unravelling the pathogenesis of inflammatory bowel disease. *Nature.* 2007;448(7152):427-434.

83. Farrokhyar F, Marshall J, Easterbrook B, Irvine E. Functional gastrointestinal disorders and mood disorders in patients with inactive inflammatory bowel disease: prevalence and impact on health. *Inflamm Bowel Dis.* 2006;12(1):38-46.

84. McLafferty L CA, Levine A, Jones N, Becker A, Szigethy E. Thematic analysis of physical illness perceptions in depressed youth with inflammatory bowel disease. *Inflamm Bowel Dis.* 2011;17(suppl 1):S54.

85. Guthrie E, Jackson J, Shaffer J, Thompson D, Tomenson B, Creed F. Psychological disorder and severity of inflammatory bowel disease predict health-related quality of life in ulcerative colitis and Crohn's disease. *Am J Gastroenterol.* 2002;97(8):1994-1999.

86. Maunder R, Greenberg G, Lancee W, Steinhart A, Silverberg M. The impact of ulcerative colitis is greater in unmarried and young patients. *Can J Gastroenterol.* 2007;21(11):715-720.

87. Saibeni S, Cortinovis I, Beretta L, et al. Gender and disease activity influence health-related quality of life in inflammatory bowel diseases. *Hepatogastroenterology.* 2005;52(62):509-515.

88. Bernklev T, Jahnsen J, Aadland E, et al. Health-related quality of life in patients with inflammatory bowel disease five years after the initial diagnosis. *Scand J Gastroenterol.* 2004;39(4):365-373.

89. Finlay D, Basu D, Sellin J. Effect of race and ethnicity on perceptions of inflammatory bowel disease. *Inflamm Bowel Dis.* 2006;12(6):503-507.

90. Tang LY, Nabalamba A, Graff LA, Bernstein CN. A comparison of self-perceived health status in inflammatory bowel disease and irritable bowel syndrome patients from a Canadian national population survey. *Can J Gastroenterol.* 2008;22(5):475-483.

91. Moreno-Jiménez B, López Blanco B, Rodríguez-Muñoz A, Garrosa Hernández E. The influence of personality factors on health-related quality of life of patients with inflammatory bowel disease. *J Psychosom Res.* 2007;62(1):39-46.

92. Mussell M, Bocker U, Nagel N, Singer MV. Predictors of disease-related concerns and other aspects of health-related quality of life in outpatients with inflammatory bowel disease. *Eur J Gastroenterol Hepatol.* 2004;16(12):1273-1280.

93. Dorrian A, Dempster M, Adair P. Adjustment to inflammatory bowel disease: the relative influence of illness perceptions and coping. *Inflamm Bowel Dis.* 2009;15(1):47-55.

94. Kinash RG, Fischer DG, Lukie BE, Carr TL. Coping patterns and related characteristics in patients with IBD. *Rehabil Nurs.* 1993;18(1):12-19.

95. Taft TH, Keefer L, Leonhard C, Nealon-Woods M. Impact of perceived stigma on inflammatory bowel disease patient outcomes. *Inflamm Bowel Dis.* 2009;15(8):1224-1232.

96. Nicholas DB, Otley A, Smith C, Avolio J, Munk M, Griffiths AM. Challenges and strategies of children and adolescents with inflammatory bowel disease: a qualitative examination. *Health Qual Life Outcomes.* 2007;5:28.

97. Nicholas DB, Swan SR, Gerstle TJ, Allan T, Griffiths AM. Struggles, strengths, and strategies: an ethnographic study exploring the experiences of adolescents living with an ostomy. *Health Qual Life Outcomes.* 2008;6:114.

98. Gasche C, Lomer MC, Cavill I, Weiss G. Iron, anaemia, and inflammatory bowel diseases. *Gut.* 2004;53(8):1190-1197.

99. Irvine EJ, Zhou Q, Thompson AK. The Short Inflammatory Bowel Disease Questionnaire: a quality of life instrument for community physicians managing inflammatory bowel disease. CCRPT Investigators. Canadian Crohn's Relapse Prevention Trial. *Am J Gastroenterol.* 1996;91(8):1571-1578.

100. Guyatt G, Mitchell A, Irvine EJ, et al. A new measure of health status for clinical trials in inflammatory bowel disease. *Gastroenterology.* 1989;96(3):804-810.

101. Otley A, Smith C, Nicholas D, et al. The IMPACT questionnaire: a valid measure of health-related quality of life in pediatric inflammatory bowel disease. *J Pediatr Gastroenterol Nutr.* 2002;35(4):557-563.

102. Sewitch MJ, Abrahamowicz M, Bitton A, et al. Psychological distress, social support, and disease activity in patients with inflammatory bowel disease. *Am J Gastroenterol.* 2001;96(5):1470-1479.

103. Buysse DJ, Reynolds CF 3rd, Monk TH, Berman SR, Kupfer DJ. The Pittsburgh Sleep Quality Index: a new instrument for psychiatric practice and research. *Psychiatry Res.* 1989;28(2):193-213.

104. Johns MW. A new method for measuring daytime sleepiness: the Epworth sleepiness scale. *Sleep.* 1991;14(6):540-545.

105. Jaff JC, Arnold J, Bousvaros A. Effective advocacy for patients with inflammatory bowel disease: communication with insurance companies, school administrators, employers, and other health care overseers. *Inflamm Bowel Dis.* 2006;12(8):814-823.

106. Moser G, Tillinger W, Sachs G, et al. Disease-related worries and concerns: a study on outpatients with inflammatory bowel disease. *Eur J Gastroenterol Hepatol.* 1995;7(9):853-858.

107. Waters B, Jensen L, Fedorak R. Effects of formal education for patients with inflammatory bowel disease: a randomized controlled trial. *Can J Gastroenterol.* 2005;19(4):235-244.

108. Robinson A, Thompson D, Wilkin D, Roberts C, Group NGR. Guided self-management and patient-directed follow-up of ulcerative colitis: a randomised trial. *Lancet.* 2001;358(9286):976-981.

109. Jackson CA, Clatworthy J, Robinson A, Horne R. Factors associated with non-adherence to oral medication for inflammatory bowel disease: a systematic review. *Am J Gastroenterol.* 2010;105(3):525-539.

110. Nigro G, Angelini G, Grosso SB, Caula G, Sategna-Guidetti C. Psychiatric predictors of noncompliance in inflammatory bowel disease: psychiatry and compliance. *J Clin Gastroenterol.* 2001;32(1):66-68.

111. Shale MJ, Riley SA. Studies of compliance with delayed-release mesalazine therapy in patients with inflammatory bowel disease. *Aliment Pharmacol Ther.* 2003;18(2):191-198.

112. Sewitch MJ, Abrahamowicz M, Barkun A, et al. Patient nonadherence to medication in inflammatory bowel disease. *Am J Gastroenterol.* 2003;98(7):1535-1544.

113. Oliveira S, Zaltman C, Elia C, et al. Quality-of-life measurement in patients with inflammatory bowel disease receiving social support. *Inflamm Bowel Dis.* 2007;13(4):470-474.

114. Nicholas D, Otley A, Smith C, Avolio J, Munk M, Griffiths A. Challenges and strategies of children and adolescents with inflammatory bowel disease: a qualitative examination. *Health Qual Life Outcomes.* 2007;5:28.

115. Karwowski CA, Keljo D, Szigethy E. Strategies to improve quality of life in adolescents with inflammatory bowel disease. *Inflamm Bowel Dis.* 2009;15(11):1755-1764.

116. Milne B, Joachim G, Niedhardt J. A stress management programme for inflammatory bowel disease patients. *J Adv Nurs.* 1986;11(5):561-567.

117. Mussell M, Bocker U, Nagel N, Olbrich R, Singer MV. Reducing psychological distress in patients with inflammatory bowel disease by cognitive-behavioural treatment: exploratory study of effectiveness. *Scand J Gastroenterol.* 2003;38(7):755-762.

118. Garcia-Vega E, Fernandez-Rodriguez C. A stress management programme for Crohn's disease. *Behav Res Ther.* 2004;42(4):367-383.

119. Diaz Sibaja MA, Comeche Moreno MI, Mas Hesse B. Protocolized cognitive-behavioural group therapy for inflammatory bowel disease. *Rev Esp Enferm Dig.* 2007;99(10):593-598.

120. Wahed M, Corser M, Goodhand J, Rampton D. Does psychological counseling alter the natural history of inflammatory bowel disease? *Inflamm Bowel Dis.* 2010;16(4):664-669.

121. Szigethy E, Kenney E, Carpenter J, et al. Cognitive-behavioral therapy for adolescents with inflammatory bowel disease and subsyndromal depression. *J Am Acad Child Adolesc Psychiatry.* 2007;46(10):1290-1298.

122. Raymer D, Weininger O, Hamilton JR. Psychological problems in children with abdominal pain. *Lancet.* 1984;1(8374):439-440.

123. Szigethy E, Carpenter J, Baum E, et al. Case study: longitudinal treatment of adolescents with depression and inflammatory bowel disease. *J Am Acad Child Adolesc Psychiatry.* 2006; 45(4):396-400.

124. O'Connor JF, Daniels G, Karush A, Moses L, Flood C, Stern LO. The effects of psychotherapy on the course of ulcerative colitis—a preliminary report. *Am J Psychiatry.* 1964;120: 738-742.

125. Jantschek G, Zeitz M, Pritsch M, et al. Effect of psychotherapy on the course of Crohn's disease. Results of the German prospective multicenter psychotherapy treatment study on Crohn's disease. German Study Group on Psychosocial Intervention in Crohn's Disease. *Scand J Gastroenterol.* 1998;33(12):1289-1296.

126. Keller W, Pritsch M, Von Wietersheim J, et al. Effect of psychotherapy and relaxation on the psychosocial and somatic course of Crohn's disease: main results of the German Prospective Multicenter Psychotherapy Treatment Study on Crohn's Disease. *J Psychosom Res.* 2004;56(6):687-696.

127. Deter H, Keller W, von Wietersheim J, et al. Psychological treatment may reduce the need for healthcare in patients with Crohn's disease. *Inflamm Bowel Dis.* 2007;13(6):745-752.

128. Maunder RG, Esplen MJ. Supportive-expressive group psychotherapy for persons with inflammatory bowel disease. *Can J Psychiatry.* 2001;46(7):622-626.

129. Loudon CP, Corroll V, Butcher J, Rawsthorne P, Bernstein CN. The effects of physical exercise on patients with Crohn's disease. *Am J Gastroenterol.* 1999;94(3):697-703.

130. Ng V, Millard W, Lebrun C, Howard J. Low-intensity exercise improves quality of life in patients with Crohn's disease. *Clin J Sport Med.* 2007;17(5):384-388.

131. Narula N, Fedorak R. Exercise and inflammatory bowel disease. *Can J Gastroenterol.* 2008;22(5):497-504.

132. Vlieger AM, Menko-Frankenhuis C, Wolfkamp SC, Tromp E, Benninga MA. Hypnotherapy for children with functional abdominal pain or irritable bowel syndrome: a randomized controlled trial. *Gastroenterology.* 2007;133(5):1430-1436.

133. Palsson OS, Turner MJ, Johnson DA, Burnett CK, Whitehead WE. Hypnosis treatment for severe irritable bowel syndrome: investigation of mechanism and effects on symptoms. *Dig Dis Sci.* 2002;47(11):2605-2614.

134. Whorwell PJ. Hypnotherapy for irritable bowel syndrome: the response of colonic and noncolonic symptoms. *J Psychosom Res.* 2008;64(6):621-623.

135. Mawdsley J, Jenkins D, Macey M, Langmead L, Rampton D. The effect of hypnosis on systemic and rectal mucosal measures of inflammation in ulcerative colitis. *Am J Gastroenterol.* 2008;103(6):1460-1469.

136. Keefer L, Keshavarzian A. Feasibility and acceptability of gut-directed hypnosis on inflammatory bowel disease: a brief communication. *Int J Clin Exp Hypn.* 2007;55(4):457-466.

137. Lix LM, Graff LA, Walker JR, et al. Longitudinal study of quality of life and psychological functioning for active, fluctuating, and inactive disease patterns in inflammatory bowel disease. *Inflamm Bowel Dis.* 2008;14(11):1575-1584.

138. Hilsden RJ, Meddings JB, Verhoef MJ. Complementary and alternative medicine use by patients with inflammatory bowel disease: an Internet survey. *Can J Gastroenterol.* 1999;13(4): 327-332.

139. Hilsden RJ, Scott CM, Verhoef MJ. Complementary medicine use by patients with inflammatory bowel disease. *Am J Gastroenterol.* 1998;93(5):697-701.

140. Hilsden RJ, Verhoef MJ. Complementary and alternative medicine: evaluating its effectiveness in inflammatory bowel disease. *Inflamm Bowel Dis.* 1998;4(4):318-323.

141. Hilsden RJ, Verhoef MJ, Best A, Pocobelli G. Complementary and alternative medicine use by Canadian patients with inflammatory bowel disease: results from a national survey. *Am J Gastroenterol.* 2003;98(7):1563-1568.

142. Hilsden RJ, Verhoef MJ, Rasmussen H, Porcino A, Debruyn JC. Use of complementary and alternative medicine by patients with inflammatory bowel disease. *Inflamm Bowel Dis.* 2011;17(2):655-662.

143. Schneider A, Streitberger K, Joos S. Acupuncture treatment in gastrointestinal diseases: a systematic review. *World J Gastroenterol.* 2007;13(25):3417-3424.

144. Campo JV, Perel J, Lucas A, et al. Citalopram treatment of pediatric recurrent abdominal pain and comorbid internalizing disorders: an exploratory study. *J Am Acad Child Adolesc Psychiatry.* 2004;43(10):1234-1242.

145. Tack J, Broekaert D, Fischler B, Van Oudenhove L, Gevers AM, Janssens J. A controlled crossover study of the selective serotonin reuptake inhibitor citalopram in irritable bowel syndrome. *Gut.* 2006;55(8):1095-1103.

146. Talley NJ, Kellow JE, Boyce P, Tennant C, Huskic S, Jones M. Antidepressant therapy (imipramine and citalopram) for irritable bowel syndrome: a double-blind, randomized, placebo-controlled trial. *Dig Dis Sci.* 2008;53(1):108-115.

147. Mikocka-Walus AA, Turnbull DA, Moulding NT, Wilson IG, Andrews JM, Holtmann GJ. Controversies surrounding the comorbidity of depression and anxiety in inflammatory bowel disease patients: a literature review. *Inflamm Bowel Dis.* 2007;13(2):225-234.

148. Walker E, Gelfand M, Gelfand A, Creed F, Katon W. The relationship of current psychiatric disorder to functional disability and distress in patients with inflammatory bowel disease. *Gen Hosp Psychiatry.* 1996;18(4):220-229.

149. Capuron L, Neurauter G, Musselman D, et al. Interferon-alpha-induced changes in tryptophan metabolism. relationship to depression and paroxetine treatment. *Biol Psychiatry.* 2003;54(9):906-914.

150. O'Connor C, Jiang W, Kuchibhatla M, et al. Safety and efficacy of sertraline for depression in patients with heart failure: results of the SADHART-CHF (Sertraline Against Depression and Heart Disease in Chronic Heart Failure) trial. *J Am Coll Cardiol.* 2010;56(9):692-699.

151. Beshay H, Pumariega A. Sertraline treatment of mood disorder associated with prednisone: a case report. *J Child Adolesc Psychopharmacol.* 1998;8(3):187-193.

152. Kane S, Altschuler EL, Kast RE. Crohn's disease remission on bupropion. *Gastroenterology.* 2003;125(4):1290.

153. Kast R, Altschuler E. Bone density loss in Crohn's disease: role of TNF and potential for prevention by bupropion. *Gut.* 2004;53(7):1056.

154. Coogan AN, Wyse CA. Neuroimmunology of the circadian clock. *Brain Res.* 2008;1232: 104-112.

155. Smith MT, Huang MI, Manber R. Cognitive behavior therapy for chronic insomnia occurring within the context of medical and psychiatric disorders. *Clin Psychol Rev.* 2005;25(5):559-592.

156. Sanchez-Barcelo EJ, Mediavilla MD, Tan DX, Reiter RJ. Clinical uses of melatonin: evaluation of human trials. *Curr Med Chem.* 2010;17(19):2070-2095.

157. Cuzzocrea S, Mazzon E, Serraino I, et al. Melatonin reduces dinitrobenzene sulfonic acid-induced colitis. *J Pineal Res.* 2001;30(1):1-12.

158. Li JH, Yu JP, Yu HG, et al. Melatonin reduces inflammatory injury through inhibiting NF-kappaB activation in rats with colitis. *Mediators Inflamm.* 2005;2005(4):185-193.

159. Sasaki M, Jordan P, Joh T, et al. Melatonin reduces TNF-a induced expression of MAdCAM-1 via inhibition of NF-kappaB. *BMC Gastroenterol.* 2002;2:9.

160. Radogna F, Diederich M, Ghibelli L. Melatonin: a pleiotropic molecule regulating inflammation. *Biochem Pharmacol.* 2010;80(12):1844-1852.

161. Allen, et al. Restless legs syndrome: diagnostic criteria, special considerations, and epidemiology. A report from the restless legs syndrome diagnosis and epidemiology workshop at the National Institutes of Health. *Sleep Med.* 2003;4(2):101-119.

162. Weinstock LB, Bosworth BP, Scherl EJ, et al. Crohn's disease is associated with restless legs syndrome. *Inflamm Bowel Dis.* 2010;16(2):275-279.

163. Hening WA, Allen RP, Chaudhuri KR, et al. Clinical significance of RLS. *Mov Disord.* 2007;22(suppl 18):S395-S400.

164. Trenkwalder C, Paulus W. Restless legs syndrome: pathophysiology, clinical presentation and management. *Nat Rev Neurol.* 2010;6(6):337-346.

165. Kennedy TM, Chalder T, McCrone P, et al. Cognitive behavioural therapy in addition to antispasmodic therapy for irritable bowel syndrome in primary care: randomised controlled trial. *Health Technol Assess.* 2006;10(19):iii-iv, ix-x, 1-67.

166. McCrone P, Knapp M, Kennedy T, et al. Cost-effectiveness of cognitive behaviour therapy in addition to mebeverine for irritable bowel syndrome. *Eur J Gastroenterol Hepatol.* 2008;20(4):255-263.

167. Moss-Morris R, McAlpine L, Didsbury LP, Spence MJ. A randomized controlled trial of a cognitive behavioural therapy-based self-management intervention for irritable bowel syndrome in primary care. *Psychol Med.* 2010;40(1):85-94.

168. Sanders MR, Rebgetz M, Morrison M, et al. Cognitive-behavioral treatment of recurrent nonspecific abdominal pain in children: an analysis of generalization, maintenance, and side effects. *J Consult Clin Psychol.* 1989;57(2):294-300.

169. Sanders MR, Shepherd RW, Cleghorn G, Woolford H. The treatment of recurrent abdominal pain in children: a controlled comparison of cognitive-behavioral family intervention and standard pediatric care. *J Consult Clin Psychol.* 1994;62(2):306-314.

170. Drossman DA, Camilleri M, Mayer EA, Whitehead WE. AGA technical review on irritable bowel syndrome. *Gastroenterology.* 2002;123(6):2108-2131.

171. Tack J, Fried M, Houghton LA, Spicak J, Fisher G. Systematic review: the efficacy of treatments for irritable bowel syndrome—a European perspective. *Aliment Pharmacol Ther.* 2006;24(2):183-205.

172. Ford AC, Talley NJ, Schoenfeld PS, Quigley EM, Moayyedi P. Efficacy of antidepressants and psychological therapies in irritable bowel syndrome: systematic review and meta-analysis. *Gut.* 2009;58(3):367-378.

SUGGESTED READINGS

Ford AC, Talley NJ, Schoenfeld PS, Quigley EM, Moayyedi P. Efficacy of antidepressants and psychological therapies in irritable bowel syndrome: systematic review and meta-analysis. *Gut.* 2009;58(3):367-378.

Goodhand J, Wahed M, Rampton D. Management of stress in inflammatory bowel disease: a therapeutic option? *Expert Rev Gastroenterol Hepatol.* 2009;3(6):661-679.

Karwowski CA, Keljo D, Szigethy E. Strategies to improve quality of life in adolescents with inflammatory bowel disease. *Inflamm Bowel Dis.* 2009;15(11):1755-1764.

Szigethy E, McLafferty L, Goyal A. Inflammatory bowel disease. *Child Adolesc Psychiatr Clin North Am.* 2010;19(2):301-318.

COMPLICATIONS DUE TO IMMUNOMODULATORS AND ANTI-TUMOR NECROSIS FACTORS

Chapter 15

Immunomodulators

Azathioprine/ 6-Mercaptopurine and Methotrexate

Miles P. Sparrow, MBBS, FRACP and David T. Rubin, MD

Treatment aims in the inflammatory bowel diseases (IBDs) are evolving beyond the induction and maintenance of corticosteroid-free remission. More recently, it has become recognized that by treating with immunomodulatory and biologic therapies earlier in the disease course, and achieving mucosal healing, the natural history of these diseases may be modified in a positive way. Despite the clear benefits of early and appropriate introduction of these therapies, the potential for risks, some of them serious, must be understood by the clinician and discussed with patients. This chapter will review the relevant adverse events associated with the use of the immunomodulatory agents azathioprine (AZA), 6-mercaptopurine (6-MP), and methotrexate (MTX).

AZATHIOPRINE AND 6-MERCAPTOPURINE

The thiopurine immunomodulators AZA and 6-MP have become the mainstay of maintenance medical therapy for many patients with Crohn's disease (CD) or ulcerative colitis (UC). In CD, meta-analyses support the use of these agents as induction and maintenance therapies and to prevent postoperative disease recurrence.[1-4] In UC, the evidence of benefit is less robust, but meta-analyses demonstrate thiopurine effectiveness as maintenance therapy, with less benefit as induction agents.[5,6] A previous retrospective referral center study in CD failed to demonstrate a reduction in surgical rates despite an increased use of thiopurines in recent decades.[7] However, a more recent prospective study of almost 400 patients in Spain demonstrated that thiopurines

Regueiro MD, Swoger JM, eds.
Clinical Challenges and Complications of IBD (pp 287-302).
© 2013 Taylor & Francis Group.

are effective in reducing hospitalizations and surgeries in both CD and UC.[8] Similarly, a recent population-based study from Wales demonstrated a reduction in surgical rates in CD patients with thiopurine therapy. These improved outcomes likely reflect the trend toward the earlier introduction of immunomodulators at a time when patients' disease phenotype is believed to be more inflammatory, before the occurrence of fibrostenotic or perforating disease complications.[9] In each patient receiving thiopurines, such benefits must be balanced against the not-infrequent potential for adverse effects, so that a favorable benefit-to-risk ratio is maintained.

Adverse Events of Thiopurine Immunomodulators

Adverse events during thiopurine therapy are not infrequent, and therefore careful monitoring is standard practice for all patients receiving these agents. Meta-analyses of induction therapies in CD reveal an odds ratio (OR) of an adverse event in patients receiving thiopurines of 3.44 (95% confidence interval [CI] 1.52 to 7.77).[2] The majority of adverse events to thiopurines can be classified as being allergic/idiosyncratic (eg, pancreatitis, flu-like syndromes) or dose-dependent (eg, myelotoxicity, hepatic transaminitis, malignancies including lymphoproliferative disease). In a New Zealand study of 216 IBD patients, 25.9% of them developed a side effect that resulted in drug cessation, the most common being allergic-type reactions, hepatitis, nausea and vomiting, myelotoxicity, and pancreatitis.[10] The most important potential side effect associated with any medication is the risk of mortality, but data regarding thiopurines and mortality are reassuring, especially in comparison to the risks with corticosteroids. A large case-control study of almost 14,500 patients demonstrated an association between mortality and current corticosteroid use (CD hazard ratio [HR] 2.48, 95% CI 1.85 to 3.31; UC HR 2.81, 95% CI 2.26 to 3.50) but not with current thiopurine use (CD HR 0.83, 95% CI 0.37 to 1.86; UC HR 0.70, 95% CI 0.29 to 1.70).[11] Similarly, recent registry data have demonstrated an increased mortality in CD associated with prednisone use (OR 2.10, 95% CI 1.15 to 3.83) but not with thiopurine exposure (OR 0.73, 95% CI 0.40 to 1.34).[12]

Allergic Adverse Events to Thiopurines

Acute Pancreatitis

The incidence of acute pancreatitis in IBD patients is 1% to 6%, with the most common cause being thiopurines, which themselves carry a risk of pancreatitis of approximately 3%.[13] The incidence appears higher in CD than UC and has variably been reported to be more common in women.[14,15] An association with pancreatitis and a deficiency in inosine triphosphate pyrophosphatase (ITPase) due to the 94C>A polymorphism has been demonstrated in some but not all studies.[16,17] Acute pancreatitis usually occurs within a few weeks of commencing AZA or 6-MP. Clinically, it is usually mild, resolves promptly on stopping the thiopurine, and inpatient admission is rarely required. Although there are case reports of successfully treating with 6-MP after an acute pancreatitis episode during AZA therapy, it is generally understood that, when drug related, there is 100% cross-reactivity for drug-related pancreatitis between the thiopurines, and therefore rechallenge is not recommended.[18]

Flu-Like Syndromes

An idiosyncratic early adverse reaction, consisting of constitutional flu-like symptoms, joint pains, rashes, and fevers, occurs not infrequently in patients exposed to thiopurines. The mechanisms of this reaction are poorly understood, although an association with the ITPase 94C>A polymorphism has again been postulated.[16] Rates of recurrence with 6-MP after hypersensitivity reactions to AZA are at least 50%, but unlike pancreatitis, rechallenge may be attempted (at a smaller initial dose) in appropriately counseled patients.

Idiopathic Cholestatic Hepatitis

An idiopathic cholestatic hepatitis associated with thiopurines is rare and usually occurs within 2 to 3 weeks of commencing thiopurines. Clinically, it is characterized by nausea, abdominal pain, and jaundice. Biochemically, increased bilirubin and alkaline phosphatase are seen along with moderate elevations of aminotransferases. Histologically, cholestasis and parenchymal cell necrosis are observed. Upon recognition and thiopurine withdrawal, the syndrome resolves clinically within weeks, although biochemical abnormalities may be present for several months. Given the potential for hepatocyte injury, switching from AZA to 6-MP should be done cautiously, if at all, after this adverse event.[19,20]

Dose-Dependent Adverse Events to Thiopurines

Myelotoxicity

Myelotoxicity is the most important potential adverse event associated with thiopurines. A recent meta-analysis reported a cumulative incidence of myelotoxicity in patients receiving thiopurines of 7%, with an incidence of 3% per patient-year. The cumulative incidence of severe myelotoxicity (defined as a neutrophil count of $< 0.5 \times 10^9$/L) is 1.1%, with an annual incidence rate of 0.9%. Myelotoxicity with thiopurines has been reported to occur in as little as days after starting, to as long as 27 years after the commencement of therapy. Of those developing myelotoxicity, only 6.5% of patients had an associated infectious complication.[21] The seemingly unpredictable nature of this complication supports the need for ongoing hematological monitoring for the duration of therapy with these agents. Myelotoxicity appears to occur, at least in part, due to the accumulation of high intracellular levels of the active metabolite 6-thioguanine nucleotide (6-TGN). The production of this metabolite is at least partially dependent on the activity of thiopurine methyltransferase (TPMT). TPMT activity is determined by a genetic polymorphism that has a trimodal distribution within the population. Eighty-nine percent of people are homozygous high, with normal enzyme activity; 11% are heterozygotes, with intermediate activity; and 0.3% are homozygous low, with negligible enzyme activity.[22] TPMT heterozygotes and homozygous low patients are at particular risk of myelotoxicity. Therefore, it is recommended that heterozygotes should receive one-third to one-half the usual thiopurine starting dose and homozygous low patients should not receive thiopurine therapy.[23] A recent meta-analysis of patients of all TPMT genotypes receiving thiopurines revealed an OR of 2.93 (95% CI 1.68 to 5.09, $P < 0.001$) for the presence of TPMT polymorphisms and any adverse drug reaction, and 5.93 (95% CI 2.96 to 11.88, $P < 0.001$) for polymorphisms and myelotoxicity.[24] Despite the importance of this pharmacogenomic relationship, the majority of patients developing myelotoxicity have normal TPMT activity, outlining the importance of regular laboratory monitoring for the duration of thiopurine therapy in all patients.[25] A suggested schedule is to monitor the white blood cell count weekly for 4 weeks, alternate weekly for 4 weeks, then at 12 weeks and every 3 months thereafter, including testing 2 weeks after any thiopurine dose escalation. More recently, there has been an appreciation of the risk of infections and vaccine-preventable illnesses with immunosuppression. Therefore, it is recommended to ensure that patients are adequately vaccinated according to routine immunization schedules for the general population in order to avoid vaccine-preventable infections prior to the commencement of thiopurines or any other immunomodulatory therapy (see Chapter 14).[26-28] In particular, in IBD patients, vaccination is recommended for the following 5 vaccines: hepatitis B virus in seronegative patients, human papillomavirus in young women, influenza virus annually (including H1N1), *Strep Pneumonia* 5 yearly, and varicella in patients without a history or serologic evidence of chickenpox or varicella zoster infection.[29] All of these are attenuated vaccines except varicella, which is a live vaccine, and should not be given to patients already on immunomodulatory agents.

Hepatotoxicity

Hepatotoxicity is a well-recognized adverse event of thiopurines; however, the prevalence varies greatly among published studies. A recent systematic review of 34 retrospective studies showed a low prevalence of hepatotoxicity of 3.3%, whereas in a prospective study of 161 patients, the rate of hepatotoxicity was as high as 23%.[30,31] Some of these differences may be due to the variety of definitions of hepatotoxicity employed—for example, abnormalities of liver function tests (LFTs) are common, while true "hepatotoxicity" is rare. In addition, hepatotoxicity appears to be less common with 6-MP compared to AZA.[32] Cases of thiopurine hepatotoxicity can be grouped into 3 types—an idiopathic cholestatic hepatitis (as discussed above), a dose-dependent transaminitis, and hepatotoxicity due to endothelial cell injury (nodular regenerative hyperplasia [NRH] and veno-occlusive disease).

The dose-dependent transaminitis seen with dose escalation of thiopurines is the most common hepatic adverse event and may be asymptomatic or may cause nausea, headaches, and malaise. It may resolve spontaneously with time, meaning that when mild (transaminase levels 2 to 3 times normal), and in an asymptomatic patient, it may be simply monitored. Alternatively, when aminotransferase elevations are moderate, or in symptomatic patients, it will reverse with dose reduction or cessation without long-term clinical sequelae. A 50% dose reduction is initially suggested, after which if LFTs normalize, cautious dose re-escalation can often be achieved successfully. Anecdotal experience and small retrospective case series have shown that more than 50% of patients intolerant of AZA may tolerate 6-MP, including those patients with AZA-induced hepatotoxicity.[33-35] Although unproven, it has been postulated that the intolerance, including hepatotoxicity associated with AZA, may be due to derivatives produced from the imidazole side chain of AZA.[36] Given the equal efficacy of AZA and 6-MP, a trial of 6-MP in patients with AZA-induced hepatotoxicity is recommended. The dose-dependent hepatitis has been variably associated with elevated levels of the end-metabolite 6-methylmercaptopurine (6-MMP), as reported in the initial pediatric studies in which 6-MMP levels >5700 pmol/8×10^8 red blood cells count were associated with biochemical hepatitis.[37] These findings have been replicated in some, but not all, studies, and the sensitivity and specificity of 6-MMP for drug-induced hepatotoxicity is low, meaning that dose reduction due to high 6-MMP levels is only recommended for patients with elevated aminotransferases.[38] More recently, it has become recognized that approximately 15% of patients preferentially metabolize thiopurines to produce 6-MMP instead of 6-TGN, predisposing them to hepatotoxicity and therapeutic inefficacy.[39] Small, retrospective, single-center studies have demonstrated that the addition of low doses of adjunctive allopurinol, in combination with thiopurine dose reduction, can be used to reverse this inefficacious metabolic profile and the associated hepatitis.[40]

The thiopurine hepatotoxicities associated with endothelial cell injury (NRH and veno-occlusive disease) are important, as they can be complicated by portal hypertension and potentially life-threatening sequelae. NRH has been associated most frequently with 6-thioguanine (6-TG) use but is also recognized to occur less commonly with AZA/6-MP, and even in thiopurine-naive IBD patients. In the initial cohort of 111 patients receiving 6-TG at high doses (80 mg daily) for a median of 9.1 months, NRH was demonstrated on liver biopsy in 76% of patients with laboratory abnormalities (elevated liver enzymes or thrombocytopenia) and 33% of patients with normal laboratory values. This finding led to the widespread recommendation that 6-TG should not be used in the treatment of IBD patients.[41] More recent European data have shown that lower doses of 6-TG (20 mg daily) may be used safely in IBD patients, although further data are required before this can be more widely recommended.[42,43] NRH has also been associated with AZA/6-MP use, especially in males and in patients with fibrostenosing small bowel disease or prior extensive small bowel resections. In one multicenter study of 37 patients with NRH, the median time to diagnosis of NRH after starting AZA was 48 months (range 6 to 187 months), and the cumulative incidence rate was 1.25% at 10 years (0.29 to 2.21). After a median follow-up of 16 months, 14 patients developed complications of portal hypertension.[44] Thrombocytopenia, with or without abnormal LFTs, should alert clinicians to the rare but potentially serious possibility of NRH in patients receiving thiopurines. Interestingly, histologic evidence of sinusoidal pathologies, including NRH, has been documented in thiopurine-naive IBD patients. In a study of 83 liver biopsy specimens from thiopurine-naive IBD patients (51 CD), sinusoidal dilation was noted in 34% and NRH in 6%, indicating that the increased frequency of NRH in IBD may not all be thiopurine related.[45] Regardless of the etiology, the natural history of NRH appears variable, with some case studies showing complete resolution and others characterized by persistence of portal hypertensive sequelae after an associated thiopurine is discontinued.[46,47]

Malignancies

As with all immunomodulatory agents, the thiopurines may be associated with an increase in the long-term risk for malignancies and are classified as carcinogens by regulatory agencies. The mechanisms for the risk of carcinogenesis may include the disruption in DNA structure, replication, and repair that occurs with the incorporation of 6-TGN into DNA, and the increased cellular sensitivity to ultraviolet radiation that occurs after thiopurine exposure. In IBD populations, thiopurines have been associated with an increased risk of lymphomas and nonmelanoma skin cancers. Data supporting an association between thiopurines and lymphoma from both referral center and population-based studies have been variable. Confounding factors including the disease itself and the underlying disease activity mean that distinction of lymphoma causality between the underlying disease or the thiopurine has been difficult. Recent, well-designed, large meta-analyses; case-control studies; and observational studies suggest that the increased risk of lymphoma associated with thiopurine exposure is real. A meta-analysis of 6 studies totaling 3891 IBD patients, yielding 11 lymphomas, revealed a pooled relative risk of 4.18 (95% CI 2.07 to 7.51) for lymphoma among patients taking thiopurines compared to patients not receiving these agents.[48] A recent case-control study of 15,471 IBD patients from the UK General Practice Research Database did not show an increased risk of developing any cancer in patients who had filled prescriptions for AZA (OR 0.92, 95% CI 0.79 to 1.06). However, patients who had never used AZA were shown to have an increased prevalence of lymphoma (OR 3.22, 95% CI 1.01 to 10.18).[49] More recently, a large French prospective observational study of 19,486 IBD patients calculated a multivariate-adjusted HR of 5.28 (95% CI 2.01 to 13.9, $P = 0.00007$) for patients currently receiving thiopurines, which reduced to baseline following treatment discontinuation. Of the 23 lymphomas reported (22 non-Hodgkin lymphoma and 1 Hodgkin lymphoma), 12 were positive for Epstein-Barr virus, an association noted in other case series of lymphomas in patients receiving thiopurines. In addition, 2 cases of fatal early postmononucleosis lymphoproliferative disease were noted in young males previously seronegative for prior Epstein-Barr virus infection.[50] More recently, the rare but almost uniformly fatal hepatosplenic T-cell lymphoma has been reported in patients receiving the combination of thiopurines and anti-tumor necrosis factor (TNF) agents. To date, 36 cases have been reported, with all patients having been exposed to thiopurines and 20 also having a history of past or present anti-TNF use. The majority of patients were males, less than 35 years of age, leading some experts to recommend avoidance of combination therapy in this patient demographic. The etiologic role of thiopurines, anti-TNFs, or combination therapy in this condition remains unknown.[51] Overall, recent data favoring the association between thiopurines and lymphomas (in particular NHL) support that patients need to be warned of this risk at the commencement of thiopurine therapy. However, absolute incidence rates remain very low, such that in the majority of cases, the benefits of immunomodulation appear to outweigh the small but discernable risks involved.

Thiopurines have been associated with an increased risk for the development of nonmelanoma skin cancers. A recent large retrospective cohort and nested case-control study revealed a background increased nonmelanoma skin cancers rate in IBD patients (incidence rate ratio 1.64, 95% CI 1.51 to 1.78). This was increased further in patients receiving thiopurines within the last 90 days (OR 3.56, 95% CI 2.81 to 4.50), or for more than 1 year (OR 4.27, 95% CI 3.08 to 5.92). Rates of nonmelanoma skin cancers were also increased, even though to a lesser extent, in patients receiving biologic therapies.[52] Otherwise, there is no evidence that thiopurines increase the incidence of solid organ tumors, while data associating their use with increased rates of cervical intraepithelial neoplasia are mixed.[53] A summary of the adverse events associated with thiopurines in IBD is presented in Table 15-1.

METHOTREXATE

MTX, a dihydrofolate reductase inhibitor, is used as both an induction and maintenance agent in CD, and less commonly in UC. In IBD, it is usually used after inefficacy or intolerance to thiopurines, in contrast to its use in rheumatological conditions in which it is the primary immunomodulatory agent. Systematic reviews support the use of MTX as both an induction and maintenance agent in CD, but only when given parenterally via either the subcutaneous or intramuscular route.[54,55] In contrast, systemic reviews do not support the use of MTX in UC, although single-center, retrospective studies have demonstrated efficacy when MTX is given parenterally.[56-58] However, the use of MTX is not infrequently limited by intolerance; in the largest randomized trial of MTX in CD, 17% of patients withdrew due to adverse effects.[59] Adverse effects can be classified into common and rare but serious events. The most common adverse events include gastrointestinal intolerance (nausea, dyspepsia, diarrhea), mild rises in aminotransferases, oral stomatitis, rashes, and neurologic effects including headache, fatigue, and reduced concentration. Rare but serious side effects include hepatotoxicity, pulmonary toxicity, and myelotoxicity.

Common Adverse Events Associated With Methotrexate

Adverse events commonly occur within 24 to 48 hours of the weekly MTX dose, especially gastrointestinal intolerance or neurologic side effects. Similarly, rashes may occur within days of a weekly dose, before fading before

Table 15-1. Adverse Events and Suggested Management Options for Thiopurines and Methotrexate in Inflammatory Bowel Disease Patients

	Adverse Event	Suggested Management
Thiopurines	Pancreatitis	Stop thiopurine
	Flu-like syndromes	If with AZA, try 6-MP
	Myelotoxicity	• Severe—withhold thiopurine ± recommence at lower dose • Mild-moderate—50% dose reduction
	Hepatotoxicity	
	• Cholestatic hepatitis	If with AZA, consider 6-MP
	• Transaminitis	• Mild and patient asymptomatic—observe • Moderate ± patient symptomatic—50% dose reduction • If with AZA and persistent, consider 6-MP
	• NRH/VOD	Stop thiopurine
	Malignancies	
	• Lymphoma	Stop thiopurine
	• Nonmelanoma skin cancer	Can continue thiopurine if strongly indicated
MTX	Hepatotoxicity	
	• Abnormal LFTs only	• Mild and patient asymptomatic—observe • Moderate ± patient symptomatic—50% dose reduction
	• Significant hepatitis or fibrosis	Stop MTX
	Pulmonary toxicity	Stop MTX
	Myelotoxicity	• Severe—withhold MTX ± recommence at lower dose • Mild-moderate—50% dose reduction

AZA = azathioprine; LFT = liver function test; 6-MP = 6-mercaptopurine; MTX = methotrexate; NRH = nodular regenerative hyperplasia; VOD = veno-occlusive disease the next dose. Stomatitis may be mild or severe and persistent enough to cause odynophagia and reduced oral intake. Concurrent use of folic acid (1 mg daily or 5 mg weekly) must be given with MTX to prevent folate depletion, and there are some, even though inconclusive, data that its use may reduce the gastro-intestinal intolerance and stomatitis associated with MTX.[60] There is a suggestion that the neurotoxicity of MTX may be due to intracellular accumulation of adenosine resulting from the inhibition of purine synthesis, and in children this has been improved with 1-hour aminophylline infusions.[61,62] Although MTX can cause drug-induced fevers, infections, including by *Pneumocystis jiroveci* and fungi, must be excluded. Intracellularly, MTX metabolism results in the progressive addition of polyglutamate residues to the base molecule. Early rheumatological studies suggested that higher MTX response rates might be associated with a higher proportion of larger polyglutamate metabolites (MTX PG_{3-5}) in an individual patient. However, these results were not replicated in a small pilot trial in IBD patients in whom, in fact, higher proportions of MTX PG_{3-5} metabolites were associated not with efficacy, but with increased adverse events.[63,64] The role of measuring MTX polyglutamate metabolites as a means of optimizing MTX dosing in individual patients awaits further research.

Rare but Serious Side Effects Associated With Methotrexate

Hepatotoxicity

MTX can cause abnormal LFTs and a variety of hepatic histologic changes including steatosis, stellate cell hypertrophy, anisonucleosis, and fibrosis. MTX-induced increases in alanine aminotransferases (ALT) and aspartate aminotransferases (AST) are seen in approximately 14% and 8% of patients, respectively.[65] All forms of hepatotoxicity appear more common in patients receiving daily rather than weekly MTX therapy, and supplemental folate may reduce aminotransferases increases, but whether it reduces histologic hepatotoxicity is unknown. Although biochemical assessment of LFTs is not predictive of hepatic histology, routine liver biopsy is no longer recommended in patients receiving MTX. However, biopsy should be considered in patients with persistently abnormal LFTs and other risk factors for hepatotoxicity, such as excessive alcohol intake or coexistent viral hepatitis B or C.[66] Reassuringly, multiple case series of IBD patients receiving MTX in whom liver biopsies were performed have shown minimal fibrosis in the majority of cases.[67,68] Despite the lack of direct correlation between hepatic biochemical and histologic findings, routine assessment of LFTs in patients receiving MTX is still recommended—a suggested regimen is to measure LFTs routinely at baseline and periodically afterward, although the appropriate interval is less well described in the existing literature (we do so at 2, 4, 8, and 12 weeks and then every 3 months thereafter), as well as 2 weeks after any MTX dose change. Recommendations from rheumatological guidelines suggest that the MTX dose should be reduced if an elevation in AST or a decrease in serum albumin is seen.[69]

Pulmonary Toxicity

Large case series, again predominantly from the rheumatological literature, suggest that MTX-induced pulmonary toxicity occurs in 2% to 8% of patients.[70] Pulmonary complications of MTX are classified as inflammatory or infectious; the role of MTX in the development of pulmonary NHL remains unconfirmed. The most common form of inflammatory toxicity is a hypersensitivity pneumonitis, although bronchiolitis obliterans with organizing pneumonia, acute lung injury (noncardiogenic pulmonary edema), pulmonary fibrosis, bronchitis, and pleuritis can occur. The mechanisms of MTX-induced pulmonary toxicity remain unknown; however, it usually develops within the first year of therapy. Predisposing risk factors include an age greater than 60 years, hypoalbuminemia, and diabetes mellitus. MTX lung disease is usually associated with higher MTX doses than are used in IBD, daily rather than weekly dosing, and is not prevented by folate repletion. The most common clinical features are of a subacute pneumonitis, presenting with dyspnea, nonproductive cough, fever, crepitations on auscultation, and cyanosis. Progression to pulmonary fibrosis occurs in 10% of patients.[71] These conditions should be suspected and diagnosed clinically, and MTX withdrawn, although occasionally bronchoalveolar lavage or lung biopsy is required to confirm the diagnosis in acutely unwell patients. Management of MTX-induced lung disease requires initial exclusion of pulmonary infection, discontinuation of MTX, and in some cases systemic corticosteroids. Most cases of pneumonitis will begin to improve within days of stopping MTX. Pulmonary infections associated with MTX include *P jiroveci* (up to 40% of cases in some series), cytomegalovirus, varicella zoster virus, nocardia, mycobacteria, or fungi.[72] Pulmonary infection must be actively excluded before MTX drug injury is assumed to be due to pneumonitis or another inflammatory cause.

Myelotoxicity

Myelotoxicity occurs more commonly with the high-dose MTX regimens used in chemotherapy than with the lower doses used to treat IBD, and it is less common than myelotoxicity due to thiopurines. Macrocytosis is common and, when myelosuppression occurs, it is usually in the form of neutropenia or thrombocytopenia, with anemia being rare.[73] As with other dose-dependent forms of MTX toxicity, myelotoxicity is more common with daily rather than weekly therapy and in the presence of renal impairment. To monitor for myelotoxicity, routine blood counts are recommended at baseline, and at 2, 4, 8, and 12 weeks after the commencement of MTX, and every 3 months thereafter, with subsequent MTX dose reduction or cessation as appropriate (Table 15-2).

Other clinically relevant serious adverse effects of MTX include its lymphoproliferative potential and teratogenicity. There are insufficient data to associate MTX use with the development of lymphomas in IBD patient populations. At present, whether this is due to a lack of data or no true association remains unknown. Large prospective studies in rheumatoid arthritis have shown a slightly increased risk of Hodgkin lymphoma in males receiving

Table 15-2. Suggested Blood Test Monitoring for All Inflammatory Bowel Disease Patients Receiving Thiopurines or Methotrexate

Duration of Immunomodulator Therapy	Suggested Blood Test Monitoring	
	AZA/6-MP	MTX
First month of therapy	Weekly	Alternate weekly
Second month of therapy	Alternate weekly	At 8 weeks
Third month of therapy	At 12 weeks	At 12 weeks
For the duration of therapy	Every 3 months	Every 3 months
After any dose escalation	2 weeks later	2 weeks later
AZA = azathioprine; 6-MP = 6-mercaptopurine; MTX = methotrexate		

MTX, suggesting that further data are required in IBD patients before it can be assumed that there is no increased risk.[74] MTX is an abortifacient and a strongly teratogenic agent (pregnancy class X) that is contraindicated in pregnant women. It should be discontinued at least 3 months prior to planned conception in women, and although there are no data in relation to the risks of males taking MTX around the time of conception, the same recommendation is usually made. A summary of the adverse events associated with MTX in IBD is presented in Table 15-2.

CONCLUSION

As with any therapy used to treat IBD, adverse events are not infrequent with the immunomodulatory agents used to treat these conditions. However, both thiopurines and MTX are effective corticosteroid-sparing agents, and by reducing corticosteroid adverse events, the overall side effect burden in an individual patient will usually be lessened with immunomodulator use. Implicit to the use of immunomodulators is the need for a clear explanation of their potential benefits and risks before they are commenced, putting into perspective their significant benefits and the low absolute risk rate of serious adverse events.[75] In this way, patients can choose to proceed with therapy if they understand that the benefits of immunomodulation outweigh the risks in their individual case. After therapy is commenced, regular monitoring for side effects both clinically and biochemically is required, more frequently initially, and then approximately every 3 months for the duration of therapy. With these measures, it can be confidently explained to patients that the risks of immunomodulation are generally smaller than the risks of not using these agents when they are indicated in the majority of cases.

☑ Key Points

☑ When clinically indicated, the benefits of immunomodulation usually outweigh the risks, but this should be assessed and discussed on a case-by-case basis with each patient.

☑ A thorough explanation of the risks of immunomodulation, including rare but serious side effects such as malignancy, must be outlined to patients prior to the commencement of therapy. These risks must be placed in context of the risks of not using immunomodulators, including greater cumulative corticosteroid exposure or disease progression.

☑ All patients on immunomodulators must be closely monitored clinically and biochemically for potential adverse events for the duration of therapy.

☑ Many adverse events to AZA may be overcome by dose reduction, slow re-escalation, or the use of 6-MP.

☑ Vaccination schedules of patients should be assessed and updated prior to the commencement of immunomodulators.

REFERENCES

1. Doherty G, Bennett G, Patil S, Cheifetz A, Moss AC. Interventions for prevention of postoperative recurrence of Crohn's disease. *Cochrane Database Syst Rev.* 2009;(4):CD006873.
2. Prefontaine E, Macdonald JK, Sutherland LR. Azathioprine or 6-mercaptopurine for induction of remission in Crohn's disease. *Cochrane Database Syst Rev.* 2010;(6):CD000545.
3. Prefontaine E, Sutherland LR, Macdonald JK, Cepoiu M. Azathioprine or 6-mercaptopurine for maintenance of remission in Crohn's disease. *Cochrane Database Syst Rev.* 2009;(1):CD000067.
4. Peyrin-Biroulet L, Deltenre P, Ardizzone S, et al. Azathioprine and 6-mercaptopurine for the prevention of postoperative recurrence in Crohn's disease: a meta-analysis. *Am J Gastroenterol.* 2009;104(8):2089-2096.
5. Timmer A, McDonald JW, Macdonald JK. Azathioprine and 6-mercaptopurine for maintenance of remission in ulcerative colitis. *Cochrane Database Syst Rev.* 2007;(1):CD000478.
6. Gisbert JP, Linares PM, McNicholl AG, Mate J, Gomollon F. Meta-analysis: the efficacy of azathioprine and mercaptopurine in ulcerative colitis. *Aliment Pharmacol Ther.* 2009;30(2):126-137.
7. Cosnes J, Nion-Larmurier I, Beaugerie L, Afchain P, Tiret E, Gendre JP. Impact of the increasing use of immunosuppressants in Crohn's disease on the need for intestinal surgery. *Gut.* 2005;54(2):237-241.
8. Gisbert JP, Nino P, Cara C, Rodrigo L. Comparative effectiveness of azathioprine in Crohn's disease and ulcerative colitis: prospective, long-term, follow-up study of 394 patients. *Aliment Pharmacol Ther.* 2008;28(2):228-238.

9. Ramadas AV, Gunesh S, Thomas GA, Williams GT, Hawthorne AB. Natural history of Crohn's disease in a population-based cohort from Cardiff (1986-2003): a study of changes in medical treatment and surgical resection rates. *Gut.* 2010;59(9):1200-1206.

10. Gearry RB, Barclay ML, Burt MJ, Collett JA, Chapman BA. Thiopurine drug adverse effects in a population of New Zealand patients with inflammatory bowel disease. *Pharmacoepidemiol Drug Saf.* 2004;13(8):563-567.

11. Lewis JD, Gelfand JM, Troxel AB, et al. Immunosuppressant medications and mortality in inflammatory bowel disease. *Am J Gastroenterol.* 2008;103(6):1428-1435.

12. Lichtenstein GR, Feagan BG, Cohen RD, et al. Serious infections and mortality in association with therapies for Crohn's disease: TREAT registry. *Clin Gastroenterol Hepatol.* 2006;4(5):621-630.

13. Rasmussen HH, Fonager K, Sorensen HT, Pedersen L, Dahlerup JF, Steffensen FH. Risk of acute pancreatitis in patients with chronic inflammatory bowel disease. A Danish 16-year nationwide follow-up study. *Scand J Gastroenterol.* 1999;34(2):199-201.

14. Bermejo F, Lopez-Sanroman A, Taxonera C, et al. Acute pancreatitis in inflammatory bowel disease, with special reference to azathioprine-induced pancreatitis. *Aliment Pharmacol Ther.* 2008;28(5):623-628.

15. van Geenen EJ, de Boer NK, Stassen P, et al. Azathioprine or mercaptopurine-induced acute pancreatitis is not a disease-specific phenomenon. *Aliment Pharmacol Ther.* 2010;31(12): 1322-1329.

16. Marinaki AM, Ansari A, Duley JA, et al. Adverse drug reactions to azathioprine therapy are associated with polymorphism in the gene encoding inosine triphosphate pyrophosphatase (ITPase). *Pharmacogenetics.* 2004;14(3):181-187.

17. Gearry RB, Roberts RL, Barclay ML, Kennedy MA. Lack of association between the ITPA 94C>A polymorphism and adverse effects from azathioprine. *Pharmacogenetics.* 2004;14(11):779-781.

18. Alexander S, Dowling D. Azathioprine pancreatitis in inflammatory bowel disease and successful subsequent treatment with mercaptopurine. *Intern Med J.* 2005;35(9):570-571.

19. Romagnuolo J, Sadowski DC, Lalor E, Jewell L, Thomson AB. Cholestatic hepatocellular injury with azathioprine: a case report and review of the mechanisms of hepatotoxicity. *Can J Gastroenterol.* 1998;12(7):479-483.

20. DePinho RA, Goldberg CS, Lefkowitch JH. Azathioprine and the liver. Evidence favoring idiosyncratic, mixed cholestatic-hepatocellular injury in humans. *Gastroenterology.* 1984;86(1):162-165.

21. Gisbert JP, Gomollon F. Thiopurine-induced myelotoxicity in patients with inflammatory bowel disease: a review. *Am J Gastroenterol.* 2008;103(7):1783-1800.

22. Weinshilboum RM, Sladek SL. Mercaptopurine pharmacogenetics: monogenic inheritance of erythrocyte thiopurine methyltransferase activity. *Am J Hum Genet.* 1980;32(5):651-662.

23. Gardiner SJ, Gearry RB, Begg EJ, Zhang M, Barclay ML. Thiopurine dose in intermediate and normal metabolizers of thiopurine methyltransferase may differ three-fold. *Clin Gastroenterol Hepatol.* 2008;6(6):654-660.

24. Dong XW, Zheng Q, Zhu MM, Tong JL, Ran ZH. Thiopurine S-methyltransferase polymorphisms and thiopurine toxicity in treatment of inflammatory bowel disease. *World J Gastroenterol.* 2010;16(25):3187-3195.

25. Colombel JF, Ferrari N, Debuysere H, et al. Genotypic analysis of thiopurine S-methyltransferase in patients with Crohn's disease and severe myelosuppression during azathioprine therapy. *Gastroenterology.* 2000;118(6):1025-1030.

26. Wasan SK, Baker SE, Skolnik PR, Farraye FA. A practical guide to vaccinating the inflammatory bowel disease patient. *Am J Gastroenterol.* 2010;105(6):1231-1238.

27. Melmed GY. Vaccination strategies for patients with inflammatory bowel disease on immunomodulators and biologics. *Inflamm Bowel Dis.* 2009;15(9):1410-1416.

28. Sands BE, Cuffari C, Katz J, et al. Guidelines for immunizations in patients with inflammatory bowel disease. *Inflamm Bowel Dis.* 2004;10(5):677-692.

29. Rahier JF, Ben-Horin S, Chowers Y, et al. European evidence-based consensus on the prevention, diagnosis and management of opportunistic infections in inflammatory bowel disease. *J Crohns Colitis.* 2009;3(2):47-91.

30. Gisbert JP, Gonzalez-Lama Y, Mate J. Thiopurine-induced liver injury in patients with inflammatory bowel disease: a systematic review. *Am J Gastroenterol.* 2007;102(7):1518-1527.

31. Bastida G, Nos P, Aguas M, et al. Incidence, risk factors and clinical course of thiopurine-induced liver injury in patients with inflammatory bowel disease. *Aliment Pharmacol Ther.* 2005;22(9):775-782.

32. Present DH, Meltzer SJ, Krumholz MP, Wolke A, Korelitz BI. 6-mercaptopurine in the management of inflammatory bowel disease: short- and long-term toxicity. *Ann Intern Med.* 1989;111(8):641-649.

33. Lees CW, Maan AK, Hansoti B, Satsangi J, Arnott ID. Tolerability and safety of mercaptopurine in azathioprine-intolerant patients with inflammatory bowel disease. *Aliment Pharmacol Ther.* 2008;27(3):220-227.

34. Kiefer K, El-Matary W. 6-mercaptopurine as an alternative to azathioprine in azathioprine-induced hepatoxicity. *Inflamm Bowel Dis.* 2009;15(2):318-319.

35. Kuriyama M, Kato J, Suzuki H, et al. Tolerability and usefulness of mercaptopurine in azathioprine-intolerant Japanese patients with ulcerative colitis. *Dig Endosc.* 2010;22(4):289-296.

36. McGovern DP, Travis SP, Duley J, Shobowale-Bakre el M, Dalton HR. Azathioprine intolerance in patients with IBD may be imidazole-related and is independent of TPMT activity. *Gastroenterology.* 2002;122(3):838-839.

37. Dubinsky MC, Lamothe S, Yang HY, et al. Pharmacogenomics and metabolite measurement for 6-mercaptopurine therapy in inflammatory bowel disease. *Gastroenterology.* 2000;118(4):705-713.

38. Shaye OA, Yadegari M, Abreu MT, et al. Hepatotoxicity of 6-mercaptopurine (6-MP) and azathioprine (AZA) in adult IBD patients. *Am J Gastroenterol.* 2007;102(11):2488-2494.

39. Ansari A, Hassan C, Duley J, et al. Thiopurine methyltransferase activity and the use of azathioprine in inflammatory bowel disease. *Aliment Pharmacol Ther.* 2002;16(10):1743-1750.

40. Sparrow MP, Hande SA, Friedman S, Cao D, Hanauer SB. Effect of allopurinol on clinical outcomes in inflammatory bowel disease nonresponders to azathioprine or 6-mercaptopurine. *Clin Gastroenterol Hepatol.* 2007;5(2):209-214.

41. Dubinsky MC, Vasiliauskas EA, Singh H, et al. 6-thioguanine can cause serious liver injury in inflammatory bowel disease patients. *Gastroenterology.* 2003;125(2):298-303.

42. van Asseldonk DP, Jharap B, Kuik DJ, et al. Prolonged thioguanine therapy is well tolerated and safe in the treatment of ulcerative colitis. *Dig Liver Dis.* 2011;43(2):110-115.

43. Seinen ML, van Asseldonk DP, Mulder CJ, de Boer NK. Dosing 6-thioguanine in inflammatory bowel disease: expert-based guidelines for daily practice. *J Gastrointestin Liver Dis.* 2010; 19(3):291-294.

44. Vernier-Massouille G, Cosnes J, Lemann M, et al. Nodular regenerative hyperplasia in patients with inflammatory bowel disease treated with azathioprine. *Gut.* 2007;56(10):1404-1409.

45. De Boer NK, Tuynman H, Bloemena E, et al. Histopathology of liver biopsies from a thiopurine-naive inflammatory bowel disease cohort: prevalence of nodular regenerative hyperplasia. *Scand J Gastroenterol.* 2008;43(5):604-608.

46. Herrlinger KR, Deibert P, Schwab M, et al. Remission maintenance by tioguanine in chronic active Crohn's disease. *Aliment Pharmacol Ther.* 2003;17(12):1459-1464.

47. Teml A, Schwab M, Harrer M, et al. A prospective, open-label trial of 6-thioguanine in patients with ulcerative or indeterminate colitis. *Scand J Gastroenterol.* 2005;40(10):1205-1213.

48. Kandiel A, Fraser AG, Korelitz BI, Brensinger C, Lewis JD. Increased risk of lymphoma among inflammatory bowel disease patients treated with azathioprine and 6-mercaptopurine. *Gut.* 2005;54(8):1121-1125.

49. Armstrong RG, West J, Card TR. Risk of cancer in inflammatory bowel disease treated with azathioprine: a UK population-based case-control study. *Am J Gastroenterol.* 2010;105(7):1604-1609.

50. Beaugerie L, Brousse N, Bouvier AM, et al. Lymphoproliferative disorders in patients receiving thiopurines for inflammatory bowel disease: a prospective observational cohort study. *Lancet.* 2009;374(9701):1617-1625.

51. Kotlyar DS, Osterman MT, Diamond RH, et al. A systematic review of factors that contribute to hepatosplenic T-cell lymphoma in patients with inflammatory bowel disease. *Clin Gastroenterol Hepatol.* 2011;9(1):36 e1-41 e1.

52. Long MD, Herfarth HH, Pipkin CA, Porter CQ, Sandler RS, Kappelman MD. Increased risk for non-melanoma skin cancer in patients with inflammatory bowel disease. *Clin Gastroenterol Hepatol.* 2010;8(3):268-274.

53. Smith MA, Irving PM, Marinaki AM, Sanderson JD. Review article: malignancy on thiopurine treatment with special reference to inflammatory bowel disease. *Aliment Pharmacol Ther.* 2010;32(2):119-130.

54. Alfadhli AA, McDonald JW, Feagan BG. Methotrexate for induction of remission in refractory Crohn's disease. *Cochrane Database Syst Rev.* 2005;(1):CD003459.

55. Patel V, Macdonald JK, McDonald JW, Chande N. Methotrexate for maintenance of remission in Crohn's disease. *Cochrane Database Syst Rev.* 2009;(4):CD006884.

56. Chande N, MacDonald JK, McDonald JW. Methotrexate for induction of remission in ulcerative colitis. *Cochrane Database Syst Rev.* 2007;(4):CD006618.

57. El-Matary W, Vandermeer B, Griffiths AM. Methotrexate for maintenance of remission in ulcerative colitis. *Cochrane Database Syst Rev.* 2009;(3):CD007560.

58. Nathan DM, Iser JH, Gibson PR. A single center experience of methotrexate in the treatment of Crohn's disease and ulcerative colitis: a case for subcutaneous administration. *J Gastroenterol Hepatol.* 2008;23(6):954-958.

59. Feagan BG, Rochon J, Fedorak RN, et al. Methotrexate for the treatment of Crohn's disease. The North American Crohn's Study Group Investigators. *N Engl J Med.* 1995;332(5):292-297.

60. Ortiz Z, Shea B, Suarez-Almazor ME, Moher D, Wells GA, Tugwell P. The efficacy of folic acid and folinic acid in reducing methotrexate gastrointestinal toxicity in rheumatoid arthritis. A meta-analysis of randomized controlled trials. *J Rheumatol.* 1998;25(1):36-43.

61. Quinn CT, Kamen BA. A biochemical perspective of methotrexate neurotoxicity with insight on nonfolate rescue modalities. *J Investig Med.* 1996;44(9):522-530.

62. Bernini JC, Fort DW, Griener JC, et al. Aminophylline for methotrexate-induced neurotoxicity. *Lancet.* 1995;345(8949):544-547.

63. Goodman S. Measuring methotrexate polyglutamates. *Clin Exp Rheumatol.* 2010;28(5 suppl 61): S24-S26.

64. Brooks AJ, Begg EJ, Zhang M, Frampton CM, Barclay ML. Red blood cell methotrexate polyglutamate concentrations in inflammatory bowel disease. *Ther Drug Monit.* 2007; 29(5):619-625.

65. Berkowitz RS, Goldstein DP, Bernstein MR. Ten year's experience with methotrexate and folinic acid as primary therapy for gestational trophoblastic disease. *Gynecol Oncol.* 1986;23(1):111-118.

66. Menter A, Korman NJ, Elmets CA, et al. Guidelines of care for the management of psoriasis and psoriatic arthritis. Section 3. Guidelines of care for the management and treatment of psoriasis with topical therapies. *J Am Acad Dermatol.* 2009;60(4):643-659.

67. Te HS, Schiano TD, Kuan SF, Hanauer SB, Conjeevaram HS, Baker AL. Hepatic effects of long-term methotrexate use in the treatment of inflammatory bowel disease. *Am J Gastroenterol.* 2000;95(11):3150-3156.

68. Fournier MR, Klein J, Minuk GY, Bernstein CN. Changes in liver biochemistry during methotrexate use for inflammatory bowel disease. *Am J Gastroenterol.* 2010;105(7): 1620-1626.

69. Kremer JM, Furst DE, Weinblatt ME, Blotner SD. Significant changes in serum AST across hepatic histological biopsy grades: prospective analysis of 3 cohorts receiving methotrexate therapy for rheumatoid arthritis. *J Rheumatol.* 1996;23(3):459-461.

70. Sostman HD, Matthay RA, Putman CE. Cytotoxic drug-induced lung disease. *Am J Med.* 1977;62(4):608-615.

71. Searles G, McKendry RJ. Methotrexate pneumonitis in rheumatoid arthritis: potential risk factors. Four case reports and a review of the literature. *J Rheumatol.* 1987;14(6):1164-1171.

72. LeMense GP, Sahn SA. Opportunistic infection during treatment with low dose methotrexate. *Am J Respir Crit Care Med.* 1994;150(1):258-260.

73. Gutierrez-Urena S, Molina JF, Garcia CO, Cuellar ML, Espinoza LR. Pancytopenia secondary to methotrexate therapy in rheumatoid arthritis. *Arthritis Rheum.* 1996;39(2):272-276.

74. Mariette X, Cazals-Hatem D, Warszawki J, Liote F, Balandraud N, Sibilia J. Lymphomas in rheumatoid arthritis patients treated with methotrexate: a 3-year prospective study in France. *Blood.* 2002;99(11):3909-3915.

75. Siegel CA. Review article: explaining risks of inflammatory bowel disease therapy to patients. *Aliment Pharmacol Ther.* 2011;33(1):23-32.

SUGGESTED READINGS

Beaugerie L, Brousse N, Bouvier AM, et al. Lymphoproliferative disorders in patients receiving thiopurines for inflammatory bowel disease: a prospective observational cohort study. *Lancet.* 2009;374(9701):1617-1625.

Colombel JF, Ferrari N, Debuysere H, et al. Genotypic analysis of thiopurine S-methyltransferase in patients with Crohn's disease and severe myelosuppression during azathioprine therapy. *Gastroenterology.* 2000;118(6):1025-1030.

Gisbert JP, Nino P, Cara C, Rodrigo L. Comparative effectiveness of azathioprine in Crohn's disease and ulcerative colitis: prospective, long-term, follow-up study of 394 patients. *Aliment Pharmacol Ther.* 2008;28(2):228-238.

Melmed GY. Vaccination strategies for patients with inflammatory bowel disease on immunomodulators and biologics. *Inflamm Bowel Dis.* 2009;15(9):1410-1416.

Ramadas AV, Gunesh S, Thomas GA, Williams GT, Hawthorne AB. Natural history of Crohn's disease in a population-based cohort from Cardiff (1986-2003): a study of changes in medical treatment and surgical resection rates. *Gut.* 2010;59(9):1200-1206.

Siegel CA. Review article: explaining risks of inflammatory bowel disease therapy to patients. *Aliment Pharmacol Ther.* 2011;33(1):23-32.

Chapter 16

Anti-Tumor Necrosis Factor Therapy
Safety and Toxicity

A. Hillary Steinhart, MD, MSc, FRCP(C)

The development of anti-tumor necrosis factor-alpha (TNF-α)–based therapies for the treatment of Crohn's disease (CD) and ulcerative colitis (UC) has been a major advance in the management of these conditions. Large randomized controlled trials have demonstrated efficacy in both CD and UC, leading to their approval for use in both conditions in many countries. Just as important as the demonstration of efficacy, these trials with few exceptions found that the use of anti-TNF-α therapy was not associated with increased risk of adverse effects or toxicity as compared to placebo (Tables 16-1 through 16-3).[1-17] Although these clinical trials did not suggest that there might be an increased risk of clinically important side effects or toxicity in the populations studied, the trials were not of sufficient size or duration of follow-up to allow for definitive conclusions regarding the true risk of toxicity and important side effects related to anti-TNF-α therapy. Medium-sized randomized trials, such as those that were part of the anti-TNF-α development programs, can provide information regarding the incidence of more common side effects of acute or short-term therapy, but they are not able to provide definitive conclusions regarding less common side effects. Additionally, these trials cannot address those side effects that might occur many years after the start of therapy or those that are associated with long-term use of anti-TNF-α agents. Describing those types of adverse events generally requires large postmarketing studies and registries involving large numbers of patients. In addition, the benefit obtained from these drugs, with respect to their disease-remitting effect and the associated potential improvements in nutritional state, improved patient well-being, and decreased rates of disease-associated complications may offset the occurrence of adverse effects that are specifically related to the use of the drug in question.

Regueiro MD, Swoger JM, eds.
Clinical Challenges and Complications of IBD (pp 303-326).
© 2013 Taylor & Francis Group.

Table 16-1. Adverse Event Reporting in Infliximab-Controlled Trials

Study	Targan et al[7]		Present et al[4]			Hanauer et al[2]			Sands et al[6]		Hyams et al[10]		Colombel et al[17]	
Drug and dose	Placebo (n = 25)	IFX All doses (n = 102)	Placebo (n = 31)	IFX 5 mg/kg (n = 31)	IFX 10 mg/kg (n = 32)	Placebo (n = 188)	IFX 5 mg/kg (n = 192)	IFX 10 mg/kg (n = 193)	Placebo (n = 99)	IFX 5 mg/kg (n = 96)	Q8 wk (n = 96)	Q12 wk (n = 92)	AZA (n = 170)	IFX 5 mg/kg (n = 169)
Follow-up (wk)	6.9	10.4	18			54			54		51.5	49.6	54	
Adverse Event														
Any AE	60	75	65	65	84	NR	NR	NR	NR	NR	96	92	89	89
SAE	NR	NR	0	3	13	29	28	22	23	14	15	14	27	24
Discontinue due to AE	NR	NR	NR	NR	NR	3	15	8	8	4	4	8	NR	NR
Infusion reaction	NR	NR	NR		6	9	23	19	3	9	17	18	6	17
ANA	NR	NR	NR		NR	NR	NR	NR	18	46	NR	NR	NR	NR
Anti-dsDNA	NR	NR	NR		NR	NR	NR	NR	6	23	NR	NR	NR	NR
All infections	NR	NR	NR		NR	37	33	27	27	34	74	38	45	46
Serious infections	NR	NR	NR		NR	4	4	3	6	3	6	8	6	5
Malignancy	NR	NR	NR		NR	1	1.5	0.5	0*	0*	NR	NR	2	0
Death	NR	NR	NR		NR	0	1.5	0	0	0	NR	NR	1	0

Event rates are presented as percentages. AE = adverse event; ANA = antinuclear antibody; AZA = azathioprine; IFX = infliximab; NR = not reported; SAE = serious adverse event.
*No malignancies occurred during the study period but were subsequently reported in 2 infliximab-treated patients during long-term follow-up.

Table 16-2. Adverse Event Reporting in Adalimumab-Controlled Trials

STUDY	HANAUER ET AL[3]				SANDBORN ET AL[16]				COLOMBEL ET AL[11]		
Drug and dose	Placebo (n = 74)	ADA 40 mg/ 20 mg (n = 74)	ADA 80 mg/ 40 mg (n = 75)	ADA 160 mg/ 80 mg (n = 76)	Placebo (n = 18)	ADA 40 mg eow (n = 19)	ADA 40 mg ew (n = 18)	ADA OL* (n = 221)	Placebo (n = 261)	ADA 40 mg eow (n = 260)	ADA 40 mg ew (n = 257)
Follow-up (wk)	4				56				56		
Adverse Event											
Any AE	74	68	68	75	100	79	78	94	85	89	86
SAE	4	0	1	4	1	5	0	17	15	9	8
Discontinue due to AE	3	1	1	0	11	5	6	18	13	7	5
Injection site reaction	16	26	24	38	12	5	0	12	0.4	4.2	5.8
All infections	16	10	17	21	83	74	33	58	37	46	44
Serious infections	0	0	0	3	0	0	0	4	3.4	2.7	2.7
Malignancy	NR	NR	NR	NR	5	0	0	0	0.4	0	0
Death	NR	NR	NR	NR	0	0	0	0	0	0	0

ADA = adalimumab; AE = adverse event; ew = every week; eow = every other week; NR = not reported; OL = open-label adalimumab; SAE = serious adverse event.
*Patients who were not in remission at week 4 of CLASSIC I trial[3] and week 4 of CLASSIC II[16] were offered open-label ADA 40 mg every other week.

Table 16-3. Adverse Event Reporting in Certolizumab-Controlled Trials

Study	Schreiber et al[13]				Sandborn et al[12]		Schreiber et al[15]		
	Placebo (n=73)	CTZ 100 mg (n=74)	CTZ 200 mg (n=72)	CTZ 400 mg (n=72)	Placebo (n=328)	CTZ 400 mg (n=331)	Induction* (n=668)	Placebo (n=212)	CTZ 400 mg (n=216)
Follow-up (wk)	12				26		26		
Adverse Event									
Any AE	70	77	76	66	79	81	59	67	65
SAE	8	10	14	8	7	10	7	7	6
Discontinue due to AE	10	12	10	10	12	11	8	13	8
Injection site reaction	3	7	6	3	14	3	2	15	3
All infections	23		26.5	NR	NR	NR	NR	NR	NR
Infectious SAE	NR	NR	NR	NR	2	4.5	2	<1	3
Nasopharyngitis	4	12	10	6	8	13	4	4	6
UTI	7	1	1	0	5	8	NR	NR	NR
Pyrexia	NR	NR	NR	NR	7	6	NR	NR	NR
Headache	NR	NR	NR	NR	16	18	13	7	7
Neoplasm	NR	NR	NR	NR	<1	<1	<1	0	0
Death	0	0	0	0	0	<1	<1	0	0

AE = adverse event; CTZ = certolizumab pegol; NR = not reported; SAE = serious adverse event; UTI = urinary tract infection
*All patients in induction phase received CTZ 400 mg at weeks 0, 2, and 4 and were assessed for adverse events to week 6.

There are accumulating data regarding complications of anti-TNF-α therapy from large registries and postmarketing surveillance programs with some suggesting that there is an increased risk of serious adverse events occurring with anti-TNF-α therapy,[18] whereas others have suggested that there is not any increased incidence relative to what is observed in a comparable population of patients not treated with anti-TNF-α therapy.[19]

This chapter will review the current state of knowledge regarding the safety and potential adverse events that have been observed in inflammatory bowel disease (IBD) patients treated with anti-TNF-α therapy (Table 16-4). However, this review will not specifically examine the safety experience of anti-TNF-α agents in patients with other conditions except as they directly relate to IBD.

INFUSION REACTIONS

Infusion reactions only occur in patients receiving intravenous anti-TNF-α therapy (eg, infliximab [IFX]). The incidence of infusion reactions in randomized controlled trials was between 1.0% and 4.5% with 5.0% to 23.0% of patients experiencing at least one reaction.[2,6,17] In open series of IFX-treated patients, infusion reactions have been reported during 6% of infusions and in up to 10% of patients.[20] Infusion reactions usually consist of one or more symptoms of flushing, fever, tachycardia, and a sense of chest tightness, and shortness of breath. There may be associated hypotension in some cases, but in most instances, there is no hemodynamic instability and no suggestion that these reactions are manifestations of anaphylactoid or type I hypersensitivity reactions.[20] However, anaphylactic reactions have been rarely reported.[21] Serious infusion reactions occur in approximately 1% of infusions.[20] Higher rates of acute infusion reactions during IFX infusions may occur in patients who have antibodies against IFX and in those who have stopped therapy and then later received a second course of therapy.

The best strategy for management of infusion reactions is preventing their occurrence before they become a problem. The use of a concomitant antimetabolite immunosuppressive, such as azathioprine, has been shown to reduce the occurrence of acute infusion reactions.[17] Acute infusion reactions can, in some instances, be prevented by giving hydrocortisone 200 mg intravenously just prior to the infusion,[22] but not all studies have been able to confirm this protective effect of glucocorticosteroid pretreatment with respect to the development of a first infusion reaction.[23] In addition, it is not clear whether a potential protective effect of intravenous hydrocortisone extends to patients who are already on an immunomodulator therapy in addition to IFX. For patients who have developed infusion reactions, pretreatment with intravenous hydrocortisone and antihistamines may reduce the incidence of subsequent acute infusion reactions.[23] It has also been the experience of some clinicians that acetaminophen can contribute to the prevention of infusion reactions.[24] Desensitization regimens may effectively prevent reactions in patients who have had anaphylactic or anaphylactoid reactions to IFX and may allow ongoing use of IFX.[25]

Table 16-4. Adverse Effects of Anti-TNF-α Therapy in Inflammatory Bowel Disease

INFUSION REACTIONS AND INJECTION SITE REACTIONS
Acute infusion reactions (infliximab)
Delayed infusion reactions (infliximab)
Injection site reactions (adalimumab and certolizumab)
INFECTIONS
Viral
• Adenovirus
• Cytomegalovirus
• Herpes simplex
• Herpes zoster
• Varicella zoster
• Hepatitis B
Bacterial
• *Salmonella* sp
• *Staphylococcus* sp
• *Legionella pneumophila*
• *Listeria moncytogenes*
• *Mycobacterium tuberculosis*
• *Clostridium difficile*
• Nocardia
Fungal
• *Candida* sp
• *Histoplasma capsulatum*
• Aspergillus
• *Pneumocystis jiroveci*
• Actinomycosis
• Mucormycosis
Protozoan and parasitic
• *Leishmania* sp
AUTOIMMUNE PHENOMENA
Drug-induced lupus erythematosus
Leukocytoclastic vasculitis
Idiopathic pericarditis
Sarcoidosis

continued

Table 16-4 (continued). Adverse Effects of Anti-TNF-α Therapy in Inflammatory Bowel Disease

SKIN LESIONS
Psoriasis
• Worsening of existing disease
• New onset of disease
Psoriaform rashes
Eczematoid rashes
HEART FAILURE
LIVER INJURY
Autoimmune (?)
HEMATOLOGIC
Thrombocytopenia
Neutropenia
Pancytopenia
NEUROLOGIC
Demyelination
• Central
• Peripheral (neuropathy)
Myelitis
Encephalopathy
MALIGNANCY
Lymphoma
• Non-Hodgkin lymphoma
• Hepatosplenic T-cell lymphoma
Skin cancers (nonmelanoma)
Other solid organ malignancies (?)

Infusion reactions, when they occur, can generally be managed effectively by temporarily stopping the infusion and treating with intravenous antihistamines and oral acetaminophen. Once symptoms have settled, the infusion can be resumed by a gradual upward titration of the infusion rate. This method of upward rate titration can also be used in patients who have had reactions severe enough to require discontinuation of IFX therapy, although some patients may still experience infusion reactions, some of which may be severe.[26] Although acute infusion reactions have been suggested to be related to the rate of infusion, more rapid infusions of IFX, over periods of as short as 30 minutes, can be given without an apparent increase in infusion reactions.[27,28] When infusion reactions do occur despite prophylactic measures, infusion reactions can be avoided by switching to a subcutaneous anti-TNF-α (eg, adalimumab or certolizumab pegol). Overall, infusion reactions are responsible for cessation of IFX in approximately 3% of patients treated but this can probably be reduced by aggressive prophylactic measures prior to starting therapy or by using the preventive and management measures described above when infusion reactions do occur. What is not entirely known is whether the occurrence of infusion reactions predict a diminished response to IFX by virtue of the fact that the presence of antibodies to IFX have been associated with an increased risk of infusion reactions and may also be associated with diminished efficacy. When IFX is discontinued due to acute infusion reactions, and adalimumab or certolizumab pegol is initiated, there is not an increased risk of adverse reaction to the subcutaneous injection, nor is there any reduction in observed effectiveness.

A second form of infusion reaction is the delayed infusion reaction or serum sickness type of reaction that typically occurs anywhere from 2 to 10 days after the infusion but can occur up to several weeks later.[29] It is characterized by diffuse arthralgias and myalgias, which can often be severe and incapacitating. Although these reactions appear clinically similar to serum sickness in their presentation, there is no end-organ involvement with IFX-related delayed infusion reactions. These infusion reactions typically respond promptly to several days of glucocorticosteroids and may be avoided by a 7- to 10-day tapering course of glucocorticosteroids started the day prior to an infusion.

Acute reactions, aside from local pain and erythema, are exceedingly rare with the subcutaneously administered anti-TNF-α agents. The local skin reactions rarely result in the need to discontinue therapy and are not associated with any reduction in efficacy.

INFECTIOUS COMPLICATIONS

As the administration of agents that interfere with the action of TNF-α and the cells that produce TNF-α have a dampening effect on certain aspects of cell-mediated immunity, it is not entirely surprising that there may be increased incidence of infections caused by microorganisms that are normally controlled or prevented by cell-mediated immunity. The best example of this is the reactivation of latent tuberculosis that was described shortly after IFX was introduced for the treatment of rheumatoid arthritis and CD.[30] Despite the fact that the association between the use of anti-TNF-α therapy and reactivation of latent tuberculosis seems well founded, a subsequent study has shown that the rate of tuberculosis was higher in the IBD patient population compared to that observed in the general population prior to the introduction of anti-TNF-α agents.[31] This suggests that the underlying IBD itself, or treatment with steroids or other immunosuppressive medications, predisposes patients to infection with the tuberculous bacillus.

Recognition of reactivation of latent tuberculosis as a potential complication has led to recommendations for pretreatment screening and introduction of prophylaxis or avoidance of anti-TNF-α therapy for at-risk individuals, with subsequent reduction in rates of tuberculosis.[30,32] It is generally recommended that all patients who are being considered for anti-TNF-α therapy be screened for latent tuberculosis according to local guidelines and adjusted according to the patient's individual demographic and clinical situation. Patients who are found to have, or are strongly suspected of having, latent tuberculosis should generally receive antituberculous prophylaxis prior to initiating anti-TNF-α therapy. The optimal duration of antituberculous therapy prior to starting anti-TNF-α therapy is not known. The decision in individual patients requires a balance between the risk of reactivation of tuberculosis if anti-TNF-α therapy is started too early in the course of prophylactic therapy versus the risk of worsening or complicated IBD if introduction of anti-TNF-α therapy is delayed too long. Antituberculous prophylaxis is not universally effective and infection can occur despite adequate prophylaxis.[33]

Although tuberculosis provided an important example of the potential risk of the immune suppression produced by blocking the action of TNF-α or by eliminating the cells producing TNF-α, the overall infection rate does not appear to be increased in patients treated with IFX or the other anti-TNF-α antibodies based upon a meta-analysis of randomized controlled trials.[34] This was confirmed by a large postmarketing registry involving 3179 patients who were treated with IFX and were compared to a similar number of patients with CD who had not received IFX or other anti-TNF-α therapies.[19] Data from a large population-based administrative health care utilization database of 10,662 IBD patients found no statistically significant increased risk of serious bacterial infection in patients treated with IFX as compared with other immunosuppressive agents.[35] Despite the absence of proof of an association between anti-TNF-α therapy and serious bacterial infection, there are a number of open or retrospective series that have reported rates of serious infection as being between 4% and 15% of patients.[36-39] Although the lack of an appropriate reference population limits the inferences that can be made from these data, these study results do argue for increased vigilance for bacterial infections in patients with IBD that is severe enough to require anti-TNF-α therapy.

Although there is no evidence from prospective controlled trials that serious bacterial infections are increased in IBD patients on anti-TNF-α therapy, there are numerous reports of opportunistic infections occurring in these patients.[40-51] The occurrence of opportunistic infections is likely an unusual event, but their detection requires careful clinical monitoring and a high index of suspicion. Although opportunistic infections appear to occur at a low level, some specific infectious agents appear to have been reported with higher than expected frequency. The Food and Drug Administration Adverse Event Reporting System registered a total of 84 cases of *Pneumocystis jiroveci* (*carinii*) pneumonia in patients with CD treated with IFX over a 5-year period, up to 2003.[42] This has led at least one organization to recommend cotrimoxazole prophylaxis against *Pneumocystis* for patients receiving anti-TNF-α therapy along with 2 or other immunosuppressive medications.[52]

The specific role of the anti-TNF-α therapy in the pathogenesis of serious bacterial infections and opportunistic infections that occur in patients receiving these agents is not completely known. In many instances, patients who develop opportunistic infections are also receiving treatment with immunosuppressives or steroids, and as such, the role of an anti-TNF-α agent in serious infections relative to that of the other pharmacotherapies is not clear. A retrospective case-control study from a tertiary care center has suggested that steroids, immunosuppressives, and anti-TNF-α agents each individually increase risk, but that the combination of any 2 or 3 further increases the risk.[40] However, the increased risk of infection with dual therapy incorporating an anti-TNF-α agent and an antimetabolite immunosuppressive drug has not been substantiated by prospective randomized controlled trials.[2,5,17,53,54]

Abscess

Although anti-TNF-α therapy does not appear to significantly increase the overall rate of serious bacterial infections seen in patients with IBD, there was some initial concern, based upon the first randomized controlled trial reported in patients with fistulizing CD, that IFX therapy was associated with an increased risk of abscess formation.[4] However, this was not substantiated by a subsequent larger randomized controlled trial.[55]

Postoperative Complications

There has also been concern that the use of anti-TNF-α therapy can increase the risk of postoperative complications, infections in particular, in patients who undergo IBD surgery while receiving anti-TNF-α therapy. However, the majority of studies have not substantiated an increased risk associated with the use of immunosuppressive therapy, including anti-TNF-α antibody therapy.[56-59] One study suggested an increased risk of postoperative complications, including septic complications, in patients who received IFX and subsequently underwent ileal pouch surgery for UC.[60] However, there was no indication as to the time between IFX therapy and the pouch surgery.

Hepatitis

The effect of TNF-α blockade on liver function and liver disease in patients with pre-existing chronic viral hepatitis appears to differ according to the type of viral hepatitis. Anti-TNF-α therapy has no apparent deleterious effect on hepatitis C viral copy levels, as measured by hepatitis C viral RNA levels in the serum of the infected host. There is no apparent deleterious effect on liver function, and anti-TNF-α therapy does not result in progression of liver damage.[61-64] In addition, anti-TNF-α therapy may actually have some degree of antiviral activity through its promotion of hepatocyte apoptosis and reduced regeneration.[65]

In patients with chronic hepatitis B, the use of anti-TNF-α therapy is generally contraindicated due to the reported occurrence of hepatitis B reactivation and acute liver damage in patients with previously quiescent hepatitis B infection.[66,67] However, therapy could be considered following the initiation of antiviral therapy directed toward the hepatitis B virus.[66]

Irrespective of a patient's viral status, caution is required whenever using an anti-TNF-α antibody-based therapy, and careful monitoring of viral loads, serum aminotransferases, and liver function are necessary.[68]

Other Viral Infections

Although the effect of TNF-α blockade could theoretically increase the severity, persistence, or reactivation of viral infections, short-term studies of viral markers, including those for Epstein-Barr virus and cytomegalovirus, have not demonstrated evidence of reactivation or other alteration in the natural history of these infections.[69,70] One case of disseminated cytomegalovirus infection has been reported in a patient who received a single dose of IFX after having been on corticosteroids and azathioprine for the treatment of CD.[50]

Fatal aseptic meningoencephalitis has been reported following IFX therapy.[71] Other severe or atypical presentations of viral infections have also been reported, including severe adenovirus pneumonia,[41] disseminated primary varicella infection,[72] an atypical rash due to varicella,[43] and herpes zoster encephalitis.[73]

Malignancy

Randomized controlled trials have not shown an increased incidence of malignancy in IBD patients treated with anti-TNF-α therapy as compared to those who received placebo. However, these trials are generally not large enough to provide sufficient power to detect a potential clinically important increase in the incidence of malignancy, and they usually do not have sufficient duration of follow-up to allow conclusions to be made about the potential long-term consequences of TNF-α blockade. In addition, in the placebo controlled trials, the patients initially randomized to placebo often crossed over to treatment with the anti-TNF-α drug being studied, thus making the number of patient-years of follow-up for patients treated with placebo alone relatively small. However, pooling the results of randomized trials of anti-TNF-α agents, such as adalimumab, has been carried out, and the overall results do not demonstrate rates of malignancy that are any higher than a reference population.[1] Further information on the risk of malignancy comes from prospective and retrospective cohorts of patients treated with anti-TNF-α therapy since the introduction of these agents in the late 1990s. These open series have generally reported an occurrence of malignancy of less than 2% to 3% but do not provide a reference population rate of malignancy with which to compare.[38,39,74-82] There have also been cohort studies that reference healthy or disease populations, and these have not shown that the overall incidence of malignancy is any higher in IBD patients treated with these drugs than in these comparator groups.[19,83-85]

Although the overall occurrence of malignancies in patients receiving anti-TNF-α therapy is not higher than what one would observe in a population of sick patients, there have been some indications that this class of drugs may increase the risk of lymphomas. Studies done in patients treated for rheumatologic conditions have suggested that the use of anti-TNF-α antibody may increase lymphoma risk above that of the increased risk seen in this same patient population in the absence of anti-TNF-α therapy.[86,87] Prior to 2002 there had been only single case reports of lymphoma occurring in patients treated with anti-TNF-α agents. In one of the earliest aggregate reports of lymphoma associated with anti-TNF-α use, Brown and colleagues reported on 26 cases of lymphoma occurring in patients treated with anti-TNF-α therapy.[86] This study used the MedWatch database, which is based upon the passive surveillance program of the US Food and Drug Administration's Adverse Event Reporting System. The study included 8 patients who developed lymphoma while on IFX and 18 patients who were on etanercept, an anti-TNF-α fusion protein that is not used in IBD. Five of the 8 patients who developed lymphoma while on IFX were being treated for CD, and the mean age of the patients was 61.8 years. In addition, in 4 of the 8 patients, the time from initiation of IFX therapy to the occurrence of lymphoma was less than 8 weeks. In a study of children with primarily rheumatologic conditions, the use of anti-TNF-α therapy was found to be associated with a higher rate of malignancies, in particular lymphoma, as compared to the background rate of malignancy and lymphoma in children.[87] In that study, which was also based upon the MedWatch Database, the results were confounded by the fact that 88% of the children who were reported to have developed malignancy were on other immunomodulatory agents, some of which are known to carry an independent risk of lymphoma. In addition, in 15 of the 48 reported cases, etanercept was the anti-TNF-α therapy that had been used.

A population-based study from Sweden found that the annual incidence of lymphoma was 1.5% in their population of 217 IBD patients treated with IFX between 1999 and 2001.[82] This incidence is 100-fold higher compared to the background risk of lymphoma in the general Swedish population. However, no disease reference population risk was provided. In addition, over 50% of patients were on concomitant AZA or 6-mercaptopurine, and the proportion who had previously been on a thiopurine analogue was not reported.

In IBD, reports of unusual and aggressive lymphomas began to appear several years after IFX was first introduced for the treatment of CD.[88,90] One type of lymphoma in particular, hepatosplenic T-cell lymphoma, has been reported much more frequently than the background rate given its rarity. In addition, it appears to occur almost exclusively in young males and is very aggressive, leading to death almost uniformly. Whether the hepatosplenic T-cell lymphoma is directly due to an anti-TNF-α agent or whether it is due to the combined use of an anti-TNF-α agent and a purine antimetabolite is not completely known, but it seems likely that purine analogue therapy is a necessary permissive factor in the development of this lymphoma.[90,91] Hepatosplenic T-cell lymphoma was first described in 1990 in individuals without IBD.[92] In the rare cases of hepatosplenic T-cell lymphoma that had occurred prior to the introduction of anti-TNF-α therapy, a history of purine antimetabolite therapy was universal.[91,93]

Liver Damage

In general, the use of anti-TNF-α agents results in no dose-related or predictable liver damage and has no negative effect on liver function. However, there have been reports of idiosyncratic liver injury secondary to IFX. The observed hepatotoxicity may be secondary to an autoimmune process, sometimes with associated antinuclear antibodies (ANAs), or due to direct hepatocyte injury, the mechanism of which is unclear.[94] IFX has been reported to produce reversible cholestasis[95] as well as acute liver injury occurring following a single infusion.[96] The presence of pre-existing liver disease, with the exception of untreated or uncontrolled hepatitis B infection, is not an absolute contraindication to the use of an anti-TNF-α agent. In addition, the safe use of IFX has been reported in a patient with UC and a previous liver transplantation for sclerosing cholangitis.[97]

AUTOIMMUNE AND INFLAMMATORY PHENOMENA

It is well known that a significant proportion of patients receiving anti-TNF-α antibody therapy develop autoantibodies. The occurrence of ANAs has been reported in between 42% to 56% of patients and the presence of anti–double-stranded DNA antibodies in up to 34% of patients treated with regularly scheduled maintenance doses of IFX.[98,99] However, in a significant proportion of patients, the presence of one or more autoantibodies may predate the use of anti-TNF-α therapy, and the new development of autoantibodies has rarely been associated with clinical autoimmune disease or a lupus-like syndrome in IBD patients.[98,99] There have been rare reports of a lupus-like syndrome occurring in patients treated with these agents, but most have been in patients with underlying rheumatologic disorders.[100-102] The rare cases of hepatotoxicity secondary to IFX may also be associated with the presence or development of ANAs and anti–double-stranded DNA antibodies and have a picture similar to autoimmune hepatitis.[94] In order to avoid confusion with the presence of pre-existing autoantibodies, it would seem to be reasonable to obtain baseline autoantibody assays prior to initiation of anti-TNF-α therapy.

It has been suggested that the development of autoantibodies, in particular ANAs, may be related to the apoptosis of TNF-α-producing cells induced by IgG1-based anti-TNF-α therapy. These antibody-based therapies, such as IFX and adalimumab, induce apoptosis by virtue of complement fixation through the Fc portion of the molecule. The occurrence of a lupus-like syndrome has been reported to have occurred with both IFX and adalimumab in a patient.[103]

However, there has also been a report of a patient who developed drug-related lupus while on IFX and did not develop it again when subsequently treated with adalimumab.[104] A subsequent series of patients with IFX-induced lupus has demonstrated that patients treated with a second anti-TNF-α agent may not necessarily have recurrence of lupus when treated with a second anti-TNF-α agent, either adalimumab or certolizumab pegol, for treatment periods of up to 5 months.[105] certolizumab pegol, which contains only the Fab9 fragment of the antibody, should, theoretically, have an advantage over the IgG1 antibodies adalimumab and IFX. A series of 8 patients who developed drug-induced lupus erythematosus on IFX and were treated with a second anti-TNF-α agent, 2 with adalimumab and 6 with certolizumab, showed that both adalimumab and certolizumab could be used without inducing recurrence of the lupus. However, recurrence was seen in one patient on each medication (adalimumab and certolizumab), suggesting that certolizumab may not be completely free of risk of drug-induced lupus erythematosus.[105]

Other autoimmune, immunologic, or idiopathic inflammatory adverse effects that have occurred in patients receiving anti-TNF-α antibody therapy include leukocytoclastic vasculitis,[106] idiopathic pericarditis,[107] and sarcoidosis.[108,109]

Heart Failure

Anti-TNF-α therapy was initially considered for development as a treatment for heart failure based on the presumed importance of TNF-α in the pathogenesis of heart failure. However, a controlled trial of IFX in heart failure patients demonstrated increased toxicity and mortality relative to placebo-treated patients. As a result, the presence of symptomatic or decompensated heart failure has generally been listed as a contraindication to the use of anti-TNF-α agents. Further case reports of heart failure in anti-TNF-α–treated patients have been published,[110] but a subsequent study in a large population of young (<50 years of age) CD and rheumatoid arthritis patients could not demonstrate any increased risk of heart failure.[111]

NEUROLOGIC COMPLICATIONS

The development of radiologically demonstrated demyelination, with associated symptoms, has been reported in patients treated with anti-TNF-α agents.[36,112-114] As a result, these agents are contraindicated in patients with a history of multiple sclerosis, optic neuritis, or other demyelinating disorders.

Peripheral neuropathy, which is likely secondary to demyelination, can also occur uncommonly as a result of anti-TNF-α therapy.[114,115] In some instances, the neuropathy can develop following discontinuation of anti-TNF-α therapy.[115]

Acute myelitis, which resulted in self-limited flaccid paralysis, has been reported in a patient shortly after initiation of IFX[116] and a reversible encephalopathy has been reported in a pediatric patient with CD treated with IFX.[117]

HEMATOLOGIC COMPLICATIONS

Anti-TNF-α agents do not produce predictable or dose-dependent effects on hematopoiesis or on the counts of blood elements such as neutrophils, lymphocytes, or platelets. Rare cases of neutropenia and thrombocytopenia,[118] thrombocytopenia,[119,120] and pancytopenia[38] have been reported, but these appear to be idiosyncratic and extremely uncommon. Hemophagocytic syndrome can also occur as a result of anti-TNF-α therapy.[121]

The lack of consistent effect of anti-TNF-α agents on bone marrow is likely partially responsible for the relatively low rates of serious bacterial infections while on these drugs. However, in some cases of reported hematologic abnormalities there has been evidence that the events may have been the result of autoimmune destruction of blood elements. This is supported by the finding of normal cell lines on bone marrow examination and the presence of platelet-associated antibodies in serum.[119,120] In one case of thrombocytopenia occurring following treatment with IFX, the platelet count fell once again after a trial of adalimumab. As with other autoimmune phenomena, it has been suggested that these events may be occurring as a result of antibody-mediated induction of apoptosis that, in turn, may result in the production of autoantibodies.

SKIN REACTIONS

Anti-TNF-α therapy can produce a number of different skin reactions. These can occur soon after initiation of therapy or can occur several years into the treatment. Skin reactions that may be observed include folliculitis, xerosis cutis, eczema, palmoplantar pustulosis, leukocytoclastic vasculitis, lichenoid drug reaction including lichen planopilaris, superficial granuloma annulare, acne vulgaris, lymphomatoid papulosis, and Stevens-Johnson syndrome.[122-128]

Although anti-TNF-α blockade has been an effective means of treating psoriasis, there have been numerous cases reported of new onset of psoriasis and other inflammatory skin conditions in individuals being treated with anti-TNF-α therapy.[128-141] This type of paradoxical reaction has been reported with IFX, adalimumab, and etanercept and involves worsening of pre-existing psoriasis in some instances, but in the majority of cases, it represents new onset of lesions in individuals without a pre-existing history of psoriasis.[142] Whether these types of paradoxical responses to anti-TNF-α therapy require cessation of the anti-TNF-α agent in order to allow resolution of the skin lesions, or whether switching from one anti-TNF-α agent to another can be an effective means of inducing improvement or resolution of the skin lesions, is not known.

A series of 922 consecutive IBD patients treated with anti-TNF-α therapy were systematically studied for the occurrence of skin lesions.[128] Out of this series of patients, 203 (22%) developed skin lesions. Of these, 74% developed on treatment with IFX whereas 26% developed after switching from IFX to adalimumab or certolizumab. The lesions described were xerosis (12.5%), eczema (22.4%), psoriasis (5.2%), psoriasiform eczema (28.6%), and palmoplantar pustulosis (2.6%). A variety of other skin conditions accounted for the other 28.6%. The development of ANAs in a titer of greater than 1:80 was found to be associated with a higher likelihood of developing skin lesions, and a specific variation of the IL23R gene was found to be associated with a lower likelihood. In that series only 6.3% of the 203 patients discontinued anti-TNF-α therapy due to a dermatologic adverse event.

CONCLUSION

Although anti-TNF-α agents have been used for less than 15 years in the treatment of IBD, the large numbers of patients treated has provided significant experience and opportunity for observation of potential complications of therapy or adverse events. As a class, the anti-TNF-α agents appear to have relatively few side effects that are consistently observed. There appear to be some occurrences that, although relatively uncommon, do appear to have a causality link with anti-TNF-α therapy. These include the occurrence of infections, particularly reactivation of latent tuberculosis or other opportunistic infections, hepatosplenic T-cell lymphoma, and psoriatic skin disorders. However, these adverse events appear to occur at relatively low rates on therapy, and given the significant benefit provided by anti-TNF-α therapy to the majority of patients, the risk-to-benefit ratio continues to be favorable when used in the appropriate clinical setting.

☑ Key Points

☑ Anti-TNF-agents that are used for the treatment of IBD (IFX, adalimumab, and CTZ) are more similar than they are different with respect to adverse event profile—the exception is the occurrence of infusion reactions that can occur with IFX.

☑ As a class, the anti-TNF-agents have relatively few predictable or dose-related side effects that are consistently observed.

☑ Anti-TNF-agents increase the risk of reactivation of tuberculosis and likely increase the risk of opportunistic infection. However, these risks are quite low, particularly if screening and prophylactic measures are employed.

☑ Anti-TNF-agents likely increase the risk of hepatosplenic T-cell lymphoma, but their impact on the incidence of other lymphomas and malignancies is not clear.

☑ Given the totality of the evidence regarding the potential adverse effects of anti-TNF-therapy and the known clinical benefit that they can provide to patients, their overall risk-to-benefit ratio is quite good.

REFERENCES

1. Colombel JF, Sandborn WJ, Panaccione R, et al. Adalimumab safety in global clinical trials of patients with Crohn's disease. *Inflamm Bowel Dis.* 2009;15(9):1308-1319.

2. Hanauer SB, Feagan BG, Lichtenstein GR, et al. Maintenance infliximab for Crohn's disease: the ACCENT I randomised trial. *Lancet.* 2002;359(9317):1541-1549.

3. Hanauer SB, Sandborn WJ, Rutgeerts P, et al. Human anti-tumor necrosis factor monoclonal antibody (adalimumab) in Crohn's disease: the CLASSIC-I trial. *Gastroenterology.* 2006;130(2):323-333.

4. Present DH, Rutgeerts P, Targan S, et al. Infliximab for the treatment of fistulas in patients with Crohn's disease. *N Engl J Med.* 1999;340(18):1398-1405.

5. Rutgeerts P, Sandborn WJ, Feagan BG, et al. Infliximab for induction and maintenance therapy for ulcerative colitis. *N Engl J Med.* 2005;353(23):2462-2476.

6. Sands BE, Anderson FH, Bernstein CN, et al. Infliximab maintenance therapy for fistulizing Crohn's disease. *N Engl J Med.* 2004;350(9):876-885.

7. Targan SR, Hanauer SB, van Deventer SJ, et al. A short-term study of chimeric monoclonal antibody cA2 to tumor necrosis factor alpha for Crohn's disease. Crohn's Disease cA2 Study Group. *N Engl J Med.* 1997;337(15):1029-1035.

8. Feagan BG, Sandborn WJ, Baker JP, et al. A randomized, double-blind, placebo-controlled trial of CDP571, a humanized monoclonal antibody to tumour necrosis factor-alpha, in patients with corticosteroid-dependent Crohn's disease. *Aliment Pharmacol Ther.* 2005;21(4):373-384.

9. Feagan BG, Sandborn WJ, Lichtenstein G, Radford-Smith G, Patel J, Innes A. CDP571, a humanized monoclonal antibody to tumour necrosis factor-alpha, for steroid-dependent Crohn's disease: a randomized, double-blind, placebo-controlled trial. *Aliment Pharmacol Ther.* 2006;23(5):617-628.

10. Hyams J, Crandall W, Kugathasan S, et al. Induction and maintenance infliximab therapy for the treatment of moderate-to-severe Crohn's disease in children. *Gastroenterology.* 2007;132(3):863-873.

11. Colombel JF, Sandborn WJ, Rutgeerts P, et al. Adalimumab for maintenance of clinical response and remission in patients with Crohn's disease: the CHARM trial. *Gastroenterology.* 2007;132(1):52-65.

12. Sandborn WJ, Feagan BG, Stoinov S, et al. Certolizumab pegol for the treatment of Crohn's disease. *N Engl J Med.* 2007;357(3):228-238.

13. Schreiber S, Rutgeerts P, Fedorak RN, et al. A randomized, placebo-controlled trial of certolizumab pegol (CDP870) for treatment of Crohn's disease. *Gastroenterology.* 2005;129(3):807-818.

14. Schreiber S, Colombel JF, Bloomfield R, et al. Increased response and remission rates in short-duration Crohn's disease with subcutaneous certolizumab pegol: an analysis of PRECiSE 2 randomized maintenance trial data. *Am J Gastroenterol.* 2010;105(7):1574-1582.

15. Schreiber S, Khaliq-Kareemi M, Lawrance IC, et al. Maintenance therapy with certolizumab pegol for Crohn's disease. *N Engl J Med.* 2007;357(3):239-250.

16. Sandborn WJ, Hanauer SB, Rutgeerts P, et al. Adalimumab for maintenance treatment of Crohn's disease: results of the CLASSIC II trial. *Gut.* 2007;56(9):1232-1239.

17. Colombel JF, Sandborn WJ, Reinisch W, et al. Infliximab, azathioprine, or combination therapy for Crohn's disease. *N Engl J Med.* 2010;362(15):1383-1395.

18. Hansen RA, Gartlehner G, Powell GE, Sandler RS. Serious adverse events with infliximab: analysis of spontaneously reported adverse events. *Clin Gastroenterol Hepatol.* 2007;5(6):729-735.

19. Lichtenstein GR, Feagan BG, Cohen RD, et al. Serious infections and mortality in association with therapies for Crohn's disease: TREAT registry. *Clin Gastroenterol Hepatol.* 2006;4(5):621-630.

20. Cheifetz A, Smedley M, Martin S, et al. The incidence and management of infusion reactions to infliximab: a large center experience. *Am J Gastroenterol.* 2003;98(6):1315-1324.

21. Stallmach A, Giese T, Schmidt C, Meuer SC, Zeuzem SS. Severe anaphylactic reaction to infliximab: successful treatment with adalimumab—report of a case. *Eur J Gastroenterol Hepatol.* 2004;16(6):627-630.

22. Farrell RJ, Alsahli M, Jeen YT, Falchuk KR, Peppercorn MA, Michetti P. Intravenous hydrocortisone premedication reduces antibodies to infliximab in Crohn's disease: a randomized controlled trial. *Gastroenterology.* 2003;124(4):917-924.

23. Jacobstein DA, Markowitz JE, Kirschner BS, et al. Premedication and infusion reactions with infliximab: results from a pediatric inflammatory bowel disease consortium. *Inflamm Bowel Dis.* 2005;11(5):442-446.

24. Sattin B, Choquette D, Bensen W, Nantel F. Reduced incidence of infusion reactions to infliximab in patients pre-medicated with acetaminophen. *Can J Gastroenterol.* 2010;24(suppl A): A228.

25. Puchner TC, Kugathasan S, Kelly KJ, Binion DG. Successful desensitization and therapeutic use of infliximab in adult and pediatric Crohn's disease patients with prior anaphylactic reaction. *Inflamm Bowel Dis.* 2001;7(1):34-37.

26. Duburque C, Lelong J, Iacob R, et al. Successful induction of tolerance to infliximab in patients with Crohn's disease and prior severe infusion reactions. *Aliment Pharmacol Ther.* 2006;24(5):851-858.

27. Clare DF, Alexander FC, Mike S, et al. Accelerated infliximab infusions are safe and well tolerated in patients with inflammatory bowel disease. *Eur J Gastroenterol Hepatol.* 2009;21(1):71-75.

28. Yeckes AR, Hoffenberg EJ. Rapid infliximab infusions in pediatric inflammatory bowel disease. *J Pediatr Gastroenterol Nutr.* 2009;49(1):151-154.

29. Gamarra RM, McGraw SD, Drelichman VS, Maas LC. Serum sickness-like reactions in patients receiving intravenous infliximab. *J Emerg Med.* 2006;30(1):41-44.

30. Keane J, Gershon S, Wise RP, et al. Tuberculosis associated with infliximab, a tumor necrosis factor alpha-neutralizing agent. *N Engl J Med.* 2001;345(15):1098-1104.

31. Aberra FN, Stettler N, Brensinger C, Lichtenstein GR, Lewis JD. Risk for active tuberculosis in inflammatory bowel disease patients. *Clin Gastroenterol Hepatol.* 2007;5(9):1070-1075.

32. Carmona L, Gomez-Reino JJ, Rodriguez-Valverde V, et al. Effectiveness of recommendations to prevent reactivation of latent tuberculosis infection in patients treated with tumor necrosis factor antagonists. *Arthritis Rheum.* 2005;52(6):1766-1772.

33. Parra RJ, Ortego CN, Raya AE. Development of tuberculosis in a patient treated with infliximab who had received prophylactic therapy with isoniazid. *J Rheumatol.* 2003;30(7):1657-1658.

34. Peyrin-Biroulet L, Deltenre P, de Suray N, Branche J, Sandborn WJ, Colombel JF. Efficacy and safety of tumor necrosis factor antagonists in Crohn's disease: meta-analysis of placebo-controlled trials. *Clin Gastroenterol Hepatol.* 2008;6(6):644-653.

35. Schneeweiss S, Korzenik J, Solomon DH, Canning C, Lee J, Bressler B. Infliximab and other immunomodulating drugs in patients with inflammatory bowel disease and the risk of serious bacterial infections. *Aliment Pharmacol Ther.* 2009;30(3):253-264.

36. Lees CW, Ali AI, Thompson AI, et al. The safety profile of anti-tumour necrosis factor therapy in inflammatory bowel disease in clinical practice: analysis of 620 patient-years follow-up. *Aliment Pharmacol Ther.* 2009;29(3):286-297.

37. de Vries HS, van Oijen MG, de Jong DJ. Serious events with infliximab in patients with inflammatory bowel disease: a 9-year cohort study in the Netherlands. *Drug Saf.* 2008; 31(12):1135-1144.

38. Seiderer J, Goke B, Ochsenkuhn T. Safety aspects of infliximab in inflammatory bowel disease patients. A retrospective cohort study in 100 patients of a German University Hospital. *Digestion.* 2004;70(1):3-9.

39. Colombel JF, Loftus EV Jr, Tremaine WJ, et al. The safety profile of infliximab in patients with Crohn's disease: the Mayo clinic experience in 500 patients. *Gastroenterology.* 2004;126(1):19-31.

40. Toruner M, Loftus EV Jr, Harmsen WS, et al. Risk factors for opportunistic infections in patients with inflammatory bowel disease. *Gastroenterology.* 2008;134(4):929-936.

41. Ahmad NM, Ahmad KM, Younus F. Severe adenovirus pneumonia (AVP) following infliximab infusion for the treatment of Crohn's disease. *J Infect*. 2007;54(1):e29-e32.

42. Kaur N, Mahl TC. *Pneumocystis jiroveci* (carinii) pneumonia after infliximab therapy: a review of 84 cases. *Dig Dis Sci*. 2007;52(6):1481-1484.

43. Choi HJ, Kim MY, Kim HO, Park YM. An atypical varicella exanthem associated with the use of infliximab. *Int J Dermatol*. 2006;45(8):999-1000.

44. Fabre S, Gibert C, Lechiche C, Dereure J, Jorgensen C, Sany J. Visceral leishmaniasis infection in a rheumatoid arthritis patient treated with infliximab. *Clin Exp Rheumatol*. 2005;23(6):891-892.

45. Seddik M, Melliez H, Seguy D, Viget N, Cortot A, Colombel JF. *Pneumocystis jiroveci* (carinii) pneumonia after initiation of infliximab and azathioprine therapy in a patient with Crohn's disease. *Inflamm Bowel Dis*. 2005;11(6):618-620.

46. Bowie VL, Snella KA, Gopalachar AS, Bharadwaj P. Listeria meningitis associated with infliximab. *Ann Pharmacother*. 2004;38(1):58-61.

47. Singh SM, Rau NV, Cohen LB, Harris H. Cutaneous nocardiosis complicating management of Crohn's disease with infliximab and prednisone. *CMAJ*. 2004;171(9):1063-1064.

48. Velayos FS, Sandborn WJ. Pneumocystis carinii pneumonia during maintenance anti-tumor necrosis factor-alpha therapy with infliximab for Crohn's disease. *Inflamm Bowel Dis*. 2004;10(5):657-660.

49. Slifman NR, Gershon SK, Lee JH, Edwards ET, Braun MM. Listeria monocytogenes infection as a complication of treatment with tumor necrosis factor alpha-neutralizing agents. *Arthritis Rheum*. 2003;48(2):319-324.

50. Helbling D, Breitbach TH, Krause M. Disseminated cytomegalovirus infection in Crohn's disease following anti-tumour necrosis factor therapy. *Eur J Gastroenterol Hepatol*. 2002;14(12):1393-1395.

51. Warris A, Bjorneklett A, Gaustad P. Invasive pulmonary aspergillosis associated with infliximab therapy. *N Engl J Med*. 2001;344(14):1099-1100.

52. Rahier JF, Ben-Horin S, Chowers Y, et al. European evidence-based Consensus on the prevention, diagnosis and management of opportunistic infections in inflammatory bowel disease. *J Crohn Colitis*. 2009;3:47-91.

53. D'Haens G, Baert F, Van Assche G, et al. Early combined immunosuppression or conventional management in patients with newly diagnosed Crohn's disease: an open randomised trial. *Lancet*. 2008;371(9613):660-667.

54. Feagan BG, McDonald JWD, Panaccione R, et al. A randomized trial of methotrexate in combination with infliximab for the treatment of Crohn's disease. *Gut*. 2007;57(suppl II):A66.

55. Sands BE, Blank MA, Diamond RH, Barrett JP, van Deventer SJ. Maintenance infliximab does not result in increased abscess development in fistulizing Crohn's disease: results from the ACCENT II study. *Aliment Pharmacol Ther*. 2006;23(8):1127-1136.

56. Kunitake H, Hodin R, Shellito PC, Sands BE, Korzenik J, Bordeianou L. Perioperative treatment with infliximab in patients with Crohn's disease and ulcerative colitis is not associated with an increased rate of postoperative complications. *J Gastrointest Surg*. 2008;12(10):1730-1736.

57. Colombel JF, Loftus EV, Jr, Tremaine WJ, et al. Early postoperative complications are not increased in patients with Crohn's disease treated perioperatively with infliximab or immunosuppressive therapy. *Am J Gastroenterol*. 2004;99(5):878-883.

58. Marchal L, D'Haens G, Van Assche G, et al. The risk of post-operative complications associated with infliximab therapy for Crohn's disease: a controlled cohort study. *Aliment Pharmacol Ther*. 2004;19(7):749-754.

59. Tay GS, Binion DG, Eastwood D, Otterson MF. Multivariate analysis suggests improved perioperative outcome in Crohn's disease patients receiving immunomodulator therapy after segmental resection and/or strictureplasty. *Surgery*. 2003;134(4):565-572.

60. Mor IJ, Vogel JD, da Luz MA, Shen B, Hammel J, Remzi FH. Infliximab in ulcerative colitis is associated with an increased risk of postoperative complications after restorative proctocolectomy. *Dis Colon Rectum*. 2008;51(8):1202-1207.

61. Abdelmalek MF, Liu C, Valentine JF. Successful treatment of chronic hepatitis C with pegylated interferon, ribavirin, and infliximab in a patient with Crohn's disease. *Am J Gastroenterol.* 2007;102(6):1333-1334.

62. Peterson JR, Hsu FC, Simkin PA, Wener MH. Effect of tumour necrosis factor alpha antagonists on serum transaminases and viraemia in patients with rheumatoid arthritis and chronic hepatitis C infection. *Ann Rheum Dis.* 2003;62(11):1078-1082.

63. Holtmann MH, Galle PR, Neurath MF. Treatment of patients with Crohn's disease and concomitant chronic hepatitis C with a chimeric monoclonal antibody to TNF-. *Am J Gastroenterol.* 2003;98(2):504-505.

64. Campbell S, Ghosh S. Infliximab therapy for Crohn's disease in the presence of chronic hepatitis C infection. *Eur J Gastroenterol Hepatol.* 2001;13(2):191-192.

65. Brenndorfer ED, Weiland M, Frelin L, et al. Anti-tumor necrosis factor alpha treatment promotes apoptosis and prevents liver regeneration in a transgenic mouse model of chronic hepatitis C. *Hepatology.* 2010;52(5):1553-1563.

66. Esteve M, Saro C, Gonzalez-Huix F, Suarez F, Forne M, Viver JM. Chronic hepatitis B reactivation following infliximab therapy in Crohn's disease patients: need for primary prophylaxis. *Gut.* 2004;53(9):1363-1365.

67. Millonig G, Kern M, Ludwiczek O, Nachbaur K, Vogel W. Subfulminant hepatitis B after infliximab in Crohn's disease: need for HBV-screening? *World J Gastroenterol.* 2006;12(6):974-976.

68. Nathan DM, Angus PW, Gibson PR. Hepatitis B and C virus infections and anti-tumor necrosis factor-alpha therapy: guidelines for clinical approach. *J Gastroenterol Hepatol.* 2006;21(9):1366-1371.

69. Lavagna A, Bergallo M, Daperno M, et al. Infliximab and the risk of latent viruses reactivation in active Crohn's disease. *Inflamm Bowel Dis.* 2007;13(7):896-902.

70. Reijasse D, Le Pendeven C, Cosnes J, et al. Epstein-Barr virus viral load in Crohn's disease: effect of immunosuppressive therapy. *Inflamm Bowel Dis.* 2004;10(2):85-90.

71. Quispel R, van der Worp HB, Pruissen M, Schipper ME, Oldenburg B. Fatal aseptic meningoencephalitis following infliximab treatment for inflammatory bowel disease. *Gut.* 2006;55(7):1056.

72. Vonkeman H, ten Napel C, Rasker H, van de LM. Disseminated primary varicella infection during infliximab treatment. *J Rheumatol.* 2004;31(12):2517-2518.

73. Buccoliero G, Lonero G, Romanelli C, Loperfido P, Resta F. Varicella zoster virus encephalitis during treatment with anti-tumor necrosis factor-alpha agent in a psoriatic arthritis patient. *New Microbiol.* 2010;33(3):271-274.

74. Hamzaoglu H, Cooper J, Alsahli M, Falchuk KR, Peppercorn MA, Farrell RJ. Safety of infliximab in Crohn's disease: a large single-center experience. *Inflamm Bowel Dis.* 2010;16:2109-2116

75. Swoger JM, Loftus EV Jr, Tremaine WJ, et al. Adalimumab for Crohn's disease in clinical practice at Mayo clinic: the first 118 patients. *Inflamm Bowel Dis.* 2010;16:1912-1921.

76. Zabana Y, Domenech E, Manosa M, et al. Infliximab safety profile and long-term applicability in inflammatory bowel disease: 9-year experience in clinical practice. *Aliment Pharmacol Ther.* 2010;31(5):553-560.

77. Ho GT, Mowat A, Potts L, et al. Efficacy and complications of adalimumab treatment for medically-refractory Crohn's disease: analysis of nationwide experience in Scotland (2004-2008). *Aliment Pharmacol Ther.* 2009;29(5):527-534.

78. Gonzalez-Lama Y, Lopez-San Roman A, Marin-Jimenez I, et al. Open-label infliximab therapy in Crohn's disease: a long-term multicenter study of efficacy, safety and predictors of response. *Gastroenterol Hepatol.* 2008;31(7):421-426.

79. Lees CW, Ali A, Thompson AI, et al. The safety profile of anti-TNF-α therapy in inflammatory bowel disease in clinical practice: analysis of 620 patient-years follow-up. *Aliment Pharmacol Ther.* 2009;29:286-297.

80. Friesen CA, Calabro C, Christenson K, et al. Safety of infliximab treatment in pediatric patients with inflammatory bowel disease. *J Pediatr Gastroenterol Nutr.* 2004;39(3):265-269.

81. Wenzl HH, Reinisch W, Jahnel J, et al. Austrian infliximab experience in Crohn's disease: a nationwide cooperative study with long-term follow-up. *Eur J Gastroenterol Hepatol*. 2004;16(8):767-773.

82. Ljung T, Karlen P, Schmidt D, et al. Infliximab in inflammatory bowel disease: clinical outcome in a population based cohort from Stockholm County. *Gut*. 2004;53(6):849-853.

83. Fidder H, Schnitzler F, Ferrante M, et al. Long-term safety of infliximab for the treatment of inflammatory bowel disease: a single-centre cohort study. *Gut*. 2009;58(4):501-508.

84. Caspersen S, Elkjaer M, Riis L, et al. Infliximab for inflammatory bowel disease in Denmark 1999-2005: clinical outcome and follow-up evaluation of malignancy and mortality. *Clin Gastroenterol Hepatol*. 2008;6(11):1212-1217.

85. Biancone L, Orlando A, Kohn A, et al. Infliximab and newly diagnosed neoplasia in Crohn's disease: a multicentre matched pair study. *Gut*. 2006;55(2):228-233.

86. Brown SL, Greene MH, Gershon SK, Edwards ET, Braun MM. Tumor necrosis factor antagonist therapy and lymphoma development: twenty-six cases reported to the Food and Drug Administration. *Arthritis Rheum*. 2002;46(12):3151-3158.

87. Diak P, Siegel J, La Grenade L, Choi L, Lemery S, McMahon A. Tumor necrosis factor alpha blockers and malignancy in children: forty-eight cases reported to the Food and Drug Administration. *Arthritis Rheum*. 2010;62(8):2517-2524.

88. Adams AE, Zwicker J, Curiel C, et al. Aggressive cutaneous T-cell lymphomas after TNF-alpha blockade. *J Am Acad Dermatol*. 2004;51(4):660-662.

89. Thayu M, Markowitz JE, Mamula P, Russo PA, Muinos WI, Baldassano RN. Hepatosplenic T-cell lymphoma in an adolescent patient after immunomodulator and biologic therapy for Crohn disease. *J Pediatr Gastroenterol Nutr*. 2005;40(2):220-222.

90. Kotlyar DS, Blonski W, Diamond RH, Wasik M, Lichtenstein GR. Hepatosplenic T-cell lymphoma in inflammatory bowel disease: a possible thiopurine-induced chromosomal abnormality. *Am J Gastroenterol*. 2010;105(10):2299-2301.

91. Kotlyar DS, Osterman MT, Diamond RH, et al. A systematic review of factors that contribute to hepatosplenic T-cell lymphoma in patients with inflammatory bowel disease. *Clin Gastroenterol Hepatol*. 2011;9:36-41.

92. Farcet JP, Gaulard P, Marolleau JP, et al. Hepatosplenic T-cell lymphoma: sinusal/sinusoidal localization of malignant cells expressing the T-cell receptor gamma delta. *Blood*. 1990;75(11):2213-2219.

93. Navarro JT, Ribera JM, Mate JL, et al. Hepatosplenic T-gammadelta lymphoma in a patient with Crohn's disease treated with azathioprine. *Leuk Lymphoma*. 2003;44(3):531-533.

94. Mancini S, Amorotti E, Vecchio S, Ponz dL, Roncucci L. Infliximab-related hepatitis: discussion of a case and review of the literature. *Intern Emerg Med*. 2010;5(3):193-200.

95. Menghini VV, Arora AS. Infliximab-associated reversible cholestatic liver disease. *Mayo Clin Proc*. 2001;76(1):84-86.

96. Ierardi E, Valle ND, Nacchiero MC, De F, V, Stoppino G, Panella C. Onset of liver damage after a single administration of infliximab in a patient with refractory ulcerative colitis. *Clin Drug Investig*. 2006;26(11):673-676.

97. Lal S, Steinhart AH. Infliximab for ulcerative colitis following liver transplantation. *Eur J Gastroenterol Hepatol*. 2007;19(3):277-280.

98. Atzeni F, Ardizzone S, Sarzi-Puttini P, et al. Autoantibody profile during short-term infliximab treatment for Crohn's disease: a prospective cohort study. *Aliment Pharmacol Ther*. 2005;22(5):453-461.

99. Rutgeerts P, Feagan BG, Lichtenstein GR, et al. Comparison of scheduled and episodic treatment strategies of infliximab in Crohn's disease. *Gastroenterology*. 2004;126(2):402-413.

100. Klapman JB, Ene-Stroescu D, Becker MA, Hanauer SB. A lupus-like syndrome associated with infliximab therapy. *Inflamm Bowel Dis*. 2003;9(3):176-178.

101. Saint MB, De Bandt M. Vasculitides induced by TNF-alpha antagonists: a study in 39 patients in France. *Joint Bone Spine*. 2006;73(6):710-713.

102. Manosa M, Domenech E, Marin L, et al. Adalimumab-induced lupus erythematosus in Crohn's disease patients previously treated with infliximab. *Gut*. 2008;57(4):559-560.

103. Zella GC, Weinblatt ME, Winter HS. Drug-induced lupus associated with infliximab and adalimumab in an adolescent with Crohn disease. *J Pediatr Gastroenterol Nutr.* 2009;49(3):355-358.

104. Kocharla L, Mongey AB. Is the development of drug-related lupus a contraindication for switching from one TNF- alpha inhibitor to another? *Lupus.* 2009;18(2):169-171.

105. Subramanian S, Yajnik V, Sands BE, Cullen G, Korzenik JR. Characterization of patients with infliximab-induced lupus erythematosus and outcomes after retreatment with a second anti-TNF-α agent. *Inflamm Bowel Dis.* 2011;17:99-104.

106. McIlwain L, Carter JD, Bin-Sagheer S, Vasey FB, Nord J. Hypersensitivity vasculitis with leukocytoclastic vasculitis secondary to infliximab. *J Clin Gastroenterol.* 2003;36(5):411-413.

107. Burke JP, Kelleher B, Ramadan S, Quinlan M, Sugrue D, O'Donovan MA. Pericarditis as a complication of infliximab therapy in Crohn's disease. *Inflamm Bowel Dis.* 2008;14(3):428-429.

108. Massara A, Cavazzini L, La Corte R, Trotta F. Sarcoidosis appearing during anti-tumor necrosis factor alpha therapy: a new "class effect" paradoxical phenomenon. Two case reports and literature review. *Semin Arthritis Rheum.* 2010;39(4):313-319.

109. Takahashi H, Kaneta K, Honma M, et al. Sarcoidosis during infliximab therapy for Crohn's disease. *J Dermatol.* 2010;37(5):471-474.

110. Kwon HJ, Cote TR, Cuffe MS, Kramer JM, Braun MM. Case reports of heart failure after therapy with a tumor necrosis factor antagonist. *Ann Intern Med.* 2003;138(10):807-811.

111. Curtis JR, Kramer JM, Martin C, et al. Heart failure among younger rheumatoid arthritis and Crohn's patients exposed to TNF-alpha antagonists. *Rheumatology (Oxford).* 2007;46(11):1688-1693.

112. Enayati PJ, Papadakis KA. Association of anti-tumor necrosis factor therapy with the development of multiple sclerosis. *J Clin Gastroenterol.* 2005;39(4):303-306.

113. Freeman HJ, Flak B. Demyelination-like syndrome in Crohn's disease after infliximab therapy. *Can J Gastroenterol.* 2005;19(5):313-316.

114. Jarand J, Zochodne DW, Martin LO, Voll C. Neurological complications of infliximab. *J Rheumatol.* 2006;33(5):1018-1020.

115. Lozeron P, Denier C, Lacroix C, Adams D. Long-term course of demyelinating neuropathies occurring during tumor necrosis factor-alpha-blocker therapy. *Arch Neurol.* 2009;66(4):490-497.

116. Vadikolias K, Kouklakis G, Heliopoulos I, et al. Acute paraplegia after the initiation of anti-tumour necrosis factor-alpha therapy for Crohn's disease. *Eur J Gastroenterol Hepatol.* 2007;19(2):159-162.

117. Zamvar V, Sugarman ID, Tawfik RF, Macmullen-Price J, Puntis JW. Posterior reversible encephalopathy syndrome following infliximab infusion. *J Pediatr Gastroenterol Nutr.* 2009;48(1):102-105.

118. Vidal F, Fontova R, Richart C. Severe neutropenia and thrombocytopenia associated with infliximab. *Ann Intern Med.* 2003;139(3):235.

119. Salar A, Bessa X, Muniz E, Monfort D, Besses C, Andreu M. Infliximab and adalimumab-induced thrombocytopenia in a woman with colonic Crohn's disease. *Gut.* 2007;56(8):1169-1170.

120. Selby LA, Hess D, Shashidar H, de Villiers WJ, Selby LA. Crohn's disease, infliximab and idiopathic thrombocytopenic purpura. *Inflamm Bowel Dis.* 2004;10(5):698-700.

121. Francolla KA, Altman A, Sylvester FA. Hemophagocytic syndrome in an adolescent with Crohn disease receiving azathioprine and infliximab. *J Pediatr Gastroenterol Nutr.* 2008;47(2):193-195.

122. Fernandez-Torres R, Paradela S, Valbuena L, Fonseca E. Infliximab-induced lichen planopilaris. *Ann Pharmacother.* 2010;44(9):1501-1503.

123. Outlaw W, Fleischer A, Bloomfeld R. Lymphomatoid papulosis in a patient with Crohn's disease treated with infliximab. *Inflamm Bowel Dis.* 2009;15(7):965-966.

124. Salama M, Lawrance IC. Stevens-Johnson syndrome complicating adalimumab therapy in Crohn's disease. *World J Gastroenterol.* 2009;15(35):4449-4452.

125. Sun G, Wasko CA, Hsu S. Acneiform eruption following anti-TNF-alpha treatment: a report of three cases. *J Drugs Dermatol.* 2008;7(1):69-71.

126. Devos SA, Van Den BN, De Vos M, Naeyaert JM. Adverse skin reactions to anti-TNF-alpha monoclonal antibody therapy. *Dermatology.* 2003;206(4):388-390.

127. Moss AC, Treister NS, Marsee DK, Cheifetz AS. Clinical challenges and images in GI. Oral lichenoid reaction in a patient with Crohn's disease receiving infliximab. *Gastroenterology.* 2007;132(2):488, 829.

128. Cleynen I, Van Moerkercke W, Juergens M, et al. Anti-TNF-α induced cutaneous lesions in IBD patients: characterization and search for predisposing factors. *Gut.* 2010;59(suppl III):A1.

129. Collamer AN, Battafarano DF. Psoriatic skin lesions induced by tumor necrosis factor antagonist therapy: clinical features and possible immunopathogenesis. *Semin Arthritis Rheum.* 2010;40:233-240.

130. Medkour F, Babai S, Chanteloup E, Buffard V, Delchier JC, Le Louet H. Development of diffuse psoriasis with alopecia during treatment of Crohn's disease with infliximab. *Gastroenterol Clin Biol.* 2010;34(2):140-141.

131. English PL, Vender R. Occurrence of plantar pustular psoriasis during treatment with infliximab. *J Cutan Med Surg.* 2009;13(1):40-42.

132. Fouache D, Goeb V, Massy-Guillemant N, et al. Paradoxical adverse events of anti-tumour necrosis factor therapy for spondyloarthropathies: a retrospective study. *Rheumatology (Oxford).* 2009;48(7):761-764.

133. Ko JM, Gottlieb AB, Kerbleski JF. Induction and exacerbation of psoriasis with TNF-blockade therapy: a review and analysis of 127 cases. *J Dermatolog Treat.* 2009;20(2):100-108.

134. Manni E, Barachini P. Psoriasis induced by infliximab in a patient suffering from Crohn's disease. *Int J Immunopathol Pharmacol.* 2009;22(3):841-844.

135. Costa-Romero M, Coto-Segura P, Suarez-Saavedra S, Ramos-Polo E, Santos-Juanes J. Guttate psoriasis induced by infliximab in a child with Crohn's disease. *Inflamm Bowel Dis.* 2008;14(10):1462-1463.

136. Richetta A, Mattozzi C, Carlomagno V, et al. A case of infliximab-induced psoriasis. *Dermatol Online J.* 2008;14(11):9.

137. Angelucci E, Cocco A, Viscido A, Vernia P, Caprilli R. Another paradox in Crohn's disease: new onset of psoriasis in a patient receiving tumor necrosis factor-alpha antagonist. *Inflamm Bowel Dis.* 2007;13(8):1059-1061.

138. Severs GA, Lawlor TH, Purcell SM, Adler DJ, Thompson R. Cutaneous adverse reaction to infliximab: report of psoriasis developing in 3 patients. *Cutis.* 2007;80(3):231-237.

139. Takahashi H, Hashimoto Y, Ishida-Yamamoto A, Ashida T, Kohgo Y, Iizuka H. Psoriasiform and pustular eruption induced by infliximab. *J Dermatol.* 2007;34(7):468-472.

140. Umeno J, Matsumoto T, Jo Y, Ichikawa M, Urabe K, Iida M. Psoriasis during anti-tumor necrosis factor-alpha therapy for Crohn's disease. *Inflamm Bowel Dis.* 2007;13(9):1188-1189.

141. Adams DR, Buckel T, Sceppa JA. Infliximab associated new-onset psoriasis. *J Drugs Dermatol.* 2006;5(2):178-179.

142. Wollina U, Hansel G, Koch A, Schonlebe J, Kostler E, Haroske G. Tumor necrosis factor-alpha inhibitor-induced psoriasis or psoriasiform exanthemata: first 120 cases from the literature including a series of six new patients. *Am J Clin Dermatol.* 2008;9(1):1-14.

Suggested Readings

Fidder H, Schnitzler F, Ferrante M, et al. Long-term safety of infliximab for the treatment of inflammatory bowel disease: a single-centre cohort study. *Gut.* 2009;58(4):501-508.

Hansen RA, Gartlehner G, Powell GE, Sandler RS. Serious adverse events with infliximab: analysis of spontaneously reported adverse events. *Clin Gastroenterol Hepatol.* 2007;5(6):729-735.

Kotlyar DS, Osterman MT, Diamond RH, et al. A systematic review of factors that contribute to hepatosplenic T-cell lymphoma in patients with inflammatory bowel disease. *Clin Gastroenterol Hepatol.* 2011;9:36-41.

Lichtenstein GR, Feagan BG, Cohen RD, et al. Serious infections and mortality in association with therapies for Crohn's disease: TREAT registry. *Clin Gastroenterol Hepatol.* 2006;4(5):621-630.

Peyrin-Biroulet L, Deltenre P, de Suray N, Branche J, Sandborn WJ, Colombel JF. Efficacy and safety of tumor necrosis factor antagonists in Crohn's disease: meta-analysis of placebo-controlled trials. *Clin Gastroenterol Hepatol.* 2008;6(6):644-653.

POSTOPERATIVE CROHN'S DISEASE AND ULCERATIVE COLITIS

Chapter 17

Postoperative Crohn's Disease Recurrence and Prevention

Miguel D. Regueiro, MD

Crohn's disease (CD) affects nearly 750,000 people in the United States and frequently requires both medical and surgical management in order to achieve disease remission.[1] Approximately 80% of CD patients will require at least one intestinal surgery in their lifetime.[2] Although surgery removes actively diseased intestine, it is not curative and recurrence is common. The endoscopic recurrence rate of CD 1 year after intestinal resection is 70% to 90%.[3,4] Only 20% to 37% of patients have clinical symptoms 1 year postoperatively, defined as *clinical recurrence*. The disconnect between clinical and endoscopic recurrence after surgery probably has to do with the fact that CD is clinically silent until a complication develops or until transmural inflammation becomes severe. The wide range of postoperative recurrence rates cited in the literature is due to the heterogeneity of the studies in terms of definitions of recurrence (clinical or endoscopic), time to recurrence, and indication for surgery (perforating or stricturing disease). The postoperative management of CD patients offers a challenge for physicians in terms of diagnosing recurrence, minimizing risk factors for recurrence, and selecting appropriate patients for prophylactic therapies to prevent recurrence.

Definition of Recurrence

Recurrence of CD can be defined by clinical symptoms or by endoscopic, radiologic, or histopathologic means. Most patients who have recurrence by these definitions will not have symptoms (ie, clinical recurrence of CD). A prospective cohort study by Rutgeerts et al[3] evaluated 89 patients who underwent ileocolonic resection in order to assess predictors of recurrent disease. This study found the strongest predictor of recurrent CD to be the severity

Regueiro MD, Swoger JM, eds.
Clinical Challenges and Complications of IBD (pp 329-344).
© 2013 Taylor & Francis Group.

Table 17-1. *Postoperative Ileal Endoscopic Recurrence Score*

ENDOSCOPIC SCORE*	DEFINITION
i0	No lesions
i1	≤5 aphthous lesions
i2	>5 aphthous lesions with normal mucosa between the lesions or skip areas of larger lesions or lesions confined to the ileocolonic anastomosis
i3	Diffuse aphthous ileitis with diffusely inflamed mucosa
i4	Diffuse inflammation with already larger ulcers, nodules, and/or narrowing
*Remission: endoscopic score of i0 or i1; recurrence: endoscopic score of i2, i3, or i4.	

of endoscopic lesions found on colonoscopy 1 year after surgery. Endoscopic recurrence after resection was graded using the scoring system devised for this study (Table 17-1 and Figure 17-1). Patients with mild or inactive endoscopic disease (i0, i1) rarely had symptoms at 1 year, and 80% of these patients continued to have mild or absent endoscopic recurrence 3 years postoperatively. Patients with severe endoscopic disease (i3, i4) at 1 year were much more likely to have clinical recurrence at 1 year, and 92% of these patients had progressive, severe endoscopic disease at 3 years. The intermediate (i2) group falls between these 2 groups clinically and endoscopically (33% of these patients progress to i4 lesions at 3 years). Patients who progress to the most severe endoscopic score of i3 or i4 often require another surgery within 5 years.

Risk Factors for Postoperative Recurrence

Several risk factors have been identified that increase the likelihood of postoperative CD recurrence[5] (Table 17-2). The 3 factors that portend the greatest risk for postoperative recurrence are as follows: (1) active tobacco smoking after surgery, especially in women and heavy smokers; (2) patients with penetrating disease (ie, fistulas, abscesses, and intestinal perforation); and (3) those with 2 or more surgeries. Although not formally studied, those patients who progress to surgery despite treatment with an immunomodulator or biologic agent probably represent a uniquely aggressive CD phenotype at high risk of postoperative recurrence. One caveat to this is that patients who require surgery, for example, for an obstructing stricture, despite the initiation of medical therapy should not be considered failure of medical therapy. Rather, these patients probably would have been best served by surgery for the complication prior to the initiation of medications. Other risk factors for postoperative recurrence include a shorter duration between the time of diagnosis and surgery

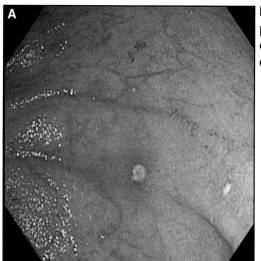

Figure 17-1. Endoscopic photos of postoperative CD recurrence in the ileum. (A) i1 disease. (B) i3 disease. (C) i4 disease.

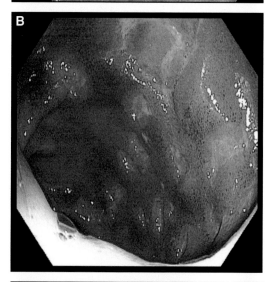

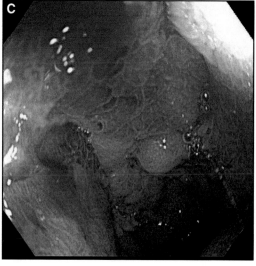

Table 17-2. Risk Factors for Postoperative Crohn's Disease Recurrence

STRONGEST RISK FACTORS
• Smoking
• Penetrating disease
• History of prior resection

STRONG RISK FACTORS
• Progression to surgery despite immunomodulators and/or biologics
• Short duration of disease prior to surgery
• Both colonic *and* small bowel involvement
• Young age at disease onset
• Perianal fistula

INCONCLUSIVE RISK FACTORS
• Family history of inflammatory bowel disease
• Type of anastomosis
• Gender
• Corticosteroids prior to surgery
• Length of diseased intestine

(<10 years), disease location in the ileum and colon (rather than ileum alone), perianal fistula, more severe disease leading to surgery, a longer segment of bowel requiring resection, and the need for corticosteroids prior to surgery.

Postoperative Crohn's Disease Surveillance

Scheduled postoperative assessment for recurrence allows for early detection and intervention. There are a range of clinical, laboratory, radiographic, and endoscopic evaluation parameters that have been evaluated. The Crohn's Disease Activity Index (CDAI) is a clinical research score that is used to define clinical activity and response to medical therapy. Although the most widely applied activity score in research studies and publications, CDAI may not accurately predict postoperative CD recurrence.[6] Regueiro et al evaluated the correlation between the CDAI and endoscopic recurrence in their postoperative CD prevention study.[7] The 1-year postoperative CDAI was identical (134) in patients with endoscopic scores of i0 or i1 compared to i2, i3, or i4. This study concluded that the CDAI did not correlate with endoscopic findings and that clinical symptoms were a poor predictor of postoperative disease recurrence. Therefore, routine colonoscopy 6 months to 1 year after intestinal resection is important for the evaluation of endoscopic recurrence, regardless of clinical symptoms.

Both ileocolonoscopy and wireless capsule endoscopy have been employed to detect the recurrence of postoperative CD. Both modalities have high specificity at identifying endoscopic recurrence, but colonoscopy has superior sensitivity.[8,9] Small intestine contrast ultrasonography (SICUS) has emerged as a noninvasive modality for detecting postoperative CD.[10] Although the sensitivity and specificity of detecting postoperative CD recurrence with SICUS are quite high, there are operability requirements and expertise most gastroenterologists currently do not have access to which.

Colonoscopy seems to be the best modality for evaluation of mucosal CD recurrence at the ileocolonic anastomosis and neoterminal ileum. Proactive evaluation for endoscopic recurrence often detects mucosal inflammatory changes that precede clinical recurrence. Effective treatment of endoscopically recurrent CD in the postoperative setting is an area of great research interest. Early treatment of mucosally evident inflammation may prove effective in altering the natural course of disease with prevention of clinical recurrence and need for future surgery. Whether prophylactic treatment immediately after surgery is more effective than treatment based on subsequent endoscopic findings is currently not known.

Medications for Postoperative Prevention

There are a number of studies that have evaluated the efficacy of medications for preventing CD recurrence after intestinal resective surgery. The medications that have been evaluated in randomized controlled trials include the 5-aminosalicylates (5-ASAs), probiotics and antibiotics, budesonide, azathioprine and 6-mercaptoputine (6-MP), and the anti-tumor necrosis factor (TNF) agents.

5-Aminosalicylates

Studies of 5-ASAs for the prevention of postoperative recurrence have failed to provide convincing evidence for benefit. A meta-analysis by the Cochrane group failed to find a benefit. However, a recent meta-analysis, which included additional studies, came to a different conclusion.[11,12] This study identified 11 randomized controlled trials for inclusion, 5 with sulfasalazine and 6 with mesalamine. Most of the studies in the analysis used clinical recurrence as an endpoint, and only a minority had radiographic or endoscopic endpoints. Sulfasalazine did not offer any benefit over placebo, but mesalamine was more effective than placebo or no therapy (RR 0.80; 95% confidence interval = 0.70 to 0.92) with a number needed to treat (NNT) of 10.

The conclusion that 5-ASAs are effective in preventing postoperative CD is questionable. The recent meta-analysis reported a small absolute treatment benefit, with a NNT = 10. This means that for every 10 patients placed on a 5-ASA postoperatively, only 1 patient will avoid a clinical recurrence. An important limitation to the 5-ASA studies is the fact that clinical recurrence, rather than endoscopic recurrence, was often the primary endpoint. As previously stated, 1-year clinical recurrence correlates poorly with the more meaningful postoperative endoscopic endpoint. Mucosal healing, or prevention of mucosally active CD, is the best predictor of long-term outcomes, such as hospitalization or surgery.[13,14] While considering postoperative endoscopic recurrence, the 5-ASAs did not prevent recurrence. Therefore, it is the author's opinion that there is no role of 5-ASAs in preventing postoperative CD.

Budesonide

Two published studies of budesonide have shown no benefit in the prevention of postoperative recurrence. In a double-blind, randomized trial with parallel groups, the frequency of endoscopic recurrence was not lower among those who received oral budesonide at 3 or 12 months.[15] In another multicenter, randomized trial, budesonide failed to statistically decrease the rates of endoscopic and/or clinical recurrence, although positive trends were seen (57% budesonide compared to 70% placebo).[16] Based on the existing data and clinical experience, budesonide should not be considered for prevention of postoperative CD.

Antibiotics and Probiotics

Two placebo-controlled trials have assessed whether nitroimidazole antibiotics can prevent postoperative CD recurrence. Metronidazole (20 mg/kg body weight) taken daily for 3 months, beginning 1 week after ileal resection and primary anastomosis, reduced recurrent lesions in the neoterminal ileum (75% versus 52%; $P = 0.09$), with clinical recurrence rates significantly reduced at 1 year (4% versus 25%).[17]

In a subsequent study of a different nitroimidazole antibiotic, 80 patients were randomized to ornidazole 1 g/day or placebo starting within 1 week of resection and continued for 1 year.[18] Ornidazole significantly reduced the clinical recurrence rates at 1 year from 37.5% among placebo-treated patients to 7.9% patients in the ornidazole group ($P = 0.003$). The actively treated group also had a significant reduction in endoscopic recurrence at 12 months (79% versus 53.6%; $P = 0.037$). Of note, however, significantly more patients dropped out of the active treatment group due to adverse effects. The positive results of the nitroimidazole antibiotics offer hope that these medications may be of benefit in preventing postoperative CD. The limitation is that the benefit is maintained only if the antibiotic is continued, and most patients do not tolerate high doses of nitroimidazole antibiotics in the long term.

The effectiveness of probiotics as postoperative CD treatment has also been studied. There was a randomized controlled trial of Synbiotic 2000, in which 30 patients were administered probiotic or placebo within 1 week of surgery.[19] There was a high drop-out rate, with only one-third of subjects completing the study, and no difference in recurrence rates, defined by C-reactive protein, CDAI, or endoscopic recurrence at 3 or 24 months.

Two similar trials studied *Lactobacillus johnsonii*. Both studies had a primary endpoint of 3-month and 6-month endoscopic recurrence. There was not a statistically significant difference in the frequency, severity, or endoscopic recurrence between the treatment and the placebo groups, with 50% of the patients having active mucosal inflammation.[20,21]

The most recent study on probiotics in the prevention of postoperative CD also did not show a benefit.[22] Patients were randomized to either VSL#3 or placebo, with a primary endpoint of endoscopic recurrence at 90 days. The endoscopic recurrence rate 3 months after surgery was low but did not differ between VSL#3 (9%) and placebo (16%) ($P = 0.36$). Patients treated with VSL#3 had significantly lower levels of ileal mucosal proinflammatory cytokines and higher levels of tumor growth factor β. Although the microflora of the intestine probably plays a role in postoperative CD recurrence, the efficacy data from the probiotic studies are currently lacking.

Azathioprine/6-Mercaptopurine

Both azathioprine and 6-MP are effective medications for maintenance of medically induced CD remission and have been considered an aggressive treatment for postoperative prevention. Two controlled trials have evaluated these agents for the prevention of postoperative CD. In a study comparing azathioprine (2 mg/kg/day) to mesalamine (3 g/day), no difference in clinical recurrence at 2 years (34% versus 46%; $P = 0.2$) was reported.[23] Endoscopic endpoints were not evaluated in this study. Another study compared 6-MP (50 mg/day) with mesalamine (3 g/day) and placebo. At 2 years, 6-MP was more effective than placebo in preventing postoperative clinical recurrence (50% versus 77%; $P = 0.045$) and endoscopic recurrence (43% versus 64%; $P = 0.03$).[24] A more recent trial evaluated 12 months of azathioprine (1.5 to 2.0 mg/kg/day) versus placebo, with each group receiving metronidazole for the immediate 3 months following surgery.[25] Significant endoscopic recurrence was low in both groups at 12 months postoperatively, with a mild decrease in severe recurrence in the azathioprine group. This indicates that azathioprine in combination with metronidazole may have additive benefit in preventing postoperative CD in a group of patients at higher risk of recurrence.[26] Another study randomized 79 patients to azathioprine (2 to 2.5 mg/kg/day) or 5-ASA and found clinical and severe endoscopic recurrence more commonly in the 5-ASA group ($P = 0.27$).[27] However, this study indicated that patients were more likely to stop the azathioprine due to adverse events ($P = 0.04$).

In a recent meta-analysis from 2009, the 4 azathioprine/6-MP studies were evaluated and compared.[28] The total analysis included 433 patients treated with azathioprine or 6-MP and compared with a control, either 5-ASAs or placebo. There was an absolute risk reduction of 8% in the azathioprine/6-MP group compared to the control group for prevention of clinical recurrence. In this case, the NNT was 13, meaning that for every 13 patients treated with azathioprine/6-MP postoperatively, only 1 did not develop a clinical recurrence. Despite these underwhelming data, the conclusion of the meta-analysis was that azathioprine/6-MP was effective in preventing postoperative recurrence. Similarly, for prevention of endoscopic recurrence, defined as an ileal score of i2, i3, or i4, azathioprine was 15% more effective than control and the NNT was 7. It is important to note that severe endoscopic recurrence (i3, i4) was not prevented by azathioprine/6-MP, which was no more effective than the control medication. Therefore, azathioprine/6-MP may have a modest

Table 17-3. Endoscopic Recurrence Rates in the Anti-Tumor Necrosis Factor Postoperative Prevention Studies

Study (Author/Medication/Duration)	Anti-TNF	Placebo/5-ASA
Sorrentino et al[29]/infliximab/2 years	0%	100%
Regueiro et al[30]/infliximab/1 year	9%	85%
Fernandez-Blanco et al[32]/adalimumab/1 year	10%	N/A
5-ASA = 5-aminosalicylates; TNF = tumor necrosis factor		

benefit in preventing 1-year clinical recurrence after CD surgery but does not appear to prevent severe endoscopic recurrence. Given the correlation of severe endoscopic recurrence with the need for future surgery and a more disabling disease course, the author recommends that patients receiving postoperative azathioprine/6-MP should undergo ileocolonoscopy 6 months after surgery to evaluate for endoscopic recurrence.

Anti-Tumor Necrosis Factor

The ability of anti-TNF therapy to induce mucosal healing in inflammatory bowel disease led to studies on the prevention of CD recurrence after bowel resection. Three anti-TNF postoperative prevention studies have been reported, 2 with infliximab and 1 with adalimumab (Table 17-3). Sorrentino et al first illustrated the potential of infliximab in the postoperative setting, with an open-label study of 23 patients who had undergone intestinal resection for CD.[29] Seven patients received infliximab (5 mg/kg every 8 weeks) and low-dose oral methotrexate (10 mg/week) beginning 2 weeks after surgery. A control group of 16 patients received 2.4 gm of mesalamine daily. Two years after surgery, the mesalamine group had a 100% endoscopic recurrence rate, while none of the 7 infliximab/methotrexate-treated patients (0%) had a recurrence.

There is only one randomized controlled trial of anti-TNF therapy for postoperative prophylaxis.[30] In this study by Regueiro et al, patients were randomized to infliximab (5 mg/kg every 8 weeks) or placebo. Patients were permitted to continue immunomodulators and 5-ASAs, but steroids and antibiotics were discontinued. Approximately 35% of the patients in each group had received infliximab prior to surgery. The treatment group contained more smokers and fewer patients on immunomodulators. One year after surgery, only 1/11 (9%) infliximab-treated patients had an endoscopic recurrence compared to 11/13 (85%) receiving placebo ($P = 0.0006$). At the end of the 1-year study, patients were offered open-label infliximab. Data of 10 patients have been presented in abstract form. The 3 infliximab responders who stopped treatment after 1 year had significant endoscopic recurrence by 2 years. Five of the 7 placebo patients with active disease at 1 year, who went on to receive open-label infliximab, entered remission by 2 years. In total, there were 48 annual endoscopies that were performed during the open-label follow-up. Of these, 88% were in endoscopic remission on infliximab compared to only 22% of patients not taking infliximab.[31] A large, international, multicenter, randomized controlled trial is underway to definitively evaluate the efficacy of infliximab in the postoperative setting.

In the only adalimumab study to date, 20 patients were treated with adalimumab after curative intestinal resection for complications of CD.[32] Sixty percent of the patients were active smokers, 35% had at least one previous CD surgery, and 65% had fistulizing disease. All patients received a standard induction adalimumab regimen with an initial 160-mg dose, 80 mg 2 weeks later, and then maintenance dosing of 40 mg every other week. After 1 year of therapy, only 2 patients (10%) had an endoscopic recurrence (>i1). There were no clinical recurrences, but 45% of the patients had at least moderate histologic recurrence.

Infliximab has also been studied in patients with established CD recurrence after surgery. Yamamoto et al studied 26 asymptomatic patients with endoscopic recurrence 6 months after ileal resection.[33] The patients were treated with mesalamine (3 g/day), azathioprine (50 mg/day), or infliximab (5 mg/kg every 8 weeks). After 6 months of treatment, endoscopic inflammation improved in none of the patients on mesalamine (0/10), 3 of 8 treated with azathioprine, and 6 of 8 on infliximab. Levels of the proinflammatory cytokines interleukin (IL)-1β, IL-6, and anti-TNF-α dropped in the infliximab group; increased in the mesalamine group; and did not change in the azathioprine group.

It is not known whether the initiation of prophylactic anti-TNF treatment following intestinal resection is more effective at preventing future surgery and clinical disease recurrence compared to waiting for the presence of endoscopic recurrence to initiate therapy. Despite impressive clinical remission results from the anti-TNF medical induction trials, the endoscopic remission/mucosal healing data were less robust (SONIC infliximab = 34%, ACCENT I infliximab 5 mg/kg = 18%, 10 mg/kg = 33%, MUSIC certolizumab = 11.5%, and EXTEND adalimumab = 27%).[34-37] Similarly, the endoscopic remission (i0, i1) results from patients treated with anti-TNF after evidence of postoperative endoscopic recurrence is not as high as the prevention data. Specifically, in the Yamamoto et al study, only 38% of patients were able to achieve endoscopic remission after the anti-TNF agent was started for established endoscopic recurrence. In the Regueiro et al postoperative prevention study, patients who received infliximab for endoscopic recurrence after 1 year of placebo treatment had modestly high endoscopic remission rates (61%), but not at the level of the patients started on an anti-TNF agent immediately after surgery Regueiro et al. When considering the totality of endoscopic remission results from the 3 anti-TNF postoperative prevention studies, the Yamamoto et al endoscopic recurrence data, and the medical induction trials of CD, endoscopic remission appears to be most complete in the prevention studies (Table 17-4). An explanation for the discrepancy between endoscopic remission results in the medical induction compared to postoperative prevention studies may have to do with irreversible tissue remodeling or permanent vascular changes that occur in patients with mucosally active CD. Therefore, preventing these changes results in sustained intestinal health, whereas treating active disease may not be able to overcome mucosal

Table 17-4. *Endoscopic Remission Rates for Anti-Tumor Necrosis Factor Crohn's Disease Studies*

STUDY TYPE	ENDOSCOPIC REMISSION (MUCOSAL HEALING)
Postoperative prevention[30,31,33]	90% to 100%
Postoperative treatment of endoscopic recurrence[32,34]	38% to 61%
Medical induction of remission trials[35-38]	11% to 34%

damage "too far gone" at the time medication is started. In order to address the optimal timing of postoperative anti-TNF therapy, a head-to-head long-term outcome study needs to be designed in which one group of postoperative CD patients are treated with postoperative prophylaxis, while a comparator group receives anti-TNF therapy only when there is evidence of endoscopic recurrence.

PROPOSED GUIDELINES FOR THE MANAGEMENT OF POSTOPERATIVE CROHN'S DISEASE

There are no formal guidelines for the prevention of postoperative CD. However, the prior discussion illustrates that, apart from the anti-TNF data, 1-year endoscopic recurrence rates are 50% or greater for most medication classes (Table 17-5). The decision on initiating postoperative medical therapy should be based on the patient's risk for postoperative recurrence. The following recommendations are the author's suggestions (Figure 17-2). Patients at low risk for postoperative recurrence include those who have had longstanding CD (>10 years) and whose indication for surgery is a short (<10 cm), fibrostenotic stricture. Given the slow progression of disease in a limited segment of bowel, these patients are less likely to have aggressive postoperative recurrence and are not routinely placed on postoperative medications. An ileocolonoscopy should be performed 6 to 12 months postoperatively, and if there is no endoscopic recurrence evident (i0, i1), no medication is started, and a colonoscopy is repeated 1 to 3 years later. If there is evidence of early endoscopic recurrence (i ≥2), an immunomodulator or anti-TNF agent is started.

Patients at moderate risk for postoperative recurrence are those naive to immunomodulators, with a relatively short duration of disease (<10 years) prior to their first surgery, who undergo resection for a long segment (>10 cm) of small bowel inflammation. These patients are started on an immunomodulator within 2 weeks of surgery. Given the compelling data on the combination of metronidazole with azathioprine for preventing postoperative CD, a nitro-imidazole antibiotic is added if possible and continued for at least 3 months. Unfortunately, most patients do not tolerate high-dose metronidazole for an

Table 17-5. Clinical and Endoscopic 1-Year Recurrence Rates From Randomized Treatment Trials

MEDICATION CLASS	CLINICAL RECURRENCE	ENDOSCOPIC RECURRENCE
Placebo	25% to 77%	53% to 79%
5-ASA	24% to 58%	63% to 66%
Budesonide	19% to 32%	52% to 57%
Nitroimidazole	7% to 8%	52% to 54%
AZA/6-MP	34% to 50%	42% to 44%
Infliximab	0%	0% to 10%
5-ASA = 5-aminosalicylates; AZA = azathioprine; 6-MP = 6-mercaptopurine.		

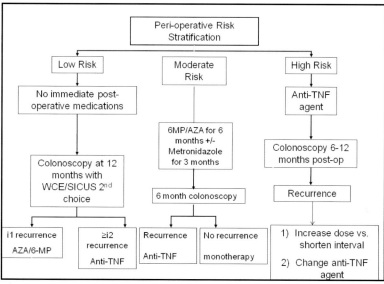

Figure 17-2. Algorithm for postoperative management of CD. AZA = azathioprine; 6-MP = 6-mercaptopurine; SICUS = small intestine contrast ultrasonography; TNF = tumor necrosis factor; WCE = wireless capsule endoscopy

extended period of time, thereby limiting this option. An ileocolonoscopy is performed 6 to 12 months postoperatively and if there is evidence of endoscopic recurrence, an anti-TNF agent is added. If the initial postoperative ileocolonoscopy shows no endoscopic recurrence, the immunomodulator is continued and a colonoscopy is repeated 1 to 3 years later.

Patients at a high risk for recurrence are those with penetrating disease (abscess, perforation, or internal fistula), smokers, patients with a prior surgery for CD, and those who progressed to surgery despite an adequate treatment trial with an immunomodulator. For these patients, an anti-TNF agent is started within 2 to 4 weeks of surgery. An ileocolonoscopy is then performed 1 year postoperatively. In those with an ileal score of i0 or i1, the anti-TNF agent is continued. If there is significant endoscopic recurrence, ≥i2, anti-TNF antibodies and serum trough levels are checked. Depending on the results, treatment options would include escalation of anti-TNF dosing, change to an alternate anti-TNF agent, and/or the addition of an immunomodulator.

TOP-DOWN THERAPY FOR POSTOPERATIVE CROHN'S DISEASE

In recent years, there has been significant controversy about the appropriate treatment paradigm for CD. Specifically, the relative merits of treatment titration (ie, "bottom-up" therapy) have been touted as a means to limit patient exposure to potentially unnecessary, toxic therapies.[38] Conversely, "top-down" therapy proposes that aggressive early intervention may in fact modify disease course and provide outcomes superior to the bottom-up approach.[35,39] Efforts to compare these approaches can be extremely challenging. Patients enrolled in such studies are, by definition, "newly diagnosed." However, it is impossible to accurately know the extent or duration of pre-existing silent CD and the extent of related tissue scarring and remodeling. Postoperative CD may provide a unique setting in which to evaluate these approaches by starting with macroscopically normal bowel at a defined point in time. It is possible that studies conducted among such patients could eventually provide missing outcome data about the impact of treatment on the natural course of the disease. Finally, there may be patients for whom primary treatment intervention is a surgical resection followed by aggressive medical therapy. It is conceivable that this approach could redefine the natural course of CD and sustain deep remission and prevention of recurrence in a manner not previously realized.

CONCLUSION

Clinical recurrence following surgery for CD is nearly universal with many patients not experiencing symptoms until a complication is present requiring additional surgery. Although some risk factors for postoperative CD recurrence have been identified, the only modifiable factor is smoking. Data on the use of antibiotics, immunomodulators, and anti-TNF agents show efficacy in preventing postoperative recurrence, although the potential risks and benefits of prophylactic therapy need to be considered in individual patients. Stratifying patients by risk factors helps to guide decision making on the timing of postoperative medical therapy and diagnostic investigations. Despite therapeutic decisions, an endoscopic evaluation within 6 to 12 months of surgery is the most accurate modality for detecting postoperative recurrence that helps to further guide medical decision making.

☑Key Points

☑ Over one-half of CD patients will require surgery in their lifetime.

☑ Postoperative CD recurrence is common and often clinically silent until a complication develops.

☑ More than 50% of patients will require additional surgery within 20 years of their initial resection.

☑ Cigarette smoking is associated with postoperative recurrence and is the only modifiable risk factor.

☑ Risk factors for postoperative recurrence should be assessed and used to determine appropriate medical treatment after surgery.

☑ Risk factors associated with a high likelihood for postoperative recurrence include cigarette smoking, penetrating disease, or more than one surgery in the patient's lifetime.

☑ Patients at low risk for recurrence do not need postoperative treatment.

☑ Patients at moderate risk for recurrence should receive azathioprine/6-MP with or without metronidazole after surgery.

☑ Patients at high risk for recurrence should receive anti-TNF after surgery.

☑ In all patients, an ileocolonoscopy should be performed 6 to 12 months after surgery and periodically thereafter to assess disease recurrence.

REFERENCES

1. Loftus EV, Schoenfeld P, Sandborn WJ. The epidemiology and natural history of Crohn's disease in population-based patient cohorts from North America: a systematic review. *Aliment Pharmacol Ther.* 2002;16:51-60.
2. Olaison G, Sjödahl R, Tagesson C. Glucocorticoid treatment in ileal Crohn's disease: relief of symptoms but not of endoscopically viewed inflammation. *Gut.* 1990;31:325-328.
3. Rutgeerts P, Geboes K, Vantrappen G, et al. Natural history of recurrent Crohn's disease at the ileocolonic anastomosis after curative surgery. *Gut.* 1984;25:665-672.
4. Olaison G, Smedh K, Sjödahl R. Natural course of Crohn's disease after ileocolonic resection: endoscopically visualised ileal ulcers preceeding symptoms. *Gut.* 1992;33:331-335.

5. Lautenbach E, Berlin JA, Lichtenstein GR. Risk factors for early post-operative recurrence of Crohn's disease. *Gastroenterology.* 1998;115:259-267.
6. Viscido A, Corrao G, Taddei G, et al. Crohn's disease activity index is inaccurate to detect the post-operative recurrence in Crohn's disease. A GISC study. *Ital J Gastroenterol Hepatol.* 1999;31:274-279.
7. Regueiro M, Kip KE, Schraut W, et al. Crohn's disease activity index does not correlate with endoscopic recurrence one year after ileocolonic resection. *Inflamm Bowel Dis.* 2011;17(1):118-126.
8. Bourreille A, Jarry M, D'Halluin P, et al. Wireless capsule endoscopy versus ileocolonoscopy for the diagnosis of post-operative recurrence of Crohn's disease: a prospective study. *Gut.* 2006;55:978-983.
9. Pons BV, Nos P, Bastida G, et al. Evaluation of postsurgical recurrence in Crohn's disease: a new indication for capsule endoscopy? *Gastrointest Endosc.* 2007;66:533-540.
10. Biancone L, Calabrese E, Petruzziello C, et al. Wireless capsule endoscopy and small intestinal contrast ultrasonography in recurrence of Crohn's disease. *Inflamm Bowel Dis.* 2007;13:1256-1265.
11. Doherty G, Bennett G, Patil S, et al. Interventions for prevention of post-operative recurrence of Crohn's disease. *Cochrane Database Syst Rev.* 2009;(4):CD006873.
12. Ford AC, Khan KJ, Talley NJ, Moayyedi P. 5-aminosalicylates prevent relapse of Crohn's disease after surgically induced remission: systematic review and meta-analysis. *Am J Gastroenterol.* 2011;106(3):413-420.
13. Rutgeerts P, Feagan BG, Lichtenstein GR, et al. Comparison of scheduled and episodic treatment strategies of infliximab in Crohn's disease. *Gastroenterology.* 2004;126:402-413.
14. Lichtenstein GR, Yan S, Bala M, et al. Infliximab maintenance treatment reduces hospitalizations, surgeries, and procedures in fistulizing Crohn's disease. *Gastroenterology.* 2005;128:862-869.
15. Hellers G, Cortot A, Jewell D, et al. Oral budesonide for prevention of postsurgical recurrence in Crohn's disease. The IOIBD Budesonide Study Group. *Gastroenterology.* 1999;116:294-300.
16. Ewe K, Böttger T, Buhr HJ, et al. Low-dose budesonide treatment for prevention of post-operative recurrence of Crohn's disease: a multicentre randomized placebo-controlled trial. German Budesonide Study Group. *Eur J Gastroenterol Hepatol.* 1999;11:277-282.
17. Rutgeerts P, Hiele M, Geboes K, et al. Controlled trial of metronidazole treatment for prevention of Crohn's recurrence after ileal resection. *Gastroenterology.* 1995;108:1617-1621.
18. Rutgeerts P, Van Assache G, Vermeire S, et al. Ordinazole for prophylaxis of post-operative Crohn's disease recurrence: a randomized, double blind, placebo-controlled trial. *Gastroenterology.* 2005;128:856-861.
19. Chermesh I, Tamir A, Reshef R, et al. Failure of Synbiotic 2000 to prevent post-operative recurrence of Crohn's disease. *Dig Dis Sci.* 2007;52:385-389.
20. Van Gossum A, Dewit O, Lewis E, et al. Multicenter randomized-controlled clinical trial of probiotics (*Lactobacillus johnsonii*, LA1) on early endoscopic recurrence of Crohn's disease after ileo-caecal resection. *Inflamm Bowel Dis.* 2007;13:135-142.
21. Marteau P, Lemann M, Seksik P, et al. Ineffectiveness of *Lactobacillus johnsonii* LA1 for prophylaxis of post-operative recurrence in Crohn's disease: a randomised, double blind, placebo controlled GETAID trial. *Gut.* 2006;55:842-847.
22. Madsen K, Backer JL, Leddin D, et al. A randomized controlled trial of VSL#3 for the prevention of endoscopic recurrence following surgery for Crohn's disease. *Gastroenterology.* 2010;138(suppl 1):A-361.
23. Ardizzone S, Maconi G, Sampietro GM, et al. Azathioprine and mesalamine for the prevention of relapse after conservative therapy for Crohn's disease. *Gastroenterology.* 2004;127:730-740.
24. Hanauer SB, Korelitz BI, Rutgeerts P, et al. Post-operative maintenance of Crohn's disease remission with 6-mercaptopurine, mesalamine, or placebo: a 2-year trial. *Gastroenterology.* 2004;127:723-729.

25. D'Haens GR, Vermiere S, Van Assche G, et al. Therapy of metronidazole with azathioprine to prevent post-operative recurrence of Crohn's disease: a controlled randomized trial. *Gastroenterology*. 2008;135:1123-1129.

26. Domènech E, Mañosa M, Bernal I, et al. Impact of azathioprine on the prevention of post-operative Crohn's disease recurrence: results of a prospective, observational, long-term follow-up study. *Inflamm Bowel Dis*. 2008;14:508-513.

27. Herfarth H, Tjaden C, Lukas M, et al. Adverse events in clinical trials with azathioprine and mesalamine for prevention of post-operative recurrence of Crohn's disease. *Gut*. 2008;55:1525-1526.

28. Peyrin-Biroulet L, Deltenre P, Ardizzone S, et al. Azathioprine and 6-mercaptopurine for the prevention of post-operative recurrence in Crohn's disease: a meta-analysis. *Am J Gastroenterol*. 2009;104(8):2089-2096.

29. Sorrentino D, Terrosu G, Avellini C, Maiero S. Infliximab with low-dose methotrexate for prevention of postsurgical recurrence of ileocolonic Crohn disease. *Arch Intern Med*. 2007;167:1804-1807.

30. Regueiro M, Schraut W, Baidoo L, et al. Infliximab prevents Crohn's disease recurrence after ileal resection. *Gastroenterology*. 2009;136:441-450.

31. Regueiro M, Kip K, Schraut W, et al. Long-term follow-up of patients enrolled in the randomized controlled trial of infliximab for prevention of post-operative Crohn's disease. *Am J Gastroenterol*. 2009;104:S459 (abstract).

32. Fernandez-Blanco I, Monturiol J, Martinez B, et al. Adalimumab in the prevention of post-operative recurrence of Crohn's disease. *Gastroenterology*. 2010;138(suppl 1):S692 (abstract).

33. Yamamoto T, Umegae S, Matsumoto K. Impact of infliximab therapy after early endoscopic recurrence following ileocolonic resection of Crohn's disease: a prospective pilot study. *Inflamm Bowel Dis*. 2009;15:1460-1466.

34. Colombel JF, Sandborn WJ, Reinisch W, et al. Infliximab, azathioprine, or combination therapy for Crohn's disease. *N Engl J Med*. 2010;362:1383-1395.

35. Rutgeerts P, Diamond RH, Bala M, et al. Scheduled maintenance treatment with infliximab is superior to episodic treatment for the healing of mucosal ulceration associated with Crohn's disease. *Gastrointest Endosc*. 2006;63:433-442.

36. Colombel JF, Hebuterne X. Endoscopic mucosal improvement in patients with active Crohn's disease treated with certolizumab pegol: first results of the MUSIC clinical trial. *Am J Gastroenterol*. 2008;103:P13.

37. Rutgeerts P. Adalimumab induces and maintains mucosal healing in patients with moderate to severe ileocolonic Crohn's disease-first results of the EXTEND Trial. *Gastroenterology*. 2009;136(suppl 1):A116 (abstract).

38. Shergill AK, Terdiman JP. Controversies in the treatment of Crohn's disease: the case for an accelerated step-up treatment approach. *World J Gastroenterol*. 2008;14:2670-2677.

39. D'Haens G, Baert F, van Assche G, et al. Early combined immunosuppression or conventional management in patients with newly diagnosed Crohn's disease: an open randomised trial. *Lancet*. 2008;371:660-667.

SUGGESTED READINGS

D'Haens GR, Vermiere S, Van Assche G, et al. Therapy of metronidazole with azathioprine to prevent post-operative recurrence of Crohn's disease: a controlled randomized trial. *Gastroenterology*. 2008;135:1123-1129.

Lautenbach E, Berlin JA, Lichtenstein GR. Risk factors for early post-operative recurrence of Crohn's disease. *Gastroenterology*. 1998;115:259-267.

Peyrin-Biroulet L, Deltenre P, Ardizzone S, et al. Azathioprine and 6-mercaptopurine for the prevention of post-operative recurrence in Crohn's disease: a meta-analysis. *Am J Gastroenterol*. 2009;104(8):2089-2096.

Regueiro M, Schraut W, Baidoo L, et al. Infliximab prevents Crohn's disease recurrence after ileal resection. *Gastroenterology.* 2009;136:441-450.

Rutgeerts P, Geboes K, Vantrappen G, et al. Natural history of recurrent Crohn's disease at the ileocolonic anastomosis after curative surgery. *Gut.* 1984;25:665-672.

Chapter 18

Ulcerative Colitis
Pouchitis and
Stoma Complications

Udayakumar Navaneethan, MD and Bo Shen, MD

Restorative proctocolectomy with ileal pouch-anal anastomosis (IPAA) is the surgical treatment of choice for patients with medically refractory ulcerative colitis (UC), colitis-associated neoplasia, or familial adenomatous polyposis (FAP).[1,2] Approximately 30% of UC patients eventually require colectomy, with the majority electing to undergo IPAA. The postoperative course may be affected by a number of inflammatory and noninflammatory complications, including pouchitis, Crohn's disease (CD) of the pouch, cuffitis, and irritable pouch syndrome. Each of these entities may adversely affect surgical outcome and health-related quality of life.[3] Pouchitis is the most frequent long-term complication of IPAA in patients with UC, with a cumulative incidence of up to 50%.[1,2,4] Chronic pouchitis, although less frequent, is one of the most difficult disorders to manage in IPAA patients.

Stomas are frequently constructed during surgical therapy for UC. Although stomas are often intended for short-term fecal diversion, some patients with pouch failure may require permanent diversion. These patients are often affected by stoma-related complications. Inflammatory bowel disease (IBD) patients with a stoma are susceptible to stoma retraction, prolapse, fistula, stenosis, necrosis, and peristomal pyoderma gangrenosum. Management of these complications can be challenging, especially if the stoma is intended for longer-term diversion.

POUCHITIS

Pouchitis is the most common long-term complication of IPAA in patients with UC.[1,2,4] Many aspects of pouchitis present clinical challenges, as the etiology and pathogenesis of this condition are not entirely clear and long-term management can be difficult.

Regueiro MD, Swoger JM, eds.
Clinical Challenges and Complications of IBD (pp 345-366).
© 2013 Taylor & Francis Group.

Etiology and Pathogenesis

Early studies demonstrated pouchitis to be associated with an increased aerobic bacterial load, including *Clostridium perfringens* and sulfate-reducing bacteria.[5-7] Gosselink et al[7] analyzed pouch bacterial content during episodes of pouchitis, both before and during treatment with ciprofloxacin or metronidazole. During a pouchitis-free period, the pouch microbiota was characterized by the presence of *Lactobacilli* and large numbers of anaerobes. However, during episodes of pouchitis, there were decreased numbers of anaerobes and *Lactobacilli*, with more aerobic bacteria and *C perfringens* being isolated.

Advances in molecular microbiology, including 16S ribosomal RNA (rRNA) techniques, have made the characterization of the gastrointestinal microbiome more feasible.[8] Utilizing a fingerprinting technique, Komanduri et al[9] studied pouch biopsy specimens from 5 patients with active pouchitis and 15 patients with normal pouches. The authors identified mucosa-associated microbiota patterns specific to each individual. Clostridium species (ie, *Clostridium paraputrificum*), Enterobacteriacae, and Streptococci were associated with healthy pouches without inflammation. Alternatively, the *Fusobacterium* species was associated with pouchitis. Adding to these findings, a recent study investigated the mucosa-associated microbiota in UC and FAP patients, with and without pouchitis, again using 16S rRNA sequencing.[10] In this study of 24 patients, there was a significant increase in *Proteobacteria* and a significant decrease in *Bacteroidetes* and *Faecalibacterium prausnitzii* in UC patients, compared to the FAP cohort. However, only limited differences were found between the UC patients with or without pouchitis and between the FAP patients with or without pouchitis. Bacterial diversity in the FAP nonpouchitis group was greater than in the UC nonpouchitis group, which, in turn, was greater than that in the UC pouchitis group. These findings suggest "dysbiosis" in the ileal pouches of UC patients, which may predispose to, but may not directly contribute to, pouchitis. At this time, molecular microbiologic analyses are limited by sampling and technical problems and the relatively broad spectrum of "normal commensal microbiota" seen in healthy individuals. Going forward, more accurate characterization of the microbiota in normal subjects and in specific disease states, using metagenomic libraries, a microbial chip, and other molecular analytical methods, may be useful.[11-13]

Comparative proteomic analysis has also been used to identify proteins critical for functional pathways in normal cells and the phenotype changes that occur during disease development. Two-dimensional polyacrylamide gel electrophoresis and matrix-assisted laser desorption/ionization-time of flight mass spectrometry are being developed to better define the differential protein displays of mucosal biopsy samples from patients with chronic refractory pouchitis before and after antibiotic treatment.[14] Results have suggested the upregulation and downregulation of certain proteins associated with glycolysis/gluconeogenesis, oxidative phosphorylation, and electron transfer chain pathways and have demonstrated the energy-deficient state of chronic pouchitis.

Table 18-1. Secondary Causes of Pouchitis
Infectious causes
• Cytomegalovirus
• *Candida* sp
• *Clostridium difficile* infection
Ischemia
Concurrent autoimmune disorders
Radiation
Chemotherapy
Collagen deposition
IgG4-associated pouchitis
Nonsteroidal anti-inflammatory drugs

An abnormal mucosal immune response, pouch dysbiosis, has been proposed to play a key role in the development of "conventional" or "idiopathic" pouchitis. Alterations in innate and adaptive mucosal immunity in the pouch, and in pouchitis, have been reported. Tissue proinflammatory cytokines, including tumor necrosis factor-α, may be increased, along with other proinflammatory cytokines. Abnormalities in immunoregulatory cytokines such as interleukin (IL)-2, interferon-γ, IL-4, and IL-10 have also been observed in pouchitis.[15,16]

A possible genetic predisposition to pouchitis was studied by evaluating the NOD2 gene in IPAA patients. NOD2 is an intracellular sensor of bacterial cell wall peptidoglycan. NOD2 mutations compromise the host response to enteric bacteria and are increased in patients with CD. Sehgal et al found NOD2 mutations to be significantly higher in patients with severe pouchitis (67%) compared with asymptomatic IPAA patients (5.4%).[17] Asymptomatic IPAA patients had NOD2 mutation profiles that were similar to both patients with mild pouchitis and healthy controls. Patients with severe pouchitis had the highest incidence of NOD2 mutations, suggesting a compromised host defense mechanism in response to enteric bacteria.

Approximately 20% to 30% of patients who present with chronic pouchitis may have clearly identifiable secondary, or modifiable, etiologies and triggering factors to explain their disease (Table 18-1). These cases of "secondary pouchitis"[18] may be secondary to cytomegalovirus (CMV), *Candida*, or *Clostridium difficile* infection (CDI), ischemia, concurrent autoimmune disorders, radiation or chemotherapy, collagen deposition in the pouch mucosa, or use of nonsteroidal anti-inflammatory drugs (NSAIDs).[18-24] An IgG4-associated pouchitis has been recently described in patients with concurrent autoimmune disorders.[25] Secondary triggering factors should be suspected in patients with pouchitis who do not respond to conventional antibiotic therapy and in patients with chronic, antibiotic-refractory pouchitis (CARP). Careful evaluation for and treatment of these secondary causes may avoid the need for pouch excision, or even permanent diversion, in these patients. The majority of patients with secondary pouchitis benefit from eradication of the causal triggering factors, with improvement in symptoms and/or pouch inflammation. However, in some patients, modulation of the secondary factors does not necessarily impact the disease course of pouchitis. For example, not all patients with CDI are symptomatic, as colonization with this bacterial agent may occur in patients with normal pouches.[20] In these cases, eradicating the bacterial pathogen may have little impact on the natural history of the pouch.

Classification and Definition

There is no uniform classification system for pouchitis. This diverse entity can be classified based on the etiology, disease duration and activity, and response to medical therapy into (1) idiopathic versus secondary, (2) acute (<4 weeks) versus chronic (≥4 weeks), and (3) infrequent (<2 acute episodes) versus relapsing (≥3 acute episodes) versus continuous.[26,27] One of the most commonly used classifications of pouchitis is based on response to antibiotics, including antibiotic-responsive, antibiotic-dependent, and antibiotic-refractory pouchitis.[28,29] Antibiotic-responsive pouchitis is characterized by infrequent episodes (<4 episodes per year), responding to a 2-week course of a single antibiotic. Patients with antibiotic-dependent pouchitis often require long-term maintenance therapy to keep the disease in remission. These patients have frequent episodes (≥4 episodes per year) of pouchitis, or persistent symptoms, which necessitate long-term, continuous antibiotic or probiotic therapy. CARP occurs when a patient fails to respond to a 4-week course of a single antibiotic (metronidazole or ciprofloxacin), requires prolonged therapy of ≥4 weeks, consisting of ≥2 antibiotics, oral or topical 5-aminosalicylates, corticosteroid therapy, or oral immunomodulator therapy. Since its introduction in 2003, the classification of pouchitis based on response to antibiotic therapy has been widely accepted and is commonly used in both clinical practice and clinical research.[27]

Pouchitis may affect up to 50% of patients who have undergone IPAA surgery for UC, and the estimated incidence within the first 12 months after ileostomy closure has been reported to be as high as 40%.[5] Common presenting symptoms include increased stool frequency, urgency, incontinence, nocturnal seepage, abdominal cramping, and pelvic discomfort. Fever, weight loss, and bloody bowel movements are less common. However, these symptoms are not specific for pouchitis and can be indicative of other inflammatory and noninflammatory disorders of the pouch. Additionally, the etiology of an individual patient's pouchitis may change over time. For example, a patient may have idiopathic pouchitis at one point, then subsequently present with CD of the pouch. Hence, periodic diagnostic endoscopic assessment, and histologic evaluation are important in differentiating among the various causes of pouch dysfunction.[29]

Various diagnostic criteria have been studied in order to diagnose and rate the severity of pouchitis, including symptom assessment alone, symptom and endoscopic assessment (modified Pouch Disease Activity Index [mPDAI]), or symptom and endoscopic assessment with histologic evaluation (PDAI, Heidelberg criteria, and St. Marks criteria).[30-33] The PDAI is the most commonly used criteria in research studies, with a score greater than or equal to 7 suggesting a diagnosis of pouchitis.[31] An overall PDAI score is calculated from 3 separate 6-point subscores for clinical symptoms, endoscopic findings, and histologic changes (Table 18-2). However, due to the cost of pouch endoscopy with histologic evaluation, the complexity in calculating PDAI scores, and the delay in determining the histologic score, the PDAI is not often applied in clinical practice. These drawbacks led to the proposal of the 12-point mPDAI, consisting of symptom (from 0 to 6) and endoscopic scores (from 0 to 6), without biopsy or histology.[30] A total mPDAI score of greater than or equal to 5 is associated with the diagnosis of pouchitis. Avoiding the need for biopsy and histologic evaluation shortens the procedure time, reduces costs, and provides immediate calculation of mPDAI scores at the time of endoscopy.[34]

Diagnosis

There is no consensus regarding the clinical diagnostic criteria and classification of pouchitis. The disease activity instruments described above have been mainly used as research tools. In symptomatic patients with IPAA, either a treat-first or test-first strategy is most often utilized in clinical practice. For patients presenting with symptoms consistent with pouchitis, empiric treatment with antibiotics is often initiated, using the treat-first strategy. Approximately 5% to 19% patients with acute pouchitis, however, will develop a refractory or rapidly relapsing form of the disease.[35] Furthermore, chronic pouchitis is one of the most common causes of pouch failure, requiring permanent ileostomy or pouch excision. Approximately 40% of patients with acute pouchitis will have a single episode that responds to treatment with antibiotics, while the remaining patients develop at least one recurrence and require further courses of maintenance antibiotics.

Pouch Endoscopy

Pouch endoscopy is the main clinical tool for the diagnosis of suspected pouch disorders. Sedated or nonsedated pouch endoscopy can be performed in an outpatient setting. The use of a gastroscope is preferred because of its flexibility and smaller caliber. Endoscopic features consistent with pouchitis include edema, erythema, granularity, loss of vascular pattern, hemorrhage, friability, ulcers, or erosions (Figure 18-1). Endoscopy also allows for the assessment of the prepouch ileum, and rectal cuff or anal transitional zone, for evidence of CD of the pouch and cuffitis. Patients with diffuse pouchitis and long segment of enteritis of the afferent limb may be suspected of having concurrent primary sclerosing cholangitis (PSC). In addition, through-the-scope therapy can be delivered during endoscopy, including endoscopic balloon

Table 18-2. The 18-Point Pouchitis Disease Activity Index

CRITERIA	SCORE
Clinical	
Stool frequency	
Usual postoperative stool frequency	0
1 to 2 stools/day > postoperative usual	1
3 or more stools/day > postoperative usual	2
Rectal bleeding	
None or rare	0
Present daily	1
Fecal urgency or abdominal cramps	
None	0
Occasional	1
Usual	2
Fever	
Absent	0
Present	1
Endoscopic inflammation	
Edema	1
Granularity	1
Friability	1
Loss of vascular pattern	1
Mucoid exudate	1
Ulceration	1
Acute histological inflammation	
Polymorphonuclear leukocyte infiltration	
Mild	1
Moderate + crypt abscess	2
Severe + crypt abscess	3
Ulceration per low-power field (mean)	
<25%	1
25% to 50%	2
>50%	3

Pouchitis is defined as a total PDAI score ≥7.
Reprinted with permission from Sandborn WJ, Tremaine WJ, Batts KP, Pemberton JH, Phillips SF. Pouchitis after ileal pouch-anal anastomosis: a Pouchitis Disease Activity Index. *Mayo Clin Proc.* 1994;69:409-415.

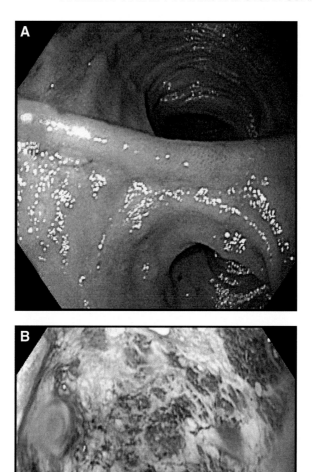

Figure 18-1. (A) Endoscopic appearance of a normal J-pouch. (B) Endoscopic appearance of pouchitis.

dilation of pouch strictures. Furthermore, surveillance biopsies for dysplasia can be obtained during endoscopic evaluation.

The presence of isolated, afferent limb ulcers should raise the suspicion of CD, NSAID-related pouchitis, or ischemia, while inflammation confined to the cuff or anal transitional zone supports a diagnosis of cuffitis.[27,36,37] Cuffitis occurs specifically in patients with a stapled IPAA, who have a retained rectal cuff. The presence of pseudomembranes, which are rarely seen in patients with IPAA, suggests CDI. Finally, an asymmetric distribution of pouch inflammation, particularly with a sharp demarcation along the suture line, between inflamed and noninflamed mucosa, suggests pouch ischemia.[22]

Histology

Histology plays a limited role in the grading of pouch inflammation, and studies have shown that a pouch endoscopy without biopsy strategy is the most cost-effective approach in the diagnosis of pouchitis.[34] Nonetheless, pouch biopsy is routinely performed during the endoscopy. Histologic features of acute inflammatory changes include ulceration, polymorphic neutrophil infiltration, and crypt abscesses.[38] Chronic histologic changes, such as villous blunting, crypt cell hyperplasia, and an increased number of mononuclear cells in the lamina propria, may be seen as a part of "normal" or "physiological" adaptive changes of pouch mucosa to fecal stasis.[37,39] These chronic histologic changes are not necessarily indicative of active pouchitis.[40] Some investigators believe that, in the background of mucosal adaptation, pouchitis is associated with increased villous atrophy, acute inflammatory infiltrates, crypt cell abscesses, and ulceration. In clinical practice, the main purposes for histologic evaluation are the detection of specific pathogens (such as CMV and *Candida*), granulomas (CD of the pouch), ischemia, mucosal prolapse, dysplasia, and other causes of secondary pouchitis.[37]

Laboratory Tests

Inflammation scores on pouch endoscopy have been an integral part of all diagnostic instruments for pouchitis, including the PDAI. However, the invasive nature and cost of endoscopy, and the frequency of episodes in some patients with pouchitis, may prevent its routine use during each episode of symptomatic exacerbation. Laboratory testing in these patients may offer a noninvasive alternative to endoscopy.[41]

The erythrocyte sedimentation rate (ESR), a nonspecific marker of inflammation, has been studied as a putative marker of pouchitis. In a study of 104 patients from Finland, there was significant correlation between the ESR and the PDAI.[42] Similarly, in a large follow-up study of biochemical parameters 10 to 20 years after pouch construction, an elevated ESR was seen in 13% of patients and was significantly correlated with episodes of pouchitis.[43]

C-reactive protein (CRP) has also been evaluated as a potential marker of pouchitis disease activity. Lu et al showed that serum CRP levels correlated with the severity of endoscopic inflammation in both the pouch and afferent limb.[44] However, CRP levels may have a limited role in distinguishing between healthy and diseased pouch conditions based on longitudinal clinical and endoscopic evaluation.

Orosomucoid and haptoglobin were also investigated in a study of biochemical parameters and were elevated in patients with pouchitis. However, the sensitivity and specificity of these markers are not clear.[13] Fecal inflammatory markers closely reflect the presence of intestinal inflammation. Fecal pyruvate kinase has been investigated in IPAA patients, with levels being significantly higher in patients with pouchitis than in patients with normal pouches.[45] Fecal calprotectin levels appear to be correlated with neutrophil-mediated inflammation in the gut and have been investigated in pouchitis, as well as in the other IBDs. Pouchitis patients have been found to have significantly higher calprotectin concentrations than those obtained from uninflamed pouches, and fecal calprotectin concentrations may correlate with PDAI scores.[46]

In a study from the Cleveland Clinic, using a quantitative enzyme-linked immunosorbent assay (ELISA) in pouchitis patients, fecal lactoferrin correlated with PDAI scores.[47] This fecal marker had a sensitivity and specificity of 100% and 85%, respectively, in diagnosing pouchitis, with a cutoff level of 7 µL/mL. In a separate study, using a modification of the quantitative ELISA in 11 pouchitis patients, the test had a sensitivity of 100% and a specificity of 86%, with a positive predictive value of 76% for diagnosing pouchitis.[48] This simple laboratory test may be cost effective, as compared with an endoscopic strategy, for the diagnosis of pouchitis. The fecal marker data are promising, and they may be used as an adjunct first-line modality to pouch endoscopy in the future.

Anti-*Saccharomyces cerevisiae* antibodies (ASCA) are directed against a cell wall component of the yeast *S cerevisiae*. The diagnostic role of ASCA has recently been evaluated in pouchitis and in CD of the pouch.[49,50] The preoperative presence of ASCA IgA antibodies in patients with UC or indeterminate colitis appears to be associated with a higher risk of developing CD of the pouch.[49] Fecal ASCA levels have also been studied in pouchitis.[50] In a recent study, qualitative fecal IgA ASCA levels were determined in patients with pouchitis, cuffitis, CD of the pouch, and normal pouches. Patients with CD of the pouch had a 3-fold higher level of fecal ASCA compared to those with non-CD pouches. However, there was no significant difference in ASCA levels between patients with pouchitis and normal pouches.

Enteric pathogens have been described in patients presenting with pouchitis, and attempts have been made to identify the pathogen responsible for triggering pouchitis. Certain pathogens, such as *C difficile*, can occasionally be detected in pouch patients, particularly in those with CARP.[37] In a study including 115 patients with IPAA, 21 patients (18.3%) tested positive for *C difficile* toxin A or B, and 3 of those 21 patients (14.2%) had CARP.[20] Although the routine quantitative and/or qualitative bacterial culture of stool is not currently a part of routine clinical practice, it may be valuable for the evaluation of patients with symptoms of general malaise and fever or suspected secondary pouchitis. Pathogenic bacteria, such as *Campylobacter jejuni* and *Salmonella typhi*, have occasionally been identified in patients with pouchitis.[51] Fecal sensitivity analysis has been evaluated as a tool for identifying the appropriate antibiotic therapy for patients with antibiotic-resistant pouchitis. McLaughlin et al analyzed fecal samples from 15 patients with active pouchitis, with a PDAI score ≥7, in iso-sensitest agar, for antibiotic sensitivity.[52] The main bacteria isolated included *Escherichia coli*, *Klebsiella*, coliforms not further classifiable, *Pseudomonas*, and *Morganella*, in isolation or in combination. Finally, in patients with persistent symptoms of pouchitis, celiac serologies and salicylate screening may be considered.[37]

Abdominal Imaging and Manometry

A water-contrast pouchogram is useful in evaluating mechanical abnormalities of the pouch, such as strictures, sinuses, fistulas, and prolapse.[53] Pelvic magnetic resonance imaging (MRI), with or without examination under anesthesia, may be performed in patients with structural lesions of the pouch or the anastomosis.[41] Pouch function can further be evaluated by defecography, MRI defecography, or pouch manometry with balloon expulsion.[54-56]

Management

Antibiotics

Broad-spectrum antibiotics are the mainstay of therapy for pouchitis. Metronidazole was the initial antibiotic to be tested in a randomized controlled trial, with 13 pouchitis patients receiving metronidazole or placebo for 2 weeks, followed by a crossover to the other treatment.[57] The overall response, defined by change in stool frequency, was 73% (8 of 11) in patients receiving metronidazole compared with 10% (1 of 10) in patients receiving placebo. The overall efficacy of metronidazole, along with the low cost, has made it the recommended first-line antibiotic for the treatment of pouchitis.

Ciprofloxacin has become a commonly prescribed antibiotic agent for the treatment of acute and chronic pouchitis. In a randomized controlled trial of 16 patients with acute pouchitis, ciprofloxacin 1000 mg/day for 2 weeks was compared to metronidazole 20 mg/kg/day for 2 weeks. There were significant decreases in the PDAI symptom, endoscopic, and histologic subscores with both antibiotics.[58] Patients in the ciprofloxacin group had greater reductions in mean total PDAI scores than those in the metronidazole group. Additionally, the long-term use of metronidazole has been associated with intolerance due to peripheral neuropathy and dysgeusia.[59] This has led to recommendations that ciprofloxacin should be considered as a first-line therapy in the treatment of active pouchitis. However, the long-term use of ciprofloxacin is also associated with a number of adverse effects, including arthropathy.[59] Achilles tendon rupture and tendinitis are unique, yet rare complications that have been reported in adults receiving this medication can occur during or after completion of a treatment course. Finally, the widespread use of ciprofloxacin has been implicated in a recent CDI epidemic.[60] The use of ciprofloxacin may result in selection of the hypervirulent CDI strain, BI/NAP/027, which may be responsible for the rising incidence of CDI. Thus, routine and long-term use of ciprofloxacin in these patients should be carefully considered.

Oral rifaximin is being evaluated as a potential treatment option for active pouchitis. In a study by Isaacs et al, patients with active pouchitis were given either rifaximin, 400 mg 3 times a day (n = 8), or placebo (n = 10), for 4 weeks.[61] Two patients (25%) in the rifaximin group achieved clinical remission (defined by the PDAI score <7 points) at week 4, compared with none in the placebo group. The low response rate to rifaximin therapy might be associated with medication underdosing. Rifaximin has also been studied as a maintenance agent in patients with antibiotic-dependent pouchitis.[62] Fifty-one patients received maintenance therapy with rifaximin (median dose 200 mg/day, maximum dose 1800 mg/day) after receiving a 2-week course of various antibiotics for induction of remission; 33 (65%) maintained remission through 3 months (primary endpoint). Of these 33 patients, 26 (79%) successfully continued maintenance for a total of 6 months, 19 (58%) successfully continued for 12 months, and 2 (6%) successfully continued for 24 months.

CARP often poses a management challenge. A controlled historical cohort study compared the efficacy of a combination of ciprofloxacin 1000 mg/day and tinidazole 15 mg/kg/day in CARP patients receiving oral (4000 mg/day), enema (8000 mg/day), or suppository (1000 mg/day) mesalamine preparations.[63] There were significant reductions in total PDAI scores, and a significant improvement in quality of life scores, in patients receiving the combination antibiotics, after 28 days.

In addition to the treatment of pouchitis, tinidazole has been investigated as primary prophylaxis against the development of pouchitis. A randomized, double-blinded, placebo-controlled clinical trial aimed to determine if tinidazole prevents an initial episode of pouchitis in UC patients 12 months after IPAA.[64] Thirty-eight UC patients were randomized in a 2:1 ratio to receive either daily tinidazole (500 mg by mouth) or placebo within 1 month after the final stage of IPAA surgery. In the tinidazole group, only 8.0% of patients developed pouchitis, compared with 38.5% of patients taking placebo. Thus, early institution of tinidazole may be an effective strategy to prevent development of pouchitis following IPAA surgery.

Probiotics

Therapeutically altering the bacterial flora in the pouch, by administering probiotics, may be effective in preventing pouchitis and/or in maintaining remission in antibiotic-dependent pouchitis. The therapeutic effect of probiotics parallels the restoration of mucosal immune response to the altered microflora in the pouch. In a randomized study comparing the probiotic VSL#3 (containing viable lyophilized bacteria including lactobacilli, bifidobacteria, and streptococcus) compared to placebo, for the prevention of an initial episode of pouchitis in patients with IPAA, the incidence of pouchitis during the first year postoperatively was 10% (versus 40% in the placebo group).[65] A randomized controlled trial of VSL#3 was conducted for maintenance therapy following induction of remission of acute pouchitis using oral antibiotics. During the 9-month trial, which included 40 patients with relapsing pouchitis, only 15% in the probiotic group relapsed, compared to 100% in the placebo group.[66] The routine use of probiotics for induction and maintenance therapy for pouchitis remains controversial. However, a pooled meta-analysis of 5 randomized controlled trials yielded an odds ratio of 0.04 in favor of probiotic treatment compared to placebo.[67] These findings further support the benefits of probiotics in the management of pouchitis, although the clinical applications of probiotics are still under investigation.

Other Treatments

Other agents, including bismuth carbomer enemas, short-chain fatty acid enemas, glutamine enemas, mesalamine enemas, 6-mercaptopurine, infliximab, and adalimumab, have been evaluated in the management of pouchitis. The authors have used a biological agent (adalimumab) in patients with CD of the pouch with a satisfactory short-term response.[68] However, the efficacy of these agents in isolated chronic pouchitis, without ileitis, is unclear.

Short-chain fatty acids play an important role in the maintenance of colonic homeostasis. Butyrate is considered to be a major energy source for colonic mucosa and contributes to the maintenance of the gut mucosal barrier. However, in a small pilot trial of butyrate suppositories in 9 patients with chronic pouchitis, only 3 of the 9 patients demonstrated a clinical response.[69] More promising was an open-label study of bismuth carbomer enemas in 12 patients with pouchitis, in which 10 patients (83%) achieved remission.[70] Finally, a double-blinded, randomized, placebo-controlled study had patients receiving either bismuth carbomer (270 mg elemental bismuth) or placebo foam enemas for 3 weeks. An identical number of patients in both groups, 9 of 20 (45%), showed improvement.[71] Thus, the evidence supporting the efficacy of glutamine, butyrate, or bismuth carbomer for the treatment of pouchitis remains weak.

Finally, AST-120 (a spherical carbon absorbent) has been evaluated in the treatment of active pouchitis.[72] AST-120 utilizes highly absorptive, porous carbon microspheres, which have the ability to absorb small-molecular-weight toxins, inflammatory mediators, and harmful bile acids. Of the 20 patients included in the pilot study, 11 (55%) had a clinical response to the therapy, defined by a decrease in PDAI ≥3 points, and 10 (50%) entered remission, defined by a PDAI <7 points. AST-120 appeared to be effective and well tolerated, although further study is required.

STOMAL COMPLICATIONS

Stomas are frequently constructed during or after colectomy for UC, either as part of the staged IPAA surgery or for permanent fecal diversion. Stoma-related complications are common and include a wide range of presentations (Table 18-3).

Early Stomal Complications

Complications of intestinal stomas may be subdivided into those occurring early in the postoperative period (<1 month postoperatively) and those occurring later.[73] Overall, between 26% and 70% of patients will experience at least one stomal complication, and most studies have found the highest complication rates to occur following creation of a loop ileostomy.[73-75] Stomal

Table 18-3. Stomal Complications
Vascular compromise with stomal necrosis
Stomal retraction
Improper stoma site location
Peristomal skin irritation and bleeding
Infection
Abscess
Fistula
Herniation—with bowel obstruction
Prolapse
Stenosis/stricture
Peristomal varices
Peristomal pyoderma gangrenosum (see Chapter 8)
Technical errors

complications may be more common in obese patients, patients without a preoperative enterostomal therapist consultation, those who require emergency stoma construction, and patients with CD.[75]

Stomal Necrosis

Stomal necrosis is one of the most serious early complications of stoma creation (Figure 18-2A).[73] Vascular compromise ranges from mild ischemia, due to operative trauma or vasospasm with mucosal sloughing, to infarction or intestinal necrosis, due to ligation of arterial supply or inadequate collateral arterial circulation. Venous outflow obstruction may lead to significant venous congestion and compromised bowel perfusion, which may also lead to stomal necrosis. The incidence of early stomal necrosis ranges from 2.3% to 20.5% in reported series.[73-78]

Insufficient vascular supply to a stoma is usually recognized at the time of initial stomal creation, and immediate surgical revision is required. Alternatively, a stoma with small areas of questionable ischemia may be followed conservatively. Poor vascular supply may also lead to delayed complications, including stomal stenosis and/or stricture.

Stomal Retraction

Stomal retraction in the early postoperative period is usually a result of tension on the bowel or its mesentery from inadequate mobilization. The stoma may retract in patients who are malnourished, obese, or receiving

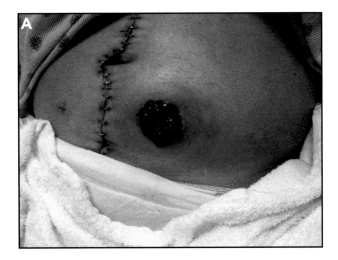

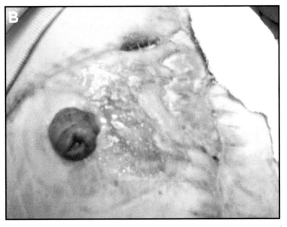

Figure 18-2. Peristomal complications. (A) Stomal necrosis. (B) Severe stomal irritation. Reprinted with permission from Jill Saltzman and Gina Conley, University of Pittsburgh Medical Center.)

corticosteroid therapy, due to poor wound healing.[73] Complete retraction can lead to subcutaneous contamination and sepsis. The majority of stomas with significant retraction eventually require surgical revision.

Peristomal Skin Irritation

The reported prevalence of peristomal skin irritation ranges from 3% to 42%. This is one of the most common complications following stomal formation and can occur both in the early and late periods.[73,74,77-80] The degree of irritation may range from a mild peristomal dermatitis to full-thickness skin necrosis and ulceration (Figure 18-2B). In most instances, peristomal skin irritation is a direct result of chemical dermatitis, resulting from exposure to the stomal effluent. In addition, patients may experience a desquamation of peristomal skin resulting from frequent appliance changes. The pouching system should ideally prevent contact of the effluent and the skin, and the appliance should not be changed too often. Due to the more liquid and irritating nature of ileostomy output, peristomal skin irritation is more commonly seen with ileostomies compared to colostomies.[73] Monitoring stoma size, patient education on stomal care and maintenance, and consultation with an enterostomal nurse are all important factors in healing the irritation.

Peristomal Skin Infection, Abscess, and Fistula

In the early postoperative period, parastomal infections and abscesses are uncommon, with a reported frequency of 2% to 14.8%.[74,77] A peristomal abscess in the immediate postoperative period often occurs in the setting of stomal revision, or the reconstruction of a stoma at the same site. The abscess is secondary to bacterial colonization on the peristomal skin in the preoperative period, along with perioperative seeding of the surgical site. Abscesses may also be due to an infected hematoma or an infected suture granuloma. Abscesses should be drained, although fistula formation following incision and drainage is not uncommon.[73]

If an abscess forms at a mature stoma site, local folliculitis or recurrent IBD should be considered in the differential diagnosis.[81] In a patient with a known history of CD, a peristomal fistula is often the result of recurrent CD, and peristomal fistulae may occur in 7% to 10% of CD patients with an ileostomy.[82,83] In patients with a presumed diagnosis of UC who develop peristomal fistula, a missed diagnosis of CD needs to be entertained. Treatment of persistent peristomal fistulae generally requires resection of the peristomal disease and construction of a new stoma, preferably at a different site. For patients with CD-associated peristomal fistulae, concurrent medical therapy for their underlying IBD is often needed.

Late Stomal Complications

Late complications are defined as occurring after the period of physiologic adjustment, which for most patients occurs 6 to 10 weeks following stomal creation. In reported series, up to 70% of patients will experience a stomal complication.[75,76,81,82] Peristomal pyoderma gangrenosum is a potential postoperative complication following stomal creation. For a complete discussion of this entity, please see Chapter 8.

Parastomal Herniation

The reported prevalence of early postoperative parastomal herniation and bowel obstruction ranges from 4.6% to 37%. Parastomal herniation may be the most common late stomal complication.[74,75,81,82,84] Older age, obesity, perioperative steroid use, prior stoma surgery, and positioning of the stoma outside the

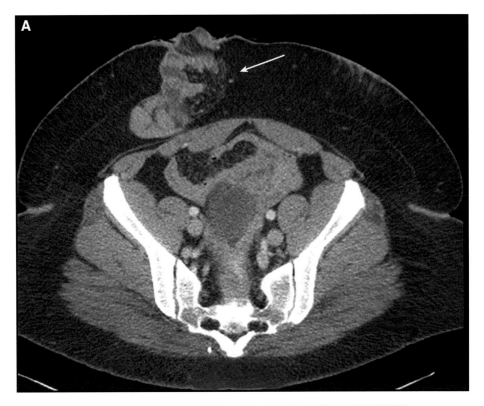

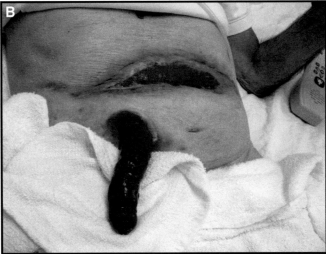

Figure 18-3. (A) Computed tomography scan showing a peristomal hernia (arrow). (B) Stomal prolapse. Reprinted with permission from Jill Saltzman and Gina Conley, University of Pittsburgh Medical Center.)

rectus muscle all may contribute to the development of parastomal herniation[81] Surgical management is required in approximately 33% of patients with herniation, with indications for surgery being incarceration, obstruction, pain, and leakage[81] (Figure 18-3A).

Stomal Prolapse

Prolapse is one of the more common late complications following stoma creation. The estimated incidence is reported to be between 2% and 26%.[85,86] Severe prolapse requires surgical correction. Risk factors include thin body habitus, stoma location within the laparotomy incision, redundant mesentery, paraplegia, and pregnancy.[81] Surgery is indicated in cases complicated by pouch leakage, incarceration, and recurrent trauma (Figure 18-3B).[81]

Stomal Retraction

Simple benign causes for stomal retraction are weight gain after stoma formation and a short length of the exteriorized segment. The incidence of retraction ranges from 3% to 17% for patients with ileostomies.[81] It is more commonly seen in obese patients.[75] Depending on the reason for creation of the stoma, a work-up for recurrent CD or ischemia may be undertaken prior to surgical revision.

Stomal Stenosis and Stricture

Ischemia is a usual underlying factor leading to stomal stenosis. This may be apparent immediately after the stomal construction or may not manifest for months later. This is thought to be secondary to retraction and circumferential scar formation, resulting from an inadequate blood supply at the stomal edges.[76] Stomal infection and retraction may also lead to stenosis, as can adhesions and volvulus.[81] The reported frequency of this complication ranges from 2% to 14%.[74,87] As part of the evaluation, recurrent CD and, in rare cases, malignancy need be ruled out.

Stomal Bleeding/Peristomal Varices

Patients presenting with stomal bleeding may have a source anywhere along the gastrointestinal tract proximal to the stoma and should be managed as any other patient with active gastrointestinal bleeding. Local trauma irritation, granular tissues is a frequent cause for visible bleeding from the mucosa of the stoma. Treatment of isolated minor trauma-related bleeding includes local pressure. Recurrent local injury is often related to trauma from a stiff appliance encroaching on the mucosa. More significant injury may require evaluation in the operating room. Significant stomal irritation can lead to exuberant granulation tissue that frequently bleeds or may have the gross appearance of recurrent CD. Once recurrent IBD has been ruled out, the granulation tissue is treated with topical application of silver nitrate or judicious electrocautery.

The presence from portal hypertension, particularly in those with concurrent PSC can lead to mucosal venous congestion and profuse gastrointestinal bleeding.[81] Furthermore, a stoma is a well-recognized ectopic site for variceal development in patients with portal hypertension. Stomal variceal bleeding is most commonly seen in patients with concomitant IBD and PSC. However, portal hypertension secondary to any etiology can result in the formation of peristomal varices.

☑ Key Points

☑ A multidisciplinary approach involving gastroenterologists and colorectal surgeons, together with a team of gastrointestinal pathologists and gastrointestinal radiologists, is necessary to successfully manage and treat patients with complex pouch disorders.

☑ Pouch endoscopy is the most valuable tool for the diagnosis and differential diagnosis of pouch complications.

☑ While the majority of patients with pouchitis respond favorably to antibiotic therapy, antibiotic-dependent and -refractory pouchitis pose therapeutic challenges.

☑ Secondary etiologies of pouchitis, such as CDI, IgG4-associated pouchitis, and CMV, should be sought if patients do not respond to first-line therapies.

☑ Technical, mechanical, and ischemic factors, along with the underlying disease process, contribute to the development of stomal complications. Topical, systemic, and sometimes surgical corrective approaches are needed.

REFERENCES

1. Fazio VW, Ziv Y, Church JM, et al. Ileal pouch-anal anastomosis: complications and function in 1005 patients. *Ann Surg.* 1995;222:120-127.
2. Sandborn WJ. Pouchitis following ileal pouch-anal anastomosis: definition, pathogenesis, and treatment. *Gastroenterology.* 1994;107:1856-1860.
3. Coffey JC, Winter DC, Neary P, et al. Quality of life after ileal pouch-anal anastomosis: an evaluation of diet and other factors using the Cleveland Global Quality of Life instrument. *Dis Colon Rectum.* 2002;45:30-38.
4. Stocchi L, Pemberton JH. Pouch and pouchitis. *Gastroenterol Clin North Am.* 2001;30:223-241.
5. Hurst RD, Molinari M, Chung TP, Rubin M, Michelassi F. Prospective study of the incidence, timing and treatment of pouchitis in 104 consecutive patients after restorative proctocolectomy. *Arch Surg.* 1996;131:497-500.
6. Ohge H, Furne JK, Springfield J, et al. Association between fecal hydrogen sulfide production and pouchitis. *Dis Colon Rectum.* 2005;48:469-475.
7. Gosselink MP, Schouten WR, van Lieshout LM, et al. Eradication of pathogenic bacteria and restoration of normal pouch flora: comparison of metronidazole and ciprofloxacin in the treatment of pouchitis. *Dis Colon Rectum.* 2004;47:1519-1525.
8. Falk A, Olsson C, Ahrne S, et al. Ileal pelvic pouch microbiota from two former ulcerative colitis patients, analysed by DNA-based methods, were unstable over time and showed the presence of *Clostridium perfringens*. *Scand J Gastroenterol.* 2007;42:973-985.
9. Komanduri S, Gillevet PM, Sikaroodi M, et al. Dysbiosis in pouchitis: evidence of unique microfloral patterns in pouch inflammation. *Clin Gastroenterol Hepatol.* 2007;5:352-360.

10. McLaughlin SD, Walker AW, Churcher C, et al. The bacteriology of pouchitis: a molecular phylogenetic analysis using 16S rRNA gene cloning and sequencing. Presented at 8th Annual BMRP Investigator Meeting, February 2010, Los Angeles, CA (abstract). Available at http://www.broadmedical.org/about/annual_meetings/2010/abstract-McLaughlin.html.

11. Ottesen EA, Hong JW, Quake SR, et al. Microfluidic digital PCR enables multigene analysis of individual environmental bacteria. *Science*. 3006;314:1464-1467.

12. Liu WT, Zhu L. Environmental microbiology-on-a-chip and its future impacts. *Trends Biotechnol*. 3005;23:174-179.

13. Marcy Y, Ouverney C, Bik EM, et al. Dissecting biological "dark matter" with single-cell genetic analysis of rare and uncultivated TM7 microbes from the human mouth. *Proc Natl Acad Sci U S A*. 2007;104:11889-11894.

14. Turroni S, Vitali B, Candela M, et al. Antibiotics and probiotics in chronic pouchitis: a comparative proteomic approach. *World J Gastroenterol*. 2010;16:30-41.

15. Kroesen AJ, Leistenschneider P, Lehmann K, et al. Increased bacterial permeation in long-lasting ileoanal pouches. *Inflamm Bowel Dis*. 2006;12:736-744.

16. DeSilva HJ, Jones M, Prince C, Kettlewell M, Mortensen NJ, Jewell DP. Lymphocyte and macrophage subpopulations in pelvic ileal reservoirs. *Gut*. 1992;32:1160-1165.

17. Sehgal R, Berg A, Hegarty JP, et al. NOD2/CARD15 mutations correlate with severe pouchitis after ileal pouch-anal anastomosis. *Dis Colon Rectum*. 2010;53:1487-1494.

18. Navaneethan U, Shen B. Secondary pouchitis: those with identifiable etiopathogenetic or triggering factors. *Am J Gastroenterol*. 2010;105:51-64.

19. Casadesus D, Tani T, Wakai T, et al. Possible role of human cytomegalovirus in pouchitis after proctocolectomy with ileal pouch-anal anastomosis in patients with ulcerative colitis. *World J Gastroenterol*. 2007;13:1085-1089.

20. Shen B, Jiang ZD, Fazio VW, et al. *Clostridium difficile* infection in patients with ileal pouch-anal anastomosis. *Clin Gastroenterol Hepatol*. 2008;6:782-788.

21. Shen B, Remzi FH, Nutter B, et al. Association between immune-associated disorders and adverse outcomes of ileal pouch-anal anastomosis. *Am J Gastroenterol*. 2009;104:655-664.

22. Shen B, Plesec TP, Remer E, et al. Asymmetric endoscopic inflammation of the ileal pouch: a sign of ischemic pouchitis? *Inflamm Bowel Dis*. 2010;16:836-846.

23. Shen B, Bennett AE, Fazio VW, et al. Collagenous pouchitis. *Dig Liver Dis*. 2006;38:704-709.

24. Shen B, Fazio VW, Bennett AE, et al. Effect of withdrawal of non-steroidal anti-inflammatory drug use in patients with the ileal pouch. *Dig Dis Sci*. 2007;52:3321-3328.

25. Navaneethan U, Bennett AE, Venkatesh PG, et al. Tissue infiltration of IgG4+ plasma cells in symptomatic patients with ileal pouch-anal anastomosis. *J Crohns Colitis*. 2011;5:570-576.

26. Sandborn WJ. Pouchitis: risk factors, frequency, natural history, classification and public health perspective. In: McLeod RS, Martin F, Sutherland LR, Wallace JL, Williams CN, eds. *Trends in Inflammatory Bowel Disease 1996*. Lancaster, UK: Kluwer Academic Publishers; 1997:51-63.

27. Pardi DS, D'Haens G, Shen B, Campbell S, Gionchetti P. Clinical guidelines for the management of pouchitis. *Inflamm Bowel Dis*. 2009;15:1424-1431.

28. Shen B. Diagnosis and management of patients with pouchitis. *Drugs*. 2003;65:453-461.

29. Shen B, Achkar JP, Lashner BA, et al. Endoscopic and histologic evaluations together with symptom assessment are required to diagnose pouchitis. *Gastroenterology*. 2001;121:261-267.

30. Shen B, Achkar JP, Connor JT, et al. Modified pouchitis disease activity index: a simplified approach to the diagnosis of pouchitis. *Dis Colon Rectum*. 2003;46:748-753.

31. Sandborn WJ, Tremaine WJ, Batts KP, Pemberton JH, Phillips SF. Pouchitis after ileal pouch-anal anastomosis: a Pouchitis Disease Activity Index. *Mayo Clin Proc*. 1994;69:409-415.

32. Moskowitz RL, Shepherd NA, Nicholls RJ. An assessment of inflammation in the reservoir after restorative proctocolectomy with ileoanal ileal reservoir. *Int J Colorectal Dis*. 1986;1:167-174.

33. Heuschen UA, Allemeyer EH, Hinz G, et al. Diagnosing pouchitis: comparative validation of two scoring systems in routine follow-up. *Dis Colon Rectum*. 2002;45:776-786.

34. Shen B, Shermock KM, Fazio VW, et al. A cost-effectiveness analysis of diagnostic strategies for symptomatic patients with ileal pouch-anal anastomosis. *Am J Gastroenterol.* 2003;98:2460-2467.

35. Lohmuller JL, Pemberton HJ, Dozois RR, Ilstrup D, van Heerden J. Pouchitis and extraintestinal manifestations of inflammatory bowel disease after ileal pouch-anal anastomosis. *Ann Surg.* 1990;211:622-629.

36. Wolf JM, Achkar JP, Lashner BA, et al. Afferent limb ulcers predict Crohn's disease in patients with ileal pouch-anal anastomosis. *Gastroenterology.* 2004;126:1686-1691.

37. Navaneethan U, Shen B. Secondary pouchitis: those with identifiable etiopathogenetic or triggering factors. *Am J Gastroenterol.* 2001;105:51-64.

38. Apel R, Cohen Z, Andrews CW Jr, McLeod R, Steinhart H, Odze RD. Prospective evaluation of early morphological changes in pelvic ileal pouches. *Gastroenterology.* 1994;107:435-443.

39. Veress B, Reinholt FP, Lindquist K, et al. Long-term histomorphological surveillance of the pelvic ileal pouch: dysplasia develops in a subgroup of patients. *Gastroenterology.* 1995;109:1090-1097.

40. Pardi DS, Sandborn WJ. Systematic review: the management of pouchitis. *Aliment Pharmacol Ther.* 2006;23:1087-1096.

41. Navaneethan U, Shen B. Laboratory tests for patients with ileal pouch-anal anastomosis: clinical utility in predicting, diagnosing, and monitoring pouch disorders. *Am J Gastroenterol.* 2009;104:2606-2015.

42. Kuisma J, Nuutinen H, Luukkonen P, et al. Long term metabolic consequences of ileal pouch–anal anastomosis for ulcerative colitis. *Am J Gastroenterol.* 2001;96:3110-3116.

43. M'koma AE. Serum biochemical evaluation of patients with functional pouches 10 to 20 years after restorative proctocolectomy. *Int J Colorectal Dis.* 2006;21:711-720.

44. Lu H, Lian L, Navaneethan U, Shen B. Clinical utility of C-reactive protein in patients with ileal pouch anal anastomosis. *Inflamm Bowel Dis.* 2010;16:1678-1684.

45. Walkowiak J, Banasiewicz T, Krokowicz P, et al. Fecal pyruvate kinase (M2-PK): a new predictor for inflammation and severity of pouchitis. *Scand J Gastroenterol.* 2005;40:1493-1494.

46. Johnson MW, Maestranzi S, Duffy AM, et al. Fecal calprotectin: a noninvasive diagnostic tool and marker of severity in pouchitis. *Eur J Gastroenterol Hepatol.* 2008;20:174-179.

47. Parsi M, Shen B, Achkar J, et al. Fecal lactoferrin for diagnosis of symptomatic patients with ileal pouch-anal anastomosis. *Gastroenterology.* 2004;126:1280-1286.

48. Lim M, Gonsalves S, Thekkinkattil D, et al. The assessment of a rapid noninvasive immunochromatographic assay test for fecal lactoferrin in patients with suspected inflammation of the ileal pouch. *Dis Colon Rectum.* 2008;51:96-99.

49. Melmed GY, Fleshner PR, Bardakcioglu O, et al. Family history and serology predict Crohn's disease after ileal pouch-anal anastomosis for ulcerative colitis. *Dis Colon Rectum.* 2008;51:100-108.

50. Tang L, Boone J, Moore L, Lopez R, Shen B. Clinical significance of stool ASCA in disorders of the ileal pouch. *Inflamm Bowel Dis.* 2008;12:S2(abstract).

51. Shen B. Campylobacter infection in patients with ileal pouches. *Am J Gastroenterol.* 2010;105:472-473.

52. McLaughlin SD, Clark SK, Shafi S, et al. Fecal coliform testing to identify effective antibiotic therapies for patients with antibiotic-resistant pouchitis. *Clin Gastroenterol Hepatol.* 2009;7:545-548.

53. Seggerman RE, Chen MY, Waters GS, Ott DJ. Radiology of ileal pouch-anal anastomosis surgery. *Am J Roentgenol.* 2003;180:999-1002.

54. Shen B, Fazio VW, Remzi FH, et al. Comprehensive evaluation of inflammatory and noninflammatory sequelae of ileal pouch-anal anastomoses. *Am J Gastroenterol.* 2005;100:93-101.

55. Shepherd NA, Hulten L, Tytgat GN, et al. Workshop: pouchitis. *Int J Colorectal Dis.* 1989;4:205-229.

56. Sagar PM, Pemberton JH. Ileo-anal pouch function and dysfunction. *Dig Dis.* 1997;15:172-188.

57. Madden MV, McIntyre AS, Nicholls RJ. Double-blind crossover trial of metronidazole versus placebo in chronic unremitting pouchitis. *Dig Dis Sci.* 1994;39:1193-1196.

58. Shen B, Achkar JP, Lashner BA, et al. A randomized clinical trial of ciprofloxacin and metronidazole to treat acute pouchitis. *Inflamm Bowel Dis.* 2001;7:301-305.
59. Navaneethan U, Shen B. Pros and cons of antibiotic therapy for pouchitis. *Expert Rev Gastroenterol Hepatol.* 2009;3:547-559.
60. Pepin J, Saheb N, Coulombe MA, et al. Emergence of fluoroquinolones as the predominant risk factor for *Clostridium difficile*–associated diarrhea: a cohort study during an epidemic in Quebec. *Clin Infect Dis.* 2005;41:1254-1260.
61. Isaacs KL, Sandler RS, Abreu M, et al. Rifaximin for the treatment of active pouchitis: a randomized, double-blind, placebo-controlled pilot study. *Inflamm Bowel Dis.* 2007;13:1250-1255.
62. Shen B, Remzi FH, Lopez AR, Queener E. Rifaximin for maintenance therapy in antibiotic-dependent pouchitis. *BMC Gastroenterol.* 2008;8:26.
63. Shen B, Fazio V, Remzi F, et al. Combined ciprofloxacin and tinidazole therapy in the treatment of chronic refractory pouchitis. *Dis Col Rectum.* 2007;50:498-508.
64. Ha CY, Bauer JJ, Lazarev M, et al. Early institution of tinidazole may prevent pouchitis following ileal-pouch anal anastomosis (IPAA) surgery in ulcerative colitis (UC) patients. *Gastroenterology.* 2010;138:S69 (abstract).
65. Gionchetti P, Rizzello F, Helwig U, et al. Prophylaxis of pouchitis onset with probiotic therapy: a double-blind, placebo-controlled trial. *Gastroenterology.* 2003;124:1202-1209.
66. Gionchetti P, Rizzello F, Venturi A, et al. Oral bacteriotherapy as maintenance treatment in patients with chronic pouchitis: a double-blind, placebo-controlled trial. *Gastroenterology.* 2000;119:305-309.
67. Elahi B, Nikfar S, Derakhshani S, Vafaie M, Abdollahi M. On the benefit of probiotics in the management of pouchitis in patients underwent ileal pouch anal anastomosis: a meta-analysis of controlled clinical trials. *Dig Dis Sci.* 2008;53:1278-1284.
68. Shen B, Remzi FH, Lavery IC, et al. Administration of adalimumab in the treatment of Crohn's disease of the ileal pouch. *Aliment Pharmacol Ther.* 2009;29:519-526.
69. Wischmeyer P, Pemberton JH, Phillips SF. Chronic pouchitis after ileal pouch-anal anastomosis: responses to butyrate and glutamine suppositories in a pilot study. *Mayo Clin Proc.* 1993;68:978-981.
70. Gioncheitti P, Rizzello F, Venturi A, et al. Long-term efficacy of bismuth carbomer enemas in patients with treatment-resistant chronic pouchitis. *Aliment Pharmacol Ther.* 1007;11:673-678.
71. Tremaine WJ, Sandborn WJ, Wolff BG, Carpenter HA, Zinsmeister AR, Metzger PP. Bismuth carbomer foam enemas for active chronic pouchitis: a randomized, double-blind, placebo-controlled trial. *Aliment Pharmacol Ther.* 1997;11:1041-1046.
72. Shen B, Pardi DS, Bennett AE, et al. The efficacy and tolerability of AST-120 (spherical carbon adsorbent) in active pouchitis. *Am J Gastroenterol.* 2009;104:1468-1474.
73. Kann BR, Cataldo TC. Early stomal complication. *Clin Colon Rectal Surg.* 2002;15:191-198.
74. Park JJ, Del Pino A, Orsay CP, et al. Stoma complications: the Cook County Hospital experience. *Dis Colon Rectum.* 1999;42:1575-1580.
75. Arumugam PJ, Bevan L, MacDonald L, et al. A prospective audit of stomas-analysis of risk factors and complication and their management. *Colorectal Dis.* 2003;5:49-52.
76. Duchesne JC, Wang Y-Z, Weintraub SL, Boyle M, Hunt JP. Stoma complications: a multivariate analysis. *Am Surg.* 2002;68:961-966.
77. Pearl RK, Prasad LM, Orsay CP, et al. Early local complications from intestinal stomas. *Arch Surg.* 1985;120:1145-1147.
78. Fasth S, Hulten L. Loop ileostomy: a superior diverting stoma in colorectal surgery. *World J Surg.* 1984;8:401-407.
79. Feinberg SM, McLeod RS, Cohen Z. Complications of loop ileostomy. *Am J Surg.* 1987;153:102-107.
80. Grobler SP, Hoise KB, Keighley MRB. Randomized trial of loop ileostomy in restorative proctocolectomy. *Br J Surg.* 1992;79:903-906.
81. Steele MCA, Wu JS. Late stomal complications. *Clin Colon Rectal Surg.* 2002;15:199-207.
82. Leong APK, Londono-Schimmer EE, Phillips RKS. Life table analysis of stomal complications following ileostomy. *Br J Surg.* 1994;81:727-729.

83. Greenstein AJ, Dicker A, Meyers S, Aufses AH. Periileostomy fistulae in Crohn's disease. *Ann Surg*. 1983;197:179-182.

84. Bass EM, Del Pino A, Tan A, Pearl RK, Orsay CP, Abcarian H. Does preoperative stoma marking and education by the enterostomal therapist affect outcome? *Dis Colon Rectum*. 1997;40:440-442.

85. Cheung MT. Complications of an abdominal stoma: an analysis of 322 stomas. *Aust N Z J Surg*. 1995;65:808-811.

86. Robertson I, Leung E, Hughes D, et al. Prospective analysis of stoma-related complications. *Colorectal Dis*. 2005;7:279-285.

87. Caricato M, Ausania F, Ripetti V, et al. Retrospective analysis of long-term defunctioning stoma complications after colorectal surgery. *Colorectal Dis*. 2007;9:559-561.

SUGGESTED READINGS

Fleshner P, Ippoliti A, Dubinsky M, et al. A prospective multivariate analysis of clinical factors associated with pouchitis after ileal pouch-anal anastomosis. *Clin Gastroenterol Hepatol*. 2007;5:952-958.

Kühbacher T, Ott SJ, Helwig U, et al. Bacterial and fungal microbiota in relation to probiotic therapy (VSL#3) in pouchitis. *Gut*. 2006;55:833-841.

McLaughlin SD, Walker AW, Churcher C, et al. The bacteriology of pouchitis: a molecular phylogenetic analysis using 16S rRNA gene cloning and sequencing. *Ann Surg*. 2010;252:90-98.

Pardi DS, D'Haens G, Shen B, Campbell S, Gionchetti P. Clinical guidelines for the management of pouchitis. *Inflamm Bowel Dis*. 2009;15:1424-1431.

Shen B, Remzi FH, Lavery IC, Lashner BA, Fazio VW. A proposed classification of ileal pouch disorders and associated complications after restorative proctocolectomy. *Clin Gastroenterol Hepatol*. 2008;6:145-158.

Financial Disclosures

Dr. Ashwin N. Ananthakrishnan has no financial or proprietary interest in the materials presented herein.

Dr. Jemilat O. Badamas has no financial or proprietary interest in the materials presented herein.

Aaron S. Bancil has no financial or proprietary interest in the materials presented herein.

Dr. David Benhayon has no financial or proprietary interest in the materials presented herein.

Dr. Adam S. Cheifetz is on the advisory boards for Abbott, Janssen, Warner Chillcot, and Prometheus.

Dr. Garret Cullen has no financial or proprietary interest in the materials presented herein.

Dr. Omer J. Deen has no financial or proprietary interest in the materials presented herein.

Dr. Monika Fischer has no financial or proprietary interest in the materials presented herein.

Dr. Mark E. Gerich has no financial or proprietary interest in the materials presented herein.

Dr. Leyla J. Ghazi has no financial or proprietary interest in the materials presented herein.

Dr. Lisa M. Grandinetti has no financial or proprietary interest in the materials presented herein.

Dr. Peter D.R. Higgins has received research funding from the NIH, the CCFA, Abbott, Janssen, UCB, Pfizer, JBR Pharma, Otsuka, and Procter & Gamble.

Dr. Kim L. Isaacs has received clinical trial support from Abbott, Centocor, Elan, UCB, Millenium, Given, and Glaxo. She is a DSMB for Centocor.

Dr. Sunanda Kane is a consultant for Abbott, Janssen, Elan, Cosmo Pharmaceuticals, Millenium, UCB, and Shire. She has received research support from Elan, Shire, and UCB.

Dr. Donald F. Kirby has no financial or proprietary interest in the materials presented herein.

Dr. Mark Lazarev has no financial or proprietary interest in the materials presented herein.

Dr. Edward V. Loftus Jr has no financial or proprietary interest in the materials presented herein.

Dr. Gil Y. Melmed is a consultant for Janssen, Celgene, Amgen, Given Imaging; a non-CME speaker for Abbott and Prometheus; and has received research support from Pfizer.

Dr. Udayakumar Navaneethan has no financial or proprietary interest in the materials presented herein.

Dr. Timothy R. Orchard acted as a speaker at meetings sponsored by Abbott, Dr Falk Pharma, Ferring, Merck, Shire, and Warner Chilcott. He has sat on advisory boards for Abbott, Dr Falk Pharma, Ferring, Merck, Shire, and Warner Chilcott. He has received research funding from Johnson and Johnson and Warner Chilcott.

Dr. Sulieman Abdal Raheem has no financial or proprietary interest in the materials presented herein.

Dr. Miguel D. Regueiro has no financial or proprietary interest in the materials presented herein.

Dr. David T. Rubin is a consultant for Prometheus Laboratories, Abbott, Janssen, and UCB and receives grant support (safety registry) from Abbott.

Dr. David A. Schwartz is a consultant for Abbott, UCB, and Braintree Labs and receives grant support from Abbott and UCB.

Dr. Bo Shen is a speaker and receives honorarium from Abbott and Aplatis. He is also on the AD board for Prometheus Labs.

Dr. Miles P. Sparrow has no financial or proprietary interest in the materials presented herein.

Dr. A. Hillary Steinhart is on the advisory board for Merck, Janssen, Abbott Laboratories, UCB, and Shire; is an investigator for Merck, Janssen, Abbott Laboratories, UCB, Millenium, Glaxo Smith Kline, Amgen, and Pfizer; and is a speaker for Merck, Janssen, Abbott Laboratories, Shire, Aptalis (Axcan Pharma), and Warner Chilcott.

Dr. Jason Swoger has no financial or proprietary interest in the materials presented herein.

Dr. Eva Szigethy receives research support from the National Institutes of Health and the National Institute of Mental Health. She also participates as a speaker for the Scripps Institute.

Dr. Fernando Velayos has not disclosed any relevant financial relationships.

Dr. David G. Walker has no financial or proprietary interest in the materials presented herein.

Index

abscess
    anti-tumor necrosis factor related, 312
    clinical presentation of, 21
    in Crohn's disease, 19
    drainage of, 52, 56
    indications for intervention in, 27–28
    management of, 32–37
    peristomal, 360
    psoas, 22
    radiographic assessment of, 22–23, 27
adalimumab
    adverse effects of, 305
    autoimmune reaction to, 315–316
    for Crohn's disease, 10
    for erythema nodosum, 147
    for eye disease, 171
    for joint disease, 137–139
    malignancy and, 313–314
    for oral Crohn's disease, 145
    for perianal fistulas, 51
    for postoperative Crohn's disease prevention, 336–338
    during pregnancy and lactation, 217
    skin reactions to, 317
adenomas, management of, 93
adenomatous polyp, 86
5-aminosalicyclic acid (5-ASA)
    for colorectal cancer prevention, 94
    for Crohn's disease, 8–10, 18
    for IBD with primary sclerosing cholangitis, 185
    for postoperative Crohn's disease prevention, 333–334
    during pregnancy and lactation, 208–211
    for pyoderma gangrenosum, 149
aminosalicylates
    during pregnancy and lactation, 208–211
    for ulcerative colitis, 66
amlexanox, 152
amoxicillin/clavulanic acid, 212
ampicillin/sulbactam, 32–33
anal canal, 45
anal sphincters, 45
analgesics, for joint disease, 136
ankylosing spondylitis, 127
    genetic markers in, 130
    treatment of, 136–138
anorexia, 235, 236–237

antibiotics
    for abdominal abscesses, 32–33, 37
    for *Clostridium difficile* infections, 106–107, 107–109
    for Crohn's disease, 9, 334–335
    for perianal fistulas, 49–50, 56
    during pregnancy and lactation, 211–212
    for ulcerative colitis, 66–67
antidiarrheals, during pregnancy and lactation, 212–213
anti-inflammatory agents
    for colorectal cancer prevention, 94
    for internal fistulas, 32
    for strictures, 29
antineutrophil cytoplasmic antibodies, 176
antinuclear antibodies, 133
antioxidant deficiencies, 234–235
antipsychotics, 273
anti-tumor necrosis factor
    in abscess formation, 19
    for perianal fistulas, 56
    for postoperative Crohn's disease prevention, 335–338
anti-tumor necrosis factor agents. *See also* tumor necrosis factor (TNF)
    abscesses and, 28
    for anal ulcers, 44
    for Crohn's disease, 10, 21
    for perianal fistulas, 51–53
    for strictures, 29
    for ulcerative colitis, 70–71
anti-tumor necrosis factor therapy, 303
    adverse effects of, 304–309
    for anti-TNF-alpha-induced psoriasis, 158–159
    autoimmune and inflammatory phenomena of, 315–316
    for *Clostridium difficile* infections, 107
    hematologic complications of, 317
    infectious risks of, 34, 310–315
    infusion reactions to, 307–310
    for joint disease, 137–138
    neurologic complications of, 316
    for perianal fistulas, 45
    skin reactions to, 317–318
anus
    fissures of, 43–44
    ulceration of, 44

Printed in the United States
by Baker & Taylor Publisher Services